The Transformation

48 Days to Eating & Living Naturally for Life™

Michele Menzel, ND, D.PSc

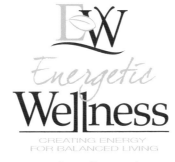

Energetic Wellness

CREATING ENERGY
FOR BALANCED LIVING

energeticwellnessok.com

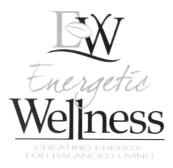

Michele Menzel, ND, D.PSc—Board Certified Naturopathic Doctor, Diplomat of Pastoral Science, Certified Nutritional Counselor, German New Medicine®, Certified Natural Health Professional
Published by Energetic Wellness, Edmond, Oklahoma, www.energeticwellnessok.com
Publishing Advisor: Mel Cohen, Inspired Authors Press, mel@inspiredauthorspress.com, 931-593-2484
Design & Layout: Karen Munger
Copy Editors: Karen Munger, Loren Paulsson, Paula Greenlaw, Robert Greenlaw, Mel Cohen, Edward Bolme, Kelli Tuter, Virginia Boyles

Dr. Menzel's intention is to reeducate and assist you with natural health information for the sole purpose of suggestion. You are responsible to research for yourself and choose the way you desire to live.

Dr. Menzel's statement regarding health: Healing is done naturally by our body. When we balance the body through lifestyle changes, including resolving conflicts, then the body has the best opportunity to repair and restore itself. This can result in complete healing.

Print: ISBN 978-0-9885602-1-5 • eBook: ISBN 978-0-9885602-2-2 • ePub: ISBN 978-0-9885602-4-6
1. Natural Health   2. Diet & Nutrition   3. Wholefood Supplements   4. Naturopathy   5. Nutrient Dense Foods
6. Health & Fitness   7. Natural Lifestyle Changes
I Michele Menzel   II *The Transformation*
Printed in China

To my husband, Steven, and our three children, Jessica, Stephen, and Michael; our son-in-law, Jordan, and our grandchildren, Serenity, Angeline, Gemma, and future grandchildren and great grandchildren. This book and my life's work is dedicated to you and to all the families who desire to live according to our Creator—for your own health and benefit, and for the hope of future, healthy generations.

This book and my journey to wellness would not have been possible without my husband, Steven—thank you for understanding the time it would take to research natural living and for encouraging me as I learned to serve our family pure, whole foods and to treat illnesses naturally. You encouraged my desire to become a naturopath and have been supportive during the writing of this book—and in the process have become quite the cook! Your support cannot be measured. I love and thank you, my dear life partner and best friend.

To my parents, Michael and Vera Angeline—words cannot express my love and gratefulness to the best parents in the world! Your continued expressions of love and support go beyond measure. You have encouraged me from the beginning of my journey and have continued to be my biggest supporters! Without your help, Energetic Wellness would not have been possible. I love you and thank you, Mom and Dad.

To my mother-in-law, Rena Menzel—thank you for your love and encouragement. And to my sister-in-law, Diana—you are a huge inspiration to me. (Diana has an amazing Italian restaurant in Lambertville, New Jersey, called DeAnna's. After 22 years of hard work and dedication, she is living her dream.)

A special thank-you to my children Jessica, Stephen and Michael, my son-in-law Jordan and grandchildren, Serenity, Angeline, and Gemma—thank you for your love and encouragement. You enjoy pure, whole foods, my cooking, and natural living. I love all of you more than you will ever know.

To My Teachers

Lee Woolley, the inventor of the SpectraVision™—you are a genius! The SpectraVision™ and your insight into the energy matrix of the body has changed my life. Thank you so much for your help with the SV section of this book. Most of all, thank you for being my teacher and friend. Your support and encouragement is a blessing to me. I am forever grateful.

Caroline Markolin, my German New Medicine® professor and dear friend—the first time I heard you speak, I was amazed at your articulate manner of teaching. I walked away in awe of the content and inspired by your passion and heart for GNM. I am grateful to you and Dr. Ryke Geerd Hamer for your unbelievable research of true, natural science.

Sally Fallon Morell, president of the Weston A. Price Foundation—although indirectly, you have been my teachers. Your book and lectures have been an integral part of learning about nutrient-dense foods and the foundation of nutrition taught in my practice. Thank you for allowing the use of your recipes and the written material you contributed to this book. The Foundation's efforts to help future generations learn the importance of nutrient-dense foods goes beyond recognition. I admire and honor your work.

To Dr. Ron Schmid—although we have only met in person a couple of times, I am extremely grateful for your knowledge and guidance through emails and telephone calls. You are the only ND I know of besides me that lives and teaches the principles of nutrient-dense foods. I am so grateful for your continued support both through your knowledge and your supplement line.

Dr. Daniel Jass and Dorie Luneski, ND—two doctors who greatly influenced my life toward natural medicine. Dr. Jass, thank you for guiding me through my own healing crisis and putting me on the path of the paleolithic diet. Dr. Dorie, thank you for introducing me to the SpectraVision™. I didn't understand my journey at the time, but a wonderful outcome was meeting you two very special people. Thank you both so much!

Mike Casey—thank you for being there to answer my questions and encourage me in my practice. I can't tell you enough how much your personal support has meant to me.

48 Days Pilot Group

My pilot group—thank you for persevering through the initial stages of this book. I will never forget your willingness to be a part of this venture! Your suggestions and input were very helpful. Thank you, Rosalie and Brenda for proofing—your corrections were much appreciated. The 48 Days classes were so much fun! You have applied many of the principles, and your testimonies are not only a blessing to me but your families. I am so proud of you. Take this wonderful awareness to your friends and families— you are a light!

Production Team

A heartfelt thank you to Karen Munger, my graphic designer. You are such a blessing to me. You inspire me with your words of encouragement and also push me with your promptings to write! You are so creative and your work reflects who you are as a person—beautiful! I'm so glad you had the intuition to approach me about organizing my patient folder. Look where it has led!

To my editor, Loren—we learned how to work together and I'm so grateful that you prompted me to follow through with my thoughts. You have helped me become a better writer. I'm still learning, but am thankful you guided me through the initial process.

Thank you, Robert and Paula, for stepping in at the very end to proof the local copy of this book. We couldn't have finished without you! Knowing you were helping with the final edits gave me confidence in the end result. Bless you!

Thank you, Paula for editing this nationwide version. You have persevered to help me in the midst of raising your family. Your encouragement and assistance in this process has helped me become a better writer. I couldn't have done it without you.

To my dear friend and publishing advisor, Mel Cohen of Inspired Authors Press—your knowledge and assistance through the writing, editing, and marketing of this book has been more than a blessing. I could not have done this without you. I am so grateful for your patience in answering my million questions! You have made this process much easier and more enjoyable than anticipated. Thank you, my dear friend.

To My Wonderful Staff

To my assistant, Kelli—you were sent from heaven! You are amazing and so supportive. I appreciate your thoroughness in your work and kindness to everyone who walks through the door. Thank you for jumping right in at the start of the 48 Days pilot group, for helping with the editing of this book, and for your willingness to do whatever is needed.

To Marion, my dear friend and colleague—thank you for shouldering extra work so I could focus on this book. You will never know how much our friendship means to me. I'm so grateful to have you as a practitioner at Energetic Wellness. You contribute a beautiful spirit to those around you.

To Virginia, my newest team member—thank you for your desire to be healthy and for supporting my work at EW. Your assistance with bookkeeping, product ordering, and our resource guide has filled a great need. Thank you for also being our staff photographer! Your creativity is much appreciated.

To my daughter, Jessica—I am so grateful for your help with the menu samples, recipes, and logo design… and for being my beautiful daughter, friend, and amazing mother to my grandchildren.

To Tammi, our wonderful cook—you started helping us with meals throughout the writing of this book, and we might never let you go. Thank you so much for your willingness to cook according to the Foods for Life. Your creative additions are delicious! All the best to you on your personal transformation journey.

The Transformation

Contents

The Transformation

Welcome to The Transformation!

Many people are searching for a path to better health for a variety of reasons. Some have been suffering a chronic illness or the symptoms of a discouraging diagnosis. Others have been trying to lose weight without success. And some just don't feel themselves, or feel older than they should. Whatever your reasons for starting on this path, you've made a wonderful decision to transform your life.

The Transformation will help you learn how to eat and live naturally—the way our Creator intended. It will be an amazing journey that will transform you for the rest of your life. And we'll be here to help you along the way.

The purpose of *The Transformation* is to take you through an amazing natural health transformation. This book was designed to be used as a reference guide on your personal wellness journey and for life.

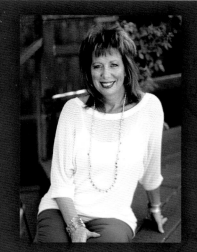

Michele Menzel, ND, D.PSc
BOARD CERTIFIED NATUROPATHIC DOCTOR
DIPLOMAT OF PASTORAL SCIENCE

Certified Nutritional Counselor
German New Medicine®
Certified Natural Health Professional

SpectraVision™ Bio-Energy
Balancing Practitioner

Going through her own major health challenges, Michele learned how to heal herself 100% naturally by assisting the body with pure whole foods and lifestyle changes. This journey has given her great insight as a naturopathic doctor and a sincere understanding and compassion for others.

After reading *The Transformation*, you will have the tools and information to begin your wellness journey. Her team at Energetic Wellness is here to empower, support, and love you every step of the way. She devotes the time needed to help you achieve **your ultimate wellness potential.**

Dear Friend,

My intention for writing this book is that you will have a clearer picture of the body's natural ability to heal. I hope you use it to find enjoyment in eating pure, whole foods and to live naturally for the rest of your life. We are creating a new generation. We have to learn the natural practices which were not handed down to us from previous healthy generations—how to conceive naturally, give birth naturally, live life naturally, and die naturally. Always be mindful that the body was designed to assist you through the challenges of life.

Although my own transformation took many years, I am encouraging you through a 48-day transformation. Take it slowly if you have to or do it several times and apply one thing at a time. You do not have to do it perfectly—it is a process. There is a lot of information in this book. Don't be overwhelmed, just apply one thing at a time. We are here to provide love and support to you along the way.

My deepest love and blessings to you as you begin or continue your healing journey,

Michele

My Story

One of the darkest times in my life also became the most transformational.
It shaped me into who I am today and continually helps me to grow, love, and
serve. I now see that time as a beautiful time of transition.

Twenty years ago I experienced a health challenge that changed the course
of my life. My husband Steven, our three children, and I returned from an
extended overseas Air Force assignment in Germany. After 12 years in the Air
Force, Steven had separated from the military. Our children Jessica, Stephen,
and Michael were still very young.

We explored living in Florida or South Carolina, but when job opportunities
did not pan out, we returned to our home state of New Jersey. Both Steven
and I grew up in New Jersey and our families were still there. After living in
many beautiful cities, this was not our first choice. There was some kicking
and even a little screaming along the way, but we finally surrendered to God
returning us home. Shortly after our move, I began having some disturbing
physical symptoms. I was only 30, and thought I was too young to be experiencing hormonal issues.

I came across some natural health medical bulletins written on the benefits
of whole grains. Although I felt we ate pretty "healthy" (*something I hear all
the time from my patients, which makes me chuckle because I was there, too*),
we were eating refined white flour products—such as bread and pasta—and
refined white sugar. Both Steven and I were raised in Italian, Catholic families—
pasta every Sunday and Wednesday!

As I changed our diet from white bread to whole wheat bread, I began to
feel better. I continued my study in natural health and slowly changed the food
we ate. I switched to using only real butter and extra virgin olive oil. Olive oil
was a staple in our Italian home, but after learning the benefits of extra virgin
olive oil, I made the switch. I am grateful my mother made home-cooked meals
and limited treats like soda and candy to birthday parties. One of my favorite
foods was an Italian hot dog (hot dog on a torpedo bun topped with potatoes,

mustard, peppers, and onions), but even they were easy to give up as I began to see the difference in how my body responded to natural, whole food. And now I enjoy a grass-fed beef hot dog with peppers and onions and no bun!

However, I became confused. The more I read, the more opinions I found. *Eat the whole egg or just the white? Grains or no grains? Red meat or vegetables? And how do you know which vitamins really work? And what about all the soy products?* The choices were overwhelming and each side had a convincing argument.

The small health-food store near our home was owned by a vegetarian. We became friends, and since she seemed to be very knowledgeable regarding health, I gravitated toward eating more grains and vegetables. Although Steven was supportive, I never took the children completely off dairy and meat—and I am so grateful I didn't. However, my children will tell you that we experimented with different dairy "alternatives" like soy and rice milk, soy and rice cheese, and soy butter. My whole family agrees that there is nothing like the real thing—real food is always better!

In 1995, we downsized to a smaller home, Steven was starting his own business (which I was helping to manage), we began homeschooling our children, and a close friend abruptly ended our relationship. I went into a severe healing crisis. There were many dark days when I wondered if I would make it. I was an emotional wreck and I was in so much pain, I couldn't sleep. Nothing I ate would stay down and my muscles and joints were always achy. This was the most fearful time of my life. I was terrified of how I felt and what was happening to me. I feared it was cancer. I was so frightened by the thought that I couldn't even say the word.

This was the most fearful time in my life.

Every test brought more anxiety and continued fear. I was seen by a medical doctor, a gynecologist, and a gastro-enterologist, and was labeled with fibromyalgia, chronic fatigue, and irritable bowel syndrome. I was fearful, but also knew in my heart that my body was created to heal itself. I stepped out in faith without medication; trusting in my body's design to heal itself.

This proved to be difficult. I was physically weak and found it overwhelming to take care of myself and my family. Jessica and Steven did all the grocery shopping and Jessica made many of the meals until I regained some strength. I fasted and prayed, did cleanses, and took enemas, but was not improving. Unable to find a naturopathic doctor, I opted for a holistic medical doctor. Dr. Daniel Jass agreed to assist me 100% naturally. After some initial tests, it was evident that I was protein and fat deficient. This did not surprise me, as I hadn't been a very good vegetarian. Grains and vegetables were my staples. Dr. Jass was the first to introduce me to the Paleolithic (hunter/gatherer) diet. This was very contrary to how I had been eating, but after learning that protein and good fats are vital to healing, I began incorporating them back into my diet. I also stopped fasting and taking enemas, which were draining my body of needed nutrients. Initially, eggs were the only food I could keep down. By giving my body the nutrients it needed to heal, I slowly regained my health and strength.

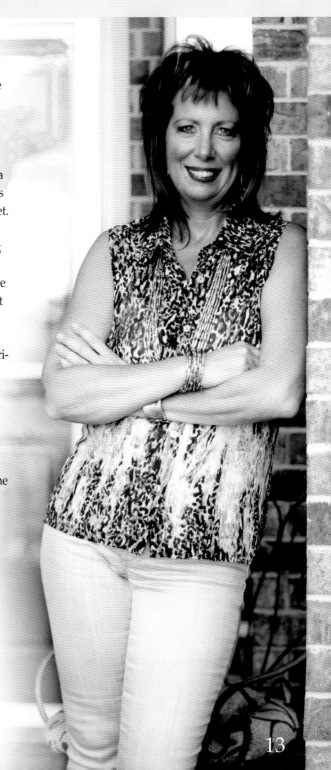

This season also caused me to go through a deep, spiritual experience and cleansing—wanting to understand what was happening to me. Years before, I had a wonderful spiritual awakening through acceptance of God's forgiveness through His Son, Jesus Christ. I felt free and was a very zealous Christian. But by this time in my life, I felt as though I was suffering through the same guilt as before my salvation. I realized that although I had received God's love and forgiveness, I had not fully forgiven myself, and could not release the shame and guilt. I began the journey of learning to love and forgive myself—working out my salvation.

Over the next several years, I grew in knowledge and wisdom regarding what we should eat, and what lifestyle changes will help the natural body recover from emotional trauma (conflicts). I realized that a vegan diet did not support the body's nutritional needs, especially when going through major healing. Animal fats and proteins are needed to support the body with nutrients that a vegetarian diet does not have. Another significant lesson I learned was that there are many diets that recommend "health food" that is just as fake as processed food. This simplified my journey as I learned to choose only pure, whole food designed by God.

From 1995 to 2005, I learned how to better my health and the health of my family through self study, research, and personal discovery. My personal 7 Laws of Wellness were developed after I attended health seminars, read over 40 books, researched, and was treated by a naturopathic doctor and clinical nutritionist. I filtered all the information through the grid of my faith, trust in God, prayer, and how the Spirit led me.

In December 2003, I turned 40. I remember telling my daughter as she brought me a birthday breakfast in bed that I thought my 40s would be better than my 30s. We don't think that it can get better as we get older, but I really felt that my body was rebuilding. I am now at the end of my 40s and I can honestly say that they have been better. If it hadn't been for the amazing transformation that took place in my life, I wouldn't have the energy to teach, run a busy practice, or write this book. I am so grateful to God and my mentors for providing me with what I need.

> "I want to guide you to an understanding of diseases, free of fear and panic."
>
> —Dr. Ryke Geerd Hamer

A great example of this guidance was a book given to me for my 40th birthday by a dear friend. This very significant book, *Nourishing Traditions*, written by Sally Fallon, introduced me to the research of Dr. Weston A. Price. This solidified what I had already come to know about whole food. The Weston A. Price Foundation has shaped the nutritional principles of my practice today.

Although never diagnosed with cancer, I sought to understand the natural body and the role of cancer and other conditions. *We fear what we do not understand, and I needed to put my fear of cancer to rest.* In 2004, while searching the web for natural cancer remedies, I came across German New Medicine® (GNM). As I began reading the compiled research of Dr. Ryke Geerd Hamer, I realized it paralleled what I believed, but had never heard it explained in such a beautiful way. Natural practitioners have been aware of the emotional mind/body connection, but Dr. Hamer's work proved it scientifically. After purchasing Dr. Hamer's published post-doctoral thesis, I became a student of GNM. I have also attended all of the GNM training seminars and incorporated its science as a foundational part of my practice. Dr. Hamer's work clarified for me God's wonderful creation of the body and its ability to support us through every challenge—as I experienced first-hand through my own healing.

We can trust this design and no longer fear symptoms. Through this understanding, my fear of cancer has completely disappeared.

My passion for natural health evolved into a passion to become a naturopathic doctor. I was toward the end of homeschooling my children and took the opportunity to return to school. After choosing The Trinity College of Natural Health, I completed my studies in nutritional counseling, then also enrolled in a Certified Natural Health Professional program. During this time I also worked in a small health-food store, a holistic pharmacy, and as an assistant to a naturopathic doctor. My message became more defined through my work and studies. I attended a training program through one of the top "pharmaceutical-grade" natural supplement companies. This solidified my conviction that vitamins made in a test tube are synthetic and should not be consumed.

The research and study I have done over the years is different from mainstream natural health practitioners. My goal is to return us to living according to nature and our design. There are many compromises to the truth of natural living. It doesn't have to be complicated and we don't have to be confused. We can have peace in knowing that we are assisting our body's natural design to follow Nature and Nature's God.

During my years of study, I visited a naturopathic doctor, Dori Luneski, who utilized an amazing technology called the SpectraVision™ (SV). The SV confirmed things about my body in a matter of minutes. Our bodies are energetic. The SV was able to measure my body's energy responses and give a clear account. This was not my first introduction to energy medicine. Having used homeopathic remedies, I was impressed with the SV's ability to help in the healing process by using a multidimensional approach to balance the body. I purchased my own device and attended the required classes to become a SpectraVision™ practitioner.

In the spring of 2008, I opened my practice, **Energetic Wellness**. I had already received my Doctor of Naturopathy, but I also became a Board Certified Naturopathic Doctor, which requires annual continuing education classes— which I do in addition to my own personal studies. My love and passion for learning and teaching will continue the rest of my life.

My hope is that this book and my practice will inspire and empower you with wisdom and understanding, and save you precious time on your journey. This book is a compilation of my personal study on health. I hope you find it to be a clear path in the world of health contradictions. You do not have to feel alone on your healing, as I felt for many years. We have the Spirit of the living God guiding us. We already have all truth at our fingertips—we have the truth written in our hearts.

Even though my initial experience was very painful, God has used it for good to help me better understand His miraculous design of creation and the human body. Finding the truth through my pain has been a miraculous journey, and facing my deepest fear has turned my life around. I hope my journey serves as a guide to help eliminate your own confusion and fear.

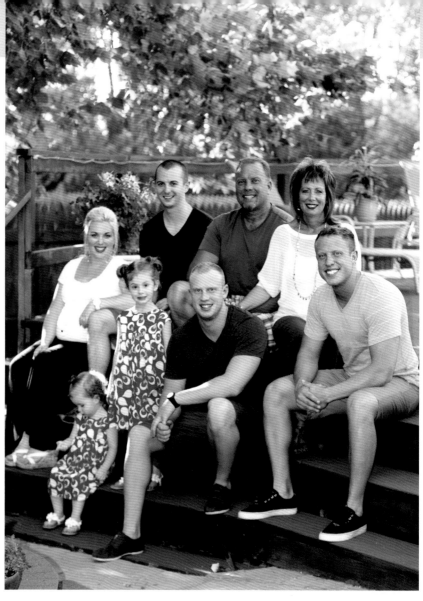

The Menzel Family
Jessica (7 months with Gemma) & Jordan Brown
with daughters Serenity and Angeline,
Steven & Michele Menzel,
Stephen Menzel, Michael Menzel

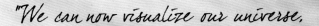

"We can now visualize our universe,

its light, gravity and heat,

its seasons, tides, and harvest,

which prepare a habitation for the universe of vital forms,

microscopic and majestic,

which fill the oceans and the forests.

We have a common denominator for universes within and around each other.

Our world, our food, and our life have potentials so vast

that we can only observe directions, not goals.

We sense human achievements

or ignominious race self-destruction.

Every creed today vaguely seeks a utopia;

all have visualized a common controlling force or deity

as the most potent force in all human affairs.

Yes, man's place is most exalted

when he obeys

Mother Nature's laws."

—Weston A. Price, DDS

The Transformation

Introduction

This book comes from my heart and is a culmination of self study, formal training, and, most of all, 20 years of my own experience!

Going through my own major healing crisis and working through it 100 percent naturally has given me the strong desire to teach others how to live naturally and assist the body in natural healing. The word *doctor* means **teacher**, so my intention is to empower you with the wisdom and the knowledge to restore your body to optimal health.

My favorite part of research is studying other cultures—how our ancestors lived, what they ate, and especially how they prepared food and why. Years ago, after reading *Nourishing Traditions* by Sally Fallon, my studies led me to The Weston A. Price Foundation. I already believed that we should eat pure whole foods, but Sally's book and Dr. Price's work delved even deeper. As you know, it can sometimes be confusing with so many options offered to us, so let's look back about 100 years, and realize that people lived on pure whole foods. Let's consider which ones and why.

The body is miraculous. We can trust the Creator and the design. The body was designed to heal naturally. You will experience changes as you go through *The Transformation* and you will discover how wonderfully your body assists you through life! Most of all, you are going to transform your life and feel amazing!

During my years of self study, I put together what I now call the **7 Laws of Wellness**. Think of them as you would the natural laws of the universe—or the natural laws of the earth. These laws of our world are precise and function automatically, and we have to pay attention to them. The human body has natural laws as well—biological laws that support the human body's existence. Our responsibility is to take care of ourselves so that our natural function can happen everyday with energy and vitality, as well as rebalance and heal itself. My seven laws of wellness came from many years of my own trial and error, as well as from researching how to live according to Nature and Nature's God.

Wellness is a way of life. We know that diets don't work, and they are hard on the body. After the diet is over, we usually go back to eating and living the way we did before, and all the weight comes back and sometimes even more than when we started. It can become a vicious, frustrating cycle. This book was designed with a plan to stop this cycle from happening again.

The Transformation takes you through an elimination diet, a transition, and by the end, you will be eating foods you can live on for life. You can use this book as a resource guide to assist you through life!

> "Let food be your medicine and medicine be your food."
> —Hippocrates

Before We Begin...

This way of eating may be a complete paradigm shift in your thinking. Three things I want you to rethink:

- **Fat does not cause you to be fat!**
- **You don't have to count calories!**
- **You can eat delicious, real food to maintain your perfect weight!**

Join me as I take you through one of the most rewarding experiences of your life!

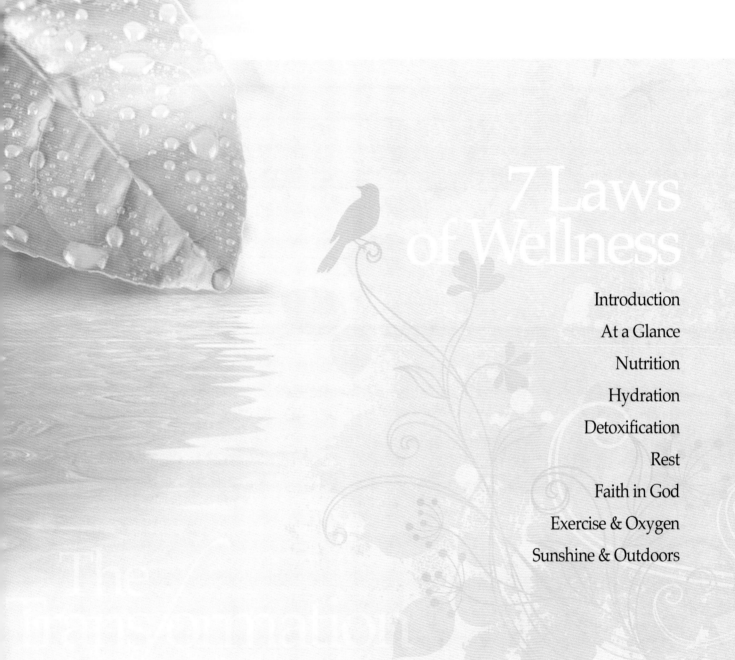

7 Laws of Wellness

The Transformation

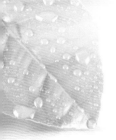

Introduction to the
7 Laws of Wellness
CREATING ENERGY FOR BALANCED LIVING

The body can never be viewed as *just* physical as many practitioners and health care professionals do today. Each individual is a whole person—including body, mind, and spirit. The whole person needs total care.

Learning how to take responsibility for our lives through natural living practices is new to us. However, natural living practices are the way we are intended to live. We were designed to live according to these practices. The body was designed with specific biological purposes to support life—to support everything about us—thought, feeling, and emotion. The foods we eat and the environment in which we live contribute to living a full and vibrant life. We are to work with nature and the design of the body, not against them. This is for our good.

Perfect Love Casts Out Fear

God is love and His design was created out of love. When we understand our design and how the body works to support us, we understand His love, and we do not need to fear.

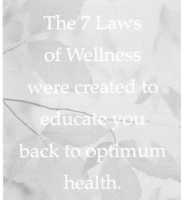

The 7 Laws of Wellness were created to educate you back to optimum health.

The world is filled with fear and most of the current medical practices are based on fear. The fear of disease and cancer has deceived us into thinking that is our fate. We don't have to expect that at a certain age we should suffer with a certain ailment. That is the expectation of modern medicine based on the standard American diet, environmental exposures, and fast-paced living.

My desire in sharing the 7 Laws of Wellness is to open your eyes to a new—actually it was the *original*—way of thinking, to live in support of the beautiful life you were given. These laws were developed to point you back to our creation and the natural design of the body. When we understand the design and the natural way the body supports us, we do not have to be afraid. Instead, we can learn to support the body and live a full and healthy life.

Throughout the last 100 years, we have been programmed to believe in the "new science" of pharmaceutical drugs, surgery, and poisonous invasive therapies. These practices are not natural; *they* are the alternative. Naturopathy is the earliest known healing system. **Foods, water, fresh air,** and **sunshine** were and still are the natural ways to heal.

I am a true naturopath and want to practice natural health care which encompasses teaching natural lifestyle changes. Understanding the biological principles of the body will always be my course of study and my subject to teach.

The Naturopathic Philosophy

These principles suggest my philosophy, not necessarily those practiced by other naturopaths. These principles were gathered from my own studies of natural health, as well as from the history of naturopathy.

"Naturopathy is a philosophy, art, and science. It recognizes the body's inherent processes of healing, and acts in no way to suppress, antagonize, or hinder these vital life forces. But rather it seeks to arouse, assist, and cooperate with the body toward a restoration to normal."

—Robert J. Thiel, PhD
Naturopathy for the 21st Century

Naturopathy is a way of healing using the body's innate ability to heal itself. This encompasses all that nature has given us—including water, air, sunlight, earthing, exercise, rest, and proper food—my 7 Laws of Wellness.

Naturopaths practice and believe in the healing power of nature. This belief includes the concept that the body can heal itself of just about anything if cleared of toxins and given proper nutrition, rest, mental outlook, and natural stimulation. It also acknowledges that no health practitioner can know everything there is to know about human health.

Thus, when in doubt, the naturopath recommends the most natural approach possible. The naturopath trusts that the natural processes within the body want it to heal! That is why I only recommend the things that I believe were intended to keep the vital energy of the body alive and functioning well.

> *"Getting well may be a matter of educating rather than medicating."*
>
> —Dr. Bernard Jenson

We work with the **cause** of symptoms. Symptoms always point to what you have just experienced. The next step is to support the body in natural healing. We need to resolve the conflict and support the healing the body is trying to do. Everything else will improve. This is truly working with the whole person.

Naturopaths believe in prevention through right living. Prevention is the best cure. Naturopaths should not use the word *cure*; naturopathic suggestions and modalities do not cure; the body "cures" itself. Naturopaths are facilitators. We identify the cause of problems, recommend ways to resolve the emotional situation, decrease and eliminate toxins, and identify foods and whole food supplements to address deficiencies and assist the body's healing abilities.

As a totally non-invasive practice, naturopathy does not make use of synthetic or inorganic vitamins or minerals—or drugs, narcotics, vaccines, etc.

All so-called "diseases" can be addressed through natural healing. In naturopathy, we work with life and the forces of life to encourage the healing process.

There are six core values that naturopathic practitioners follow. The exact wording varies, but the basic oath is in bold print below. My additions follow.

1. Do no harm; naturopaths should provide the best care possible with the least exposure to risk for their patients. Natural recommendations include counseling in lifestyle changes, whole food nutrition, whole food supplementation, and holistic therapies that support the body's natural function.

2. Promote the self-healing nature of all humans. Assist the patient in recognizing the natural causes of symptoms and assist the body in natural self-healing.

3. Identify and remove the causes of an illness instead of suppressing them. Together we will identify and creatively remove stress that is contributing to your symptoms, always allowing the body to go through the healing process to obtain full recovery.

4. Educate and inspire people to be responsible for their own health. Education and inspiration are key! I will share with you my 7 Laws of Wellness which will empower you with resources, information, hope, and the assurance you need to take your health into your own hands.

5. Treat each person according to his or her individual needs. An extensive health history review, an evaluation on the SpectraVision™, and individual time spent with each client allows me to meet your personal needs.

6. Promote good health to help prevent disease in the individual, the community, and the world. At Energetic Wellness, we are committed to help you achieve a life full of energy and balanced living. One by one, we can change our mindset and teach our children; making a difference in our communities and throughout the world! We can live a healthy, natural lifestyle!

Wellness is a way of life. The body was designed to thrive. The 7 Laws of Wellness will guide you to eating and living naturally so that you can achieve energy and vitality into old age. We don't have to believe that we will get a certain ailment because we are a certain age. That is modern-medicine thinking based on the standard American diet, environmental toxins, and fast-paced living.

I chose to list seven laws of wellness because seven is God's perfect number. The root of the word *seven* means perfect, complete, or satisfied. God marked the Bible with the number seven because it is the fullness of His revelation! It is perfection. I hope these 7 Laws of Wellness are a revelation to you of the wonder of our creation and how we can live and thrive naturally in today's world.

We can totally rebalance the body by applying the principles explained in the 7 Laws. Throughout *The Transformation*, I'll teach the fundamental laws of natural living and their application in your daily life. We have the responsibility to take care of ourselves from within—and that begins at home. **You are the only one who can heal your body and life.**

"Naturopathy is the mother, all-inclusive,

of natural therapy. It is the science of nature,

the biological way of living right,

the natural way to cure….

All the other systems,

if they are biologically correct,

must belong to naturopathy or nature cure…."

— *Dr. Benedict Lust (1925)*

Please see the Source Acknowledgments on page 272 for a list of research, books, and websites used for this section.

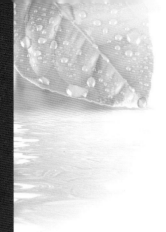

7 Laws
of Wellness *at a Glance*

CREATING ENERGY FOR BALANCED LIVING

These are short definitions of the 7 Laws of Wellness. In the following pages and in the Daily Routine section, you will find more ideas for how to apply them to your life. Helpful books, websites, DVDs, and CDs are listed in the Resource section of this book.

Nutrition

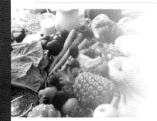

Food was created to be our medicine and medicine our food.

We should be able to obtain our nutrients from foods if we choose properly! Organic, pure, nutrient-dense whole foods are the traditional foods enjoyed by our ancestors such as grass-fed meat, pastured chicken and pork, wild-caught fish, sprouted grains, and raw dairy. When you begin to transform your life with these foods, you will see and feel the difference.

Hydration

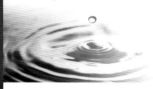

A good rule of thumb is to drink half your weight in ounces of water daily.

Do not drink or bathe in tap water. Install shower filters and use a bath ball in tubs. A reverse osmosis system (whole-house or under-the-counter) is ideal. FIJI and VOSS are good bottled water choices. The GIA Wellness iH2O hydration system energizes reverse osmosis water that lacks energy. We have to add nutrients to energize filtered water for it to hydrate the cells of the body.

Detoxification

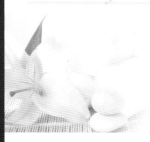

The body has a natural process. We don't have to tell the body to detoxify.

We only have to assist the body's design by eating nutrient-dense foods and whole-food supplements so that the body has what it needs to function and detox naturally. Expect the colon to eliminate daily before noon. Drink the correct amount of water for the kidneys. Keep the lymphatic system moving through exercise like rebounding and walking; this will also greatly benefit the liver.

Rest
The body has a daily two-phase cycle.

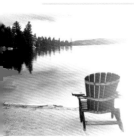

The daytime active phase and the nighttime healing phase. It is essential to our wellbeing that we allow the body the opportunity to go into the nighttime healing phase. This has to be a daily practice—probably the most important of the 7 Laws. The purpose of sleep is to heal from activities and stressors of the day. Rest enables rebuilding, regenerating, and repairing the body—giving us renewed energy in the morning. We need 6–9 hours of uninterrupted sleep per night in complete darkness, no electronic devices. Down by 10, up at 6!

Faith in God
Studies show a remarkable difference in people with a strong spiritual belief.

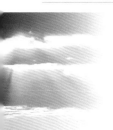

Indigenous peoples studied by Dr. Weston A. Price had a strong belief system that aided in vibrant health. Emotional perceptions also play a large role in our health. Experts say 99 percent of all illness is due to an emotional conflict or prolonged stress. German New Medicine® reveals that our bodies were created with "significant biological purposeful responses," initiated from the psyche, designed to assist the body at all times. Try to resolve conflicts in the day they happen. Pray, meditate, and surrender.

Exercise / Oxygen
A minimum of 30 minutes a day, every day, for the rest of your life!

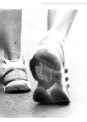

The body was designed to move! Rebounding, walking, and treadmill (in that order) are the best for the lymphatic system—which needs to be moved every day since it does not have a pump like the heart. Before cars, people walked an average of 3–6 miles a day. Resistance exercise is recommended at least three times a week. Yoga for relaxation and breathing will increase oxygen absorption. Core strengthening exercises for women are essential.

Sunshine / Outdoors
Get at least 20 minutes of sunshine a day.

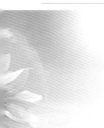

Sunshine on your skin with most of the body exposed will provide the vitamin D the body needs during different times of the year. In the fall and winter, take cod liver oil and use vitamin D-Lite therapy. Spend as much time outdoors as possible for *earthing* and fresh air, especially after a rain storm. Open windows to freshen and circulate indoor air.

Nutrition

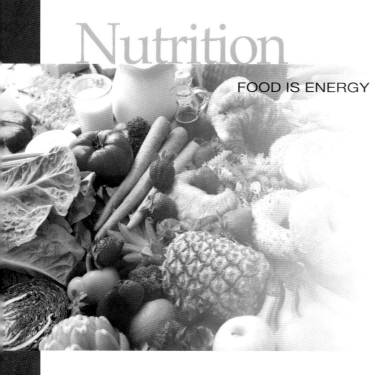

FOOD IS ENERGY

"Let food be your medicine

and medicine your food." —Hippocrates

Many centuries have passed since Hippocrates in 400 B.C.

He wrote about preventative medicine and

is known as the "Father of Medicine."

Hippocrates and his followers were very concerned about preserving health through proper diet, exercise, and rest. He is possibly the best-known naturopathic scientist.

"Throughout his professional life, he exhibited the greatest respect and reverence for nature, and taught his followers, students, and initiates that the healing of all diseases was 'up to' nature…. He stated that only nature could cure, and that the province of the physician was merely to assist, to make the healing more pleasant or less painful." —Robert J. Thiel, PhD, *Naturopathy for the 21st Century*

We have drifted so far from eating natural, pure, whole food. Today we have little understanding and connection with the foods we eat and how they affect us. Today our children have little idea of where food comes from or how it is grown. They know only that they can go to a drive-thru window and get great-tasting food really fast.

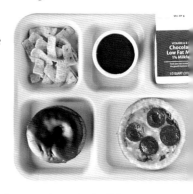

We have to understand how food changes the body, supplying the building blocks for healing and replacing old tissue with new. Food was created to sustain and rebuild. **The foods we eat have a direct correlation to the way we feel, the way we look, our ability to rest, and our ability to stay healthy.** Foods are the primary source of energy and are designed to assist the body in natural healing.

Nutrient Levels in Traditional Diets

Dr. Weston A. Price was a dentist, and, after practicing for 30 years in the United States, he began to see changes in his patients' dental and overall health. He believed these changes were a direct result of the changes happening to our food. Modern processing had begun, and he felt that the refining of our food was causing nutritional deficiencies—leading to deformed dental arches and resulting in crowded, crooked teeth.

Dr. Price and his wife, who was a nurse, traveled to isolated parts of the world for over a decade to study the health of populations untouched by Western processed food. The groups Dr. Price studied included remote villages in Switzerland, Gaelic communities in the Outer Hebrides, indigenous peoples of North and South America, Melanesian and Polynesian South Sea Islanders, African tribes, Australian Aborigines, and New Zealand Maori. Wherever he went, he found that beautiful straight teeth, freedom from decay, good physiques, resistance to disease, and fine characters (people of good character) were typical of native groups on their traditional diets, rich in essential nutrients.

When he analyzed the foods used by isolated peoples he found that, in comparison to the American diet of his day, they provided:

- Calcium and other minerals— at least 4 times higher than the modern diet.
- Vitamins A, D, and K2—10 times higher than the modern diet.

These vitamins and minerals are rich in foods such as butter, fish eggs, shellfish, organ meats, eggs, and animal fats— the very cholesterol-rich foods now shunned by Americans as unhealthy.

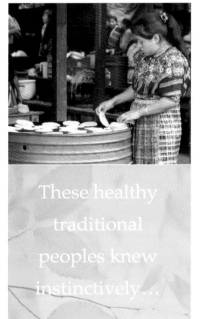

These healthy traditional peoples knew instinctively...

These healthy, traditional people knew instinctively what scientists of Dr. Price's day had recently discovered— that fat-soluble vitamins were vital to health because they acted as catalysts to mineral absorption and protein utilization. Without them, we cannot absorb minerals, no matter how abundant they may be in our food.

Price discovered an additional fat-soluble nutrient, which he labeled "Activator X," present in fish livers, shellfish, organ meats, and butter from cows eating rapidly growing green grass in the spring and fall. All primitive groups had a source of Activator X, now thought to be vitamin K2, in their diets.

The following is a summary of Dr. Price's findings that we should incorporate in our diet today. America is a melting pot of all the cultures Price studied. We have to go back to our traditional way of eating.

Characteristics of Traditional Diets

- The diets of healthy, non-industrialized people contain no refined or denatured foods or ingredients, such as refined sugar or high fructose corn syrup, white flour, canned foods, pasteurized/homogenized/skim/low-fat milk, refined or hydrogenated vegetable oils, protein powders, synthetic vitamins, toxic additives, and artificial colorings.

- All traditional cultures consume some sort of animal food, such as fish and shellfish, land and water fowl, land and sea mammals, eggs, milk and milk products, reptiles, and insects. The whole animal is consumed—muscle meat, organs, bones and fat, with the organ meats and fats preferred.

- The diets of healthy, non-industrialized people contain at least four times the minerals and water-soluble vitamins, and ten times the fat-soluble vitamins found in animal fats (vitamin A, vitamin D, and Activator X, now thought to be vitamin K2) as the average American diet.

- All traditional cultures cooked some of their food but all consumed a portion of their animal foods raw.

- Primitive and traditional diets have a high content of food enzymes and beneficial bacteria from lacto-fermented vegetables, fruits, beverages, dairy products, meats, and condiments.

- Seeds, grains, and nuts are soaked, sprouted, fermented, or naturally leavened to neutralize naturally occurring anti-nutrients such as enzyme inhibitors, tannins, and phytic acid.

Nutrition, cont.

- Total fat content of traditional diets varies from 8–30% of total calories consumed, but only about 4% of calories come from polyunsaturated oils naturally occurring in grains, legumes, nuts, fish, animals fats, and vegetables. The balance of fat calories are in the form of saturated and monounsaturated fatty acids.

- Traditional diets contain nearly equal amounts of omega-6 and omega-3 essential fatty acids.

- All traditional diets contain salt.

- All traditional cultures make use of animal bones, usually in the form of gelatin-rich bone broths.

- Traditional cultures make provisions for the health of future generations by providing special nutrient-rich animal foods for parents-to-be, pregnant women, and growing children; by adequate spacing of children; and by teaching the principles of a correct diet to the young.

I learned about Dr. Price through Sally Fallon and her book, *Nourishing Traditions*. After reading her book and purchasing Dr. Price's book, *Nutrition and Physical Degeneration*, my journey toward understanding foods began. The teaching of Dr. Price is now the foundation of my nutrition practice.

A Simpler Time

My grandmother was 97 when she passed. She took no medication, was active into her 90s, had all her faculties, and was very alert. She was born in 1902, and was breastfed. In that time people were still getting fresh milk delivered to their homes or else they owned a cow themselves. They had fresh meat that they raised or purchased from the local butcher. They grew their own vegetables or bought them at the local market from local producers. They received a very good foundation nutritionally.

There was very little processed food. White flour was new to the United States and, from what I've read, it was

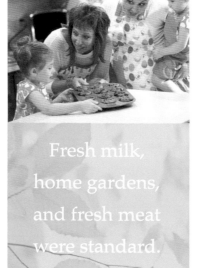

Fresh milk, home gardens, and fresh meat were standard.

very costly. In order to stretch a dollar, food was made from scratch, and the whole animal was used. Even the bones were used to make stock for soups, sauces, and gravies. There was no waste.

These pure, whole foods were alive and gave that generation the foundation and energy to live into their 90s and even 100s. My father will hopefully follow. My parents are 79 and 80. My father is in very good health and still works part-time. He remembers a lot of what I have described to you.

From Simple to Empty

Many chemical substitutes replaced real food with no thought of the consequences to the human body and the effect this would have on our children.

In 1911, Crisco replaced lard and butter. Crisco stands for "crystallized cottonseed oil." It was made from leftover seeds from the cotton industry. Proctor and Gamble was trying to be resourceful with their leftovers, but I don't think they really understood what this would mean to the health of the body. This hydrogenated oil was marketed as healthier than lard and butter with no studies!

In the last 50 years things have changed dramatically. My generation was raised on white flour, hot dogs, pasteurized milk, cupcakes, etc. Fifty years ago the average American ate 12 pounds of sugar a year. Today it is 12 pounds eaten per month! Refined grains were virtually unknown in the human diet before 1600 and never used in great quantities before the 20th century.

Dr. David Katz at Yale Preventive Medicine Research Center predicts that children born after the year 2000 may be the first generation in modern history to die before their parents. He also states that there will be more premature deaths from poor eating, obesity, and lack of activity among our youth than from smoking, drugs, and alcohol combined. I call this the generational effect of processed foods. That is a pretty profound statement and one we all should be concerned about. The children that are being born today do not have the same chance for an abundant life as their parents and grandparents.

On the Bright Side

The good news is we don't have to succumb to this effect if we change our way of eating. This country is beginning the fourth or fifth generation consuming processed foods. My grandmother was first generation, my father's the 2nd, I'm the 3rd, and my children are the 4th in our family. My new granddaughter is the 5th generation. The switch to whole foods started with my embracing change about 18 years ago when I eliminated white flour from our diet. Although my children consumed white flour and white sugar on occasion, we did not have it in our home. I am so thankful that my daughter is raising her family on whole nutrient-dense foods.

The isolated groups Dr. Price studied understood the importance of preconceptual nutrition for both parents. Many tribes required a period of special feeding before conception, in which nutrient-dense animal foods were given to young men and women. These same foods were considered important for pregnant and lactating women and growing children. Price discovered the foods to be particularly rich in minerals and in the fat-soluble activators found only in animal fats. (I guess you have realized by now that I'm not going to advise vegetarianism!)

Price also observed that they had ease in reproduction, emotional stability, and freedom from degenerative disease. In his book, *Nutrition and Physical Degeneration*, Price photographed these beautiful people with their fine bodies in contrast to civilized moderns subsisting on the "displacing foods of modern commerce, including sugar, white flour, pasteurized milk, lowfat foods, vegetable oils, and convenience items filled with extenders and additives."

If we want to reproduce healthy generations, then we must learn from these groups the importance of a nutrient-dense diet. If not, as Dr. Katz stated, this will be the generation that does not outlive their parents.

What is a Pure Whole Food?

The widespread study of nutrition by people in all walks of life is a fairly new development in our culture. It began with the need to study deficiencies aggravated by processed food, as we have just learned from Dr. Price's studies. We do not have to be confused any longer.

My own journey in discovering the best foods to eat has been a long one. For the past 20 years, I tried many different "diets" such as vegetarian, vegan, raw, food combinations, and the blood type diet. It can become very confusing to decide which one to follow.

Through this experience and many years of study, I found a good balance of the foods God created for us and also discovered ways to consume them in their natural state. Experiences of trial and error always lead me back to the foods that were created for us from the beginning.

We should eat the food God created for us, but this is a difficult task when eating the standard American diet of devitalized food. Modern agriculture, determined to see maximum harvests, has totally changed the nature of what is presented to us as food.

A pure whole food is a food that has not been changed from its original state.

31

Nutrition, cont.

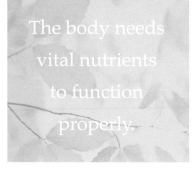

The body needs vital nutrients to function properly.

A pure, whole food is a food that has not been changed from its original state. It is unprocessed and unrefined. Whole foods do not contain added ingredients. Foods should have life. Live food has been grown or raised outdoors and has not been altered in any way. This includes fruits, vegetables, raw dairy products, grass-fed meat, pasture-raised eggs, pastured chickens, wild fish, and grains that are organic and prepared properly.

Choosing Whole Foods

The body is energetic and needs vital nutrients to function properly. One of my favorite teachers—although I only know him through his textbooks—Dr. Bernard Jensen, understood the ability of foods to heal the body. Dr. Jensen had over 50 years of experience using nutrition to restore patients to normal health. He believed in whole foods and, through his experience, learned how each food and its nutrients could be used to heal the individual. I often refer to Dr. Jensen's textbook when I see a significant deficiency and want to recommend the right foods.

If we choose properly, we should be able to obtain the nutrients we need from the foods we eat. Because of our non-whole-food foundation, it might also be beneficial to include whole-food supplements. The basic supplements outlined in this book are ones I recommend to all of my patients. They supply the body with the needed cellular nutrients to restore life and rebuild the body.

I like to use the example of an apple. An apple is a pure, whole food. It has over 2,000 nutrients in it. It is complex—consisting of vitamins, minerals, enzymes, and natural sugar. It is called a complex carbohydrate.

Now if you take that apple and squeeze it, what is extracted is apple juice, one simple part of the complexity. Fruit juice is very sweet because it is pure fructose. It could be assumed that fructose, or fruit

sugar, would be good for us. And, yes, when it is part of the apple, it is good for us. But when we separate it and only consume the juice, it affects the body very differently than a whole apple.

When we eat the whole apple, it has all that is needed for us to digest and assimilate its content. Fruit juice, on the other hand, affects your blood sugar as refined granular sugar does and, therefore, could cause problems when you consume a lot of it.

Isolated, Empty & Fake

Any one single vitamin, mineral, or sugar that we isolate will have a very different effect on the body than when we consume it as part of a whole food. Processed foods have had the nutrients removed through refinement. We can apply this principle to anything created to be our food. When the food is stripped of the vital nutrients, the body will not have the necessary catalysts of enzymes and minerals it needs to digest the food properly.

Grain is a healthy food when prepared correctly. However, when refined or processed, it is left devitalized and denatured. White flour has been stripped of its nutrients through the refining process.

Pasteurization of dairy products by high temperatures leaves little nutrient value left in the milk. The live enzymes, good bacteria, vitamins, and minerals are altered, which leave dairy products very difficult to digest. Even though vitamin D is added to the processed milk, the body cannot absorb it. Americans consume more dairy products than any other country in the world and yet are still nutritionally deficient.

Most people are running on empty. Deficiencies are a problem in the day we live because of the food we were raised on and the food that we continue to eat. We cannot expect to be well when we are putting fake food into the body. This includes such foods as white flour products, white sugar products (including artificial sweeteners), high fructose corn syrup, hydrogenated and partially hydrogenated oils, and dairy products that contain synthetic hormones, antibiotics, are ultra pasteurized, and homogenized. Our physical nature is such that we need foods that are whole—not refined and denatured—to grow, prosper, and reproduce!

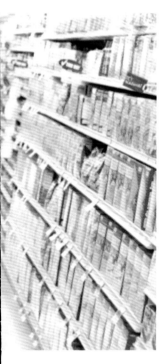

Unfortunately, our grocery store shelves are filled with refined, processed, fake food affecting the natural function and balance of the body. Food manufacturers continue to supply us with cheap imitations. If you are wondering what a fake food is, just read the label. If you can't pronounce the words, it probably contains a chemical or synthetic additive. This food has little nutritional value, is foreign to the body, and will bring the energy of the body down. It can also cause deficiencies, hormonal imbalances, and mood changes.

The rise of obesity and diabetes is also a direct result of fake food. When we consume empty calories from white flour and white sugar, the body does not process them, but instead stores them as fat. Empty calories also cause your blood sugar to rise and create an imbalance.

Carbohydrates

Carbohydrates are naturally occurring complex sugars. In nature, these energy providers are linked together with vitamins, minerals, enzymes, protein, fat, and fiber—the body-building components of the diet. In whole form, starches support life!

But refined carbohydrates have an adverse effect because they are devoid of body-building elements. Digestion of refined carbohydrates calls on the body's own store of vitamins, minerals, and enzymes for proper metabolization. When B vitamins are absent, for example, the breakdown of carbohydrates cannot take place, yet most B vitamins are removed during the refining process. The refining process strips grains of both their vitamin and mineral components.

Refined carbohydrates have been called *empty* calories. *Negative* calories is a more appropriate term because consumption of refined calories depletes the body's precious reserves. All calories are not considered equal!

The Effects of Refined Carbohydrates on Blood Sugar, Adrenals & Thyroid

The level of glucose in the blood is regulated by a finely tuned mechanism involving insulin secretions from the pancreas and hormones from several glands, including the adrenal glands and the thyroid. When you eat sugars and starches in their natural, unrefined form as part of a meal containing nourishing fats and protein, they are digested slowly and enter the bloodstream at a moderate rate over a period of several hours. If the body goes a long time without food, this mechanism will call upon reserves stored in the liver.

When working properly, this marvelous blood sugar regulation process provides our cells with a steady, even supply of glucose. The body is kept on an even keel, both physically and emotionally! But when we consume refined sugars and starches—particularly alone, without fats or protein—they enter the bloodstream in a rush, causing a sudden increase in blood sugar! The body's regulation mechanism kicks into high gear, flooding the blood with insulin and other hormones to bring blood sugar levels down to acceptable levels.

Repeated onslaughts of sugar will eventually disrupt this finely tuned process, causing some elements to remain in a constant state of activity and others to become worn out and inadequate to do the job. This situation is exacerbated because a diet high in refined carbohydrates will also be deficient in vitamins, minerals, and enzymes—those elements that keep the glands and organs in good repair.

> When we consume refined sugars and starches, they enter the bloodstream in a rush.

Nutrition, cont.

Eliminate Processed Foods

I believe strict abstinence from refined carbohydrates is very good advice for everyone.

Sugar is the number one legal drug in America. More Americans are addicted to sugar than anything else. Our bodies were not designed to thrive on "junk food." Refined sugar is mood altering, behavior altering, and disrupts hormonal balance in the body and overall homeostasis. A 2007 University of Bordeaux study revealed that white sugar has been proven to be four times more addictive than cocaine. Today the average American consumes 150 pounds of sugar per year.

Dr. David Lustig, a Pediatric Endocrinologist at the University of California in San Francisco, has been studying the effects of sugar on children and adults. In April 2012, he was interviewed on *60 Minutes*. The topic: "Is Sugar Toxic?" He also has a YouTube video that is rather lengthy (90 minutes) called "Sugar: The Bitter Truth."

When biochemical balance is thrown off by eating processed foods, the body is no longer functioning harmoniously. *Consumption of white sugar contributes indirectly to all diseases caused by a deficiency of protein, minerals, or vitamins.* So-called energy drinks are especially dangerous to the body.

Possible disruptions in natural function due to processed foods include:

- Disturbed endocrine system (hormones / glands)
- Mood swings
- Learning disabilities in children and adults
- Behavioral problems in children and adults
- Obesity
- Lowered vitality
- Reduced ability to handle everyday stress
- Diabetes, especially among children

We Live in a "Supersize Me" Society!

In the West, we are eating much more than we used to—and so much more than we need to. Your stomach is the size of your fist and that is the amount of food required in a typical meal. But the stomach is a muscular sac that can expand to hold a greater amount of food. In fact, it can expand up to three times its size after a large meal.

Stuffing ourselves causes a variety of consequences:
- nausea
- heartburn
- discomfort
- belching

Overeating can cause weight gain, especially if you are eating the wrong foods. Here are a few ways you can prevent yourself from overeating:

- **Eat slowly** and stop just before you think you are full. If you sit back and wait about 20 minutes before your second helping, you will realize that you have had enough.

- **Chew your food well** and slowly, putting the fork down in between bites. Digestion begins in the mouth.

- **Be mindful of portion size.** Fist-sized portions are usually best. Using a side plate instead of a dinner plate might be helpful.

- **Don't eat at all-you-can-eat buffets,** which contribute to America's overeating. We think that since we are paying for our buffet meal, we have to eat a lot to get our money's worth. We are paying for it—at the restaurant and in the consequences to our health.

- **Don't eat excessively,** even to prevent food waste. Most food can be refrigerated for a day or so and still keep its nutritional content.

- **Don't eat when you are angry, sad, scared, or anxious.** These emotions shut down digestion. When you are angry, your support system can be depressed for six hours, and half your day is ruined! Another reason to avoid sugar is that it can also depress your system for up to six hours.

- **Enjoy your meal**! Eat with family or friends, talk about your day, and relax.

If we eat too much, it is hard for the digestive system to handle the overload. We need sufficient digestive juices to digest properly. When we overeat, the body requires more energy to handle the excess, which depletes our energy resources.

Another reason for depleted energy is that we eat too much processed food. The top three foods consumed in America are: **hot dogs, white bread, and coffee.** In 1970, we spent 6 billion dollars on fast food. Today, we spend over 110 billion dollars. Our lifestyles are so consumed with work and activities that we have forgotten to take care of these wonderful creations—our bodies!

We cannot continue to eat the way we do and expect to be well. We have to eat real food—food that gives the body energy and vitality and leads to a long and healthy life. We have to lose our old habits and develop new ones. Foods that are pure, whole, alive, and nutrient-dense will always get the body back on track!

Recommended Foods

Buy locally grown foods directly from the farm, your farmers' market, organic foods from the grocery store, or start to grow your own food! These foods contain up to 60 percent higher nutritional value. Raw goat milk, yogurt, and kefir are alive and high in enzymes, probiotics, vitamins, and minerals. These foods energize the body, nourish the body, and ultimately keep the body in balance.

The foods recommended for the 48 Days are dense in nutrition and ideal to enjoy for life. When you start to transform your life with these foods, you will see and feel the difference.

I live according to this philosophy every day. In my pantry, you will not find a single processed food item. In fact, I don't have any boxed food. Instead, I choose foods that give the body energy and life!

PLEASE SEE THE SOURCE ACKNOWLEDGMENTS ON PAGE 272 FOR A LIST OF RESEARCH, BOOKS, AND WEBSITES USED FOR THIS SECTION.

Refrigerator – fruits, vegetables, farm-fresh, non-genetically modified eggs, raw cheeses, yogurt, kefir, kombucha, and raw milk.

Pantry – Onions, garlic, red potatoes, sweet potatoes, glass jars of dry beans, whole grains, raw nuts, coconut oil, olive oil, dried herbs, local honey, Rapunzel whole cane sugar, and maple syrup.

Freezer – Grass-fed beef and lamb, pastured pork, organ meats, pastured organic chickens, fresh-water and wild-caught fish, homemade bone broths, bones and feet for stock.

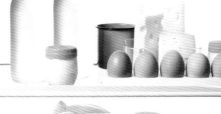
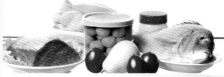
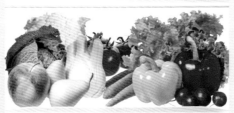

Start by Stocking Your Kitchen

• Foods free of pesticides, hormones, and antibiotics

• Foods perfect in balance of omega-3 fatty acids, such as grass-fed beef, organic free-range chicken, organic free-range eggs, and wild-caught fish

• Foods high in fiber, such as whole grains prepared correctly—brown rice, millet, and spelt (one of the healthiest grains that dates back to the book of Exodus in the Bible)

• Goat dairy products, such as raw milk, yogurt, and kefir

"Nutrition is probably the greatest of all the health arts…. Without a balanced diet of wholesome, nutritious foods, wellness cannot be achieved and sustained, no matter what else we do." —Dr. Bernard Jensen, PhD

Hydration
ESSENTIAL FOR LIFE

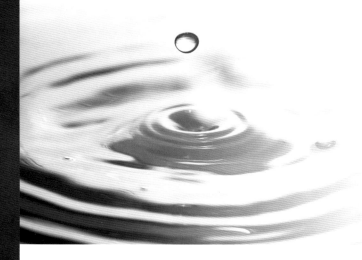

Water is essential for healing,

for vibrant health, and to sustain life!

Water is of major importance to all living things.

No living organisms would exist without the existence

of an ample water supply on Earth.

The cells in our bodies are full of water.
Muscles are 75% water;
blood is 82% water;
lungs are 90% water;
the brain, the control center
of your body, is 76% water;
and even bones are 25% water.

The unique qualities of water make it so essential to life. Its ability to dissolve so many substances allows our cells to use valuable nutrients, minerals, and chemicals in biological processes. The water in the bloodstream helps transport oxygen to the cells, removes waste, and protects and lubricates joints and organs.

Water is one of the most important *nutrients* that the body needs. When you drink plenty of water, every single system, organ, and cell in the body benefits. The health benefits of water include the following:

- More energy
- Better performance
- Weight loss
- Fewer headaches & dizziness
- Improved digestion and elimination of waste

What Causes Dehydration?

Taking in too little water or losing too much water leads to dehydration. Symptoms of mild dehydration include thirst, pains in joints and muscles, lower back pain, headaches, and constipation. In the book *Your Body's Many Cries For Water*, Dr. Batmanghelidj states that almost all conditions in the body are a result of our need for water. He explains that "unintentional chronic dehydration" contributes to and even produces many degenerative conditions that could be treated by increasing water intake on a regular basis.

I believe unintentional chronic dehydration is largely related to the type of water we drink. Many people who come to my office claim to drink "a ton of water," and yet the results of the SpectraVision™ scan and their particular symptoms suggest they are dehydrated. The quality of water we drink is critical to the effect that it will have on our body—especially the ability for the water to penetrate at the cellular level to keep you hydrated.

The Mounting Concerns with Tap Water

My patients understand that my approach to wellness is based out of love and not fear. I don't want to cause fear, but I do want you to be informed so that you have the knowledge to make wise choices when it comes to your health and the health of your family. There is a great need to tell you of the dangers of substances that the body has to contend with today.

Tap water is not clean water. It is chemically treated. It has residues of hormones, antibiotics, and drugs. It is fluoridated. A growing body of evidence indicates that fluorine is a neurotoxin that affects the central nervous system.

Fluoride is a soluble salt, not a heavy metal. There are two basic types of fluoride: calcium fluoride and sodium fluoride. Calcium fluoride appears naturally in underground water sources and even seawater. An excess can cause skeletal or dental fluorosis, which weakens bone and dental matter, but it is not nearly as toxic as sodium fluoride. This type of fluoride is a synthetic waste product of nuclear, aluminum, and phosphate fertilizer industries, and is added to many water supplies. This type of fluoride can affect the body negatively, causing many health issues.

The fluoride found in our water has an amazing capacity to combine and increase the potency of other toxic materials. When obtained from industrial waste and added to water supplies, it is already contaminated with lead, aluminum, and cadmium.

Fluoride has the potential to damage the liver and kidneys, to weaken the immune system, and possibly lead to cancer. It creates symptoms of muscle weakness and fatigue, and acts as a carrier of aluminum across the blood-brain barrier. It causes me to wonder if this is a main contributor of lower IQs and Alzheimer's disease. The evidence is mounting.

The pineal gland, located in the middle of the brain, can become calcified from fluoride, inhibiting its function as a producer of melatonin. Melatonin is needed for sound, deep sleep. The lack of it contributes to thyroid problems that affect the entire endocrine system. The pineal gland is also considered the physical link to the upper chakras or third eye for spiritual and intuitive openings.

If a child swallows a pea-size amount of toothpaste, as recommended on the tube, the FDA recommends calling Poison Control. Yet that is the same amount of fluoride in one 8-ounce glass of fluoridated water. It is very dangerous! It is a chemical and can cause neurological and brain disorders, kidney issues, thyroid problems, arthritis, bone cancer, migraines, and infertility. Fluoride is stored in the body from high amounts in our water supply, toothpaste, mouth rinses, and drops. Fluoride is not as safe as we have been told.

Another main problem with tap water is the combination of unhealthy chemicals used to purify it from pathogens.

Chlorine is a municipal additive and is perhaps one of the most dangerous poisons in our water supply. Water treatment facilities use chlorine as a powerful disinfectant to kill or inactivate biological water contaminants. But that same chlorine, that is so toxic to biological contaminants, is also poisonous to our bodies. Drinking chlorinated water and swimming in chlorinated pools can cause many problems with the natural functions of the body.

Health officials are concerned with the chlorination byproducts, also known as "chlorinated hydrocarbons" or trihalomethanes (THMs). Most THMs are formed in drinking water when chlorine reacts with naturally occurring substances such as decomposing plant and animal materials. Risk for certain types of cancer are now being correlated to the consumption of chlorinated drinking water. The President's Council on Environmental Quality states that "there is increased evidence for an association between rectal, colon, and

Hydration, cont.

bladder cancer and the consumption of chlorinated drinking water." Suspected carcinogens make the human body more vulnerable through repeated ingestion. Research indicates the incidence of cancer is 44% higher among those using chlorinated water.

Even though the Environmental Protection Agency adopted new regulations in 1980 for cities to lower the chlorination byproducts in water to a level not exceeding 100 parts per billion, experts believe that it still doesn't provide proper safeguards and should be strengthened. Unfortunately, there is little likelihood that the use of chlorine will be discontinued since it is currently the most economically acceptable chemical for bacterial control. It is ironic that the process of chlorination, by which we cleanse our water of infectious organisms, can create cancer-causing substances from otherwise innocent chemicals in water.

Drinking chlorinated water diminishes much of the intestinal flora, the friendly bacteria that help in the digestion of food and support your immune system. Chlorine can aggravate asthma, especially in children who swim in chlorinated pools. Several studies also link chlorine and chlorinated byproducts to a greater incidence of melanoma and bladder, breast, and bowel cancers.

The dangers of fluoride and chlorine are extensive, and I chose not to include *all* the dangers known to exist in this section. But it is well worth your study and investigation. Much of the information gathered for this section was found at www.naturalnews.com. You can search for related articles on fluoride and chlorine.

Better methods of water treatment exist, such as ozonation. Many alternatives are already used throughout the world. In the meantime, we now know that action is required by us, the consumer.

What Type of Water Is Best?

We should be drinking pristine, mineral-rich water. Minerals give the water life energy. Recently, I visited Hot Springs, Arkansas, and enjoyed some mountain spring water. Many areas of the country have natural springs we can enjoy. Spring water contains health-restoring minerals like lithium, calcium, and magnesium.

Additionally, spring water contains a great deal of sulphur, which has a therapeutic overall effect on the body, especially the skin. To find a spring near you, visit www.findaspring.com.

Unfortunately, many of us do not have a spring nearby. So whether we have city water or well water, we should consider installing a 5-stage reverse osmosis (RO) filtration system. Look for a unit that removes fluoride. This can be a whole-house unit or one that fits under the kitchen sink. Because the skin is the largest organ and will absorb water when bathing, it is also vital to install shower and bath filters if there is no whole-house unit.

Refer to the Resource Section on page 263 for filter recommendations.

How You Can Achieve Proper Hydration

Reverse-osmosis (RO) water is very clean, however, the filters leave behind very little life energy. We have to add minerals back into the water. **Fulvic acid**, an organic mineral supplement, is the most recommended by natural health professionals today. Fulvic acid is a part of the humic structure of rich, composting soil. It is created by microbes working on decaying matter in a soil environment. It exists in all rich soils which have not been degraded through improper farming methods, modern chemical fertilizers, and pesticides. Fulvic acid is also found in plants, which consume it, and use it for their metabolism. It then becomes available to us when we eat plants rich in fulvic acid. Fulvic acid from humic deposits usually carry 60 or more minerals and trace elements in organic complexes that are necessary for life.

Fulvic acid mineral complexes are the world's finest electrolytes. Adding this mineral complex to water helps to improve energy function, increases assimilation, stimulates metabolism, restores electrochemical balance, reduces high blood pressure, enhances nutrients, and helps rebuild the immune system. My recommendation for fulvic acid is found in **Energy Boost** by Morningstar Minerals— 100% plant-derived organic minerals. Add 1 Tbsp. Energy Boost to an 8-oz glass of RO water.

Mineral-rich water will be absorbed well by the body.

Another one of my favorites is **Master Cell Rejuvenator** (MCR). MCR is a combination of Chinese and Ayurvedic herbs that will energize your RO water. For a complete understanding of MCR, refer to page 93 of the Suggested Supplements section. Use 1 tsp. in an 8 oz. glass of water, with a maximum of 4 tsp. a day.

Or use fresh organic **lemon or lime**, which will provide your water with natural vitamin C and other vitamins and minerals that will give your water life.

Ideally, if you can purchase an **iH2O Hydration System** to go with your reverse osmosis system, its activation process will transform the triangular structure of water molecules into a single-file alignment, creating an ultra-hydrating super liquid.

When purchasing water on the go, my first recommendation is **Artesian FIJI Water**. FIJI Water comes from the remote Yaqara Valley of Viti Levu—one of Fiji's two principal islands. Here, hundreds of feet below an ancient rainforest, is a vast geologically unique underground aquifer from which the water is drawn. The Yaqara aquifer was actually a volcano which became dormant and, over time, built up layers of rock and sediment. Over thousands of years, countless tropical rainfalls soaked through these sedimentary strata, giving birth to the aquifer below.

My second recommendation is **Artesian VOSS Water** from Norway. VOSS is bottled at an artesian source in the pristine wilderness of Southern Norway, naturally filtered and protected from pollutants. The water is generated and pumped from the artesian well deep beneath the ground. The unprocessed nature of the water gives it its fresh, clean taste. Unfiltered water of this quality is rare.

It is essential that your water be pure water:
- A good rule of thumb is to drink half of your weight in ounces every day. Always drink before you become thirsty.

- Prepare water bottles with minerals at home when on the go and even when staying at home to guarantee you are drinking your required amount. Glass water bottles are best. Stainless steel is the best choice for an unbreakable container.
- Shower and bathe in filtered water.
- Do not ever swim in chlorinated water.
- Drink at least 16 ounces (about 2 cups) of water with 2 Tbsp. Energy Boost up to 2 hours before an endurance event or hard training session. Your kidneys require 60–90 minutes to process excess liquid, so you'll be able to eliminate excess before your event.
- Drink 4–8 ounces of water with 2 Tbsp. Energy Boost 5–10 minutes before starting your event.
- During the event or workout, drink fluids early to prevent dehydration. Ideally, drink 8–10 ounces, or as much as you can tolerate, every 15–20 minutes during strenuous exercise.

Water, Consciousness & Intent

We often pray before we eat, thanking God for our food. The same should be our practice before we drink water. Give thanks and be grateful for this life-giving substance.

Dr. Masaru Emoto is a Japanese author and entrepreneur who suggests that **human consciousness has an effect on the molecular structure of water.** His hypothesis has evolved over the years from his research. Initially, his studies revealed that high-quality water forms beautiful and intricate crystals, while low-quality water has difficulty forming crystals. Accordingly, an ice crystal of distilled water exhibits a basic hexagonal structure with no intricate branching. His experiments reveal that positive changes to water crystals can be achieved through prayer, music, or by attaching written words to a container of water.

To understand more of this fascinating phenomena, read Dr. Emoto's book, *The Hidden Messages in Water.*

Drink for Life

If you are committed to a healthy lifestyle, make drinking enough natural water a habit in your life. It won't take long for you to feel the benefit. Water is a survival essential, but proper hydration can help you thrive.

PLEASE SEE THE SOURCE ACKNOWLEDGMENTS ON PAGE 272 FOR A LIST OF RESEARCH, BOOKS, AND WEBSITES USED FOR THIS SECTION.

Detoxification

MINIMIZE EXPOSURE & ELIMINATE TOXINS

We don't have to tell our bodies to detoxify.

They are designed with a miraculous system

of elimination. However, we *do* have to care for

our bodies so that this natural function can

happen the way it was intended.

We live in a world where the body has to work

very hard to function naturally. The good news is that

the body responds beautifully when we give it what

it needs to thrive.

"Whether you live next to an oil refinery or on a pristine mountaintop in the Rockies, you carry environmental toxins in your tissues. From heavy metals like arsenic, lead, mercury, and cadmium emitted from smokestacks and vehicle exhaust; to pesticides, fertilizers, and PCBs released into rivers and soil, and phthalates that off-gas from household plastic products, we are all swimming in a soup of toxic chemicals."
—Jeffrey Rossman, PhD

Studies have shown that toxins reside in the fat cells of everyone's body, even newborn infants. Over 300 toxins have been reported in umbilical cord studies of pregnant women.

There has never been a time when our bodies have been so overwhelmed.

According to the Environmental Protection Agency, the United States is the only country that allows 87,000+ chemicals into its food supply and environment.

70–75% of all food in the grocery store contains products derived from a genetically modified organism (GMO).

70–75% of the food in restaurants contains some product derived from a GMO.

Our milk is processed.

Our grain is refined.

Our animals are factory farmed.

Our water is chemically treated.

The body is bombarded with electromagnetic radiation from computers, cell phones, communication towers, etc.

Environmental toxins affect all bodily systems and have been linked to endocrine, immune, reproductive, metabolic, cardiovascular, cognitive, and behavioral disorders.

Because most environmental toxins are lipid-soluble—dissolving easily in lipids—and brain tissue is primarily made up of lipids, the nervous system is especially vulnerable to toxic exposure. A number of neurodegenerative ailments have been linked to toxin exposure, including Parkinson's disease, Amyotrophic lateral sclerosis (ALS), learning disabilities, conduct disorders, and certain dementias—not to mention the effects of toxins associated with vaccinations in children and adults.

Many neurological symptoms of toxic exposure are common and not linked to a specific condition. These include headaches, fatigue, insomnia, impaired concentration, and memory loss.

The Body's Amazing Channels of Elimination

The liver, kidneys, lungs, colon, skin, and lymphatic system were designed to assist the body's detoxification.

Liver

The liver is the largest glandular organ in the body. It secretes bile, a fluid that helps digest fats and carry toxins to the bowel for disposal. When the liver is overloaded and exhausted, every part of the body is compromised.

Kidneys

The kidneys filter out drugs and heavy metals, as well as toxins made water soluble by the liver. In addition, kidneys manufacture hormones and are responsible for electrolyte balance in the blood. The kidneys work constantly and need clean, fresh water daily.

Colon

Besides acting as the channel to eliminate semisolid remains from the diet, the colon conserves fluids and electrolytes and sustains the population of intestinal microbes. Sometimes toxins are reabsorbed by the colon. A toxic, poorly functioning bowel causes the other channels of elimination to become overworked, particularly the liver.

Lungs

Breath is essential not only to maintain life but also for the healthy function of all internal organs. The lungs expel carbon dioxide and waste material during respiration. They also excrete accumulated wastes via mucous. With insufficient oxygen, the body experiences low energy and emaciation. Air pollution and respiratory conditions impede the proper function of the lungs.

Skin

The skin is the largest organ in the body. It regulates temperature, protects the internal organs, and eliminates toxins through perspiration. When the liver is overburdened, skin conditions such as eczema, rashes, and increased sweating may result. When healthy, the skin eliminates two quarts of fluid per day. The skin's health and appearance depend on proper nourishment, digestion, assimilation, and elimination. As back-up to the kidneys, the skin also helps maintain the blood pH.

Blood

The blood supplies oxygen to all cells and communicates with the body via the hormones it carries. As it circulates, it carries away toxins that are then filtered out by the kidneys and liver.

Lymphatic System

Twice as extensive as the circulatory system, the lymphatic system picks up fluid, pathogens, and waste products from spaces between the cells, and it moves them through a series of vessels similar to blood vessels. These vessels carry the lymph into areas of concentrated lymphoid tissue called nodes. In these lymph nodes, the pathogens and waste products are captured and removed by specialized lymphocytes, especially T cells, that circulate continuously throughout the lymphatic and circulatory systems. The lymphatic fluid eventually re-enters the bloodstream through the subclavian veins.

The lymphatic fluid does not move actively through the system, but relies on the physical action of the skeletal muscles and diaphragm for transport. This emphasizes the importance of physical activity in maintaining overall health.

Detoxification, cont.

How to Support the Body in Natural Detoxification

Detoxing has become a popular word. Most of my patients come to see me with a sincere desire to detoxify their bodies; they understand the need. What they do not understand is that our bodies were naturally designed to eliminate wastes and toxins. But the means by which we attempt to detoxify can be counterproductive.

Harsh detoxification diets and cleanses can cause more problems than what you anticipate when you start. In other words, if the channels of elimination are not open, then toxins can be displaced to other parts of the body and can cause more discomfort, even extreme symptoms. You could feel really bad. Further, if you go right back to the same lifestyle and diet after the cleanse, then you end up right back where you started.

My approach is gentle and flows with the natural function of the body. Since the body has a natural design to eliminate, our responsibility is to give the body what it needs **on a regular basis** so that it can do so naturally.

Here are a few ways to reduce the impact of food and environmental toxins on your health:

1. Minimize your exposure.

The lighter the toxic load on your body, the better it can function naturally to handle those toxins that we can't avoid.

• **Eat organic food and drink pure water.** By eliminating all processed food from the diet and eating high-quality pure whole foods, you allow your body to begin to clean house naturally. Essential fats, vegetables and especially greens that are high in chlorophyll will help rid the body of harmful environmental toxins.

• **Use nontoxic, environmentally friendly cleaning products.** This will benefit the planet as well as the quality of air in your home and the negative effects on the body.

• **Use organic fertilizers** and **natural pesticides**. Do not spray your lawn and garden with toxic chemicals.

• **Don't put anything on your body that you would not eat!** Your skin is your largest organ and will absorb any substance applied to it within 15-20 minutes. This includes personal care products.

• **Minimize exposure to electromagnetic radiation sources** such as computers, cell phones, and cell phone towers. EMRs shut down our cell receptor sites so that nutrients cannot get in or out of our cells. See giawellness.com.

2. Develop a routine to naturally detoxify your body on a regular basis.

• **This is the purpose of *The Transformation*.**

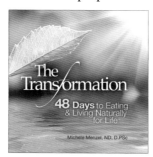

If you follow the daily way of eating outlined in this book, you will allow your body to detoxify naturally on a regular basis. The 48 Days allow a steady, natural cleanse to take place with the least amount of negative symptoms.

Use the recommended basic supplements for the most benefit. These support the body's natural detoxification process. In addition, using the cleansing products twice a year will provide the deep internal cleanse necessary.

Using Lymph Care will help to open your lymphatic system, which is the master drain of your body. Walking and rebounding are the perfect exercises to keep the lymph moving.

• **Use whole-food antioxidant supplements.** If you take the supplements for the 48 Days, you are taking an abundance of whole-food antioxidants!

• **Daily exercise** encourages the body to produce sweat, increases circulation, moves the lymph, and assists the organs in elimination.

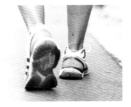

• **Exercise the lungs through deep-breathing techniques.** The way you breathe affects your whole body. Deep breathing exercises will help you relax and release stress and tension being held in the body. They can be done at any time during the day, especially first thing in the morning and at bedtime.

• **Drink mineral-rich water each day.** The combination of good hydration and frequent perspiration helps to flush your system of toxins.

• **Have a regular bowel movement** every day before noon. Twice a day is even better. This helps to decrease the reabsorption of toxins. Consistent exercise, hydration, and probiotic foods helps to keep you regular.

• **Give the body a break through periodic fasts** (p. 130).

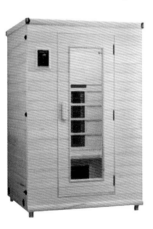

• **Natural detoxification therapies** assist in natural detoxification and include the following:

Use a far infrared sauna frequently. Perspiring is one of your body's best ways of releasing toxins.

Body Balance foot bath

Magnesium crystal baths

Dry skin brushing

• **If you are trying to lose weight,** do the detox practices listed here. As you shed fat, toxins stored in adipose tissue (fat cells) are released. It is essential to cleanse those toxins from your body, rather than reabsorb them.

3. Make a wellness appointment and take advantage of the SpectraVision™ technology.
(See Therapies on page 242.)

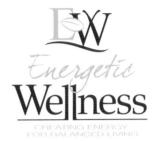

• **Determine specific areas of concern.**

• **Find out what chemicals,** heavy metals, vaccinations, old medications, etc., are resonating in the body and how they are impacting you.

• **See specifically what the body needs for support.**

• **Receive a low-level laser treatment** and create an energetic blueprint to imprint into specific homeopathic remedies to match the needed change in the body.

• **Return the body to homeostasis/balance.**

By eliminating all processed food from the diet and eating high-quality pure, whole foods, your body begins to clean house naturally. Essential fats, vegetables, and especially greens that are high in chlorophyll will help rid the body of harmful toxins. The basic supplements support the body's natural detoxification process on a regular basis. Using the cleansing products will provide a deep internal cleanse necessary twice a year.

You will see remarkable results when applying the principles outlined in this book for natural detoxification. You will feel amazing and your body will be very happy. Natural living is fun and very beneficial.

PLEASE SEE THE SOURCE ACKNOWLEDGMENTS ON PAGE 272 FOR A LIST OF RESEARCH, BOOKS, AND WEBSITES USED FOR THIS SECTION.

Rest

IN RHYTHM WITH THE EARTH

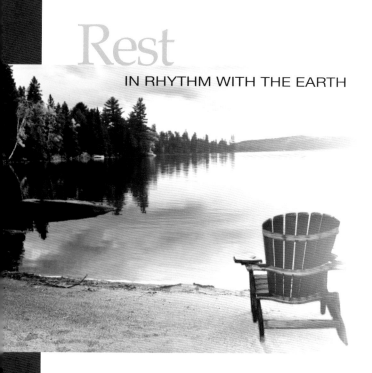

To everything there is a season,

A time for every purpose under heaven....

When we can truly relax and rest,

we know we are taking full care of the body.

We are all very busy. While writing this book, I was taking a pilot group through the *The Transformation*, working on architectural plans and zoning changes for a new wellness center and cafe, seeing patients daily, and creating an updated patient folder. I am also a wife, a daughter, a sister, a mother, a grandmother, and a friend.

A good friend of mine, Marion, said, "You take on so much, you put so much on yourself. You're so busy now. What about when the new place opens? You want to be involved in everything."

I had to really ponder her question. On the outside, it does look like I'm crazy busy. But, in my reality, I'm caring for myself while creating my dream. I love my work. I love this dream and have visualized it for years. I am at a place in my life that I can accomplish it. My kids are grown and out of the house, and I have a very supportive, loving husband.

You might have to make adjustments to accomplish your dreams. I'm constantly readjusting rather than getting frustrated. If we create our own reality, then we create our frustration. It's not the situation. It's not the other person; it's us. If we create frustration in our lives, we will constantly be frustrated. So think and do the things you want, not the things you don't want!

In order for me to make things work during the writing of this book, I made a few adjustments that might be helpful to you:

• By eating my bigger meal at lunch, I avoided the pressure to cook after I got home, saving two hours of preparation and clean up. Now we eat a light meal. And I have more time to write.

• My daughter prepared meals for the weekends.

• I had to recheck my attitude to make sure I was not getting frustrated and giving off negative energy because that is what would come back to me.

What stage of life are you in? Are you happy with the time of your life? Enjoy where you are in life, and be happy! Visualize where you want to be, and surrender to the process of getting there. Prepare and make adjustments to accomplish what you want to do. Visualize how it will play out. Be creative, solve problems, be resourceful, and repurpose areas of your life to be happy.

Choose to think good thoughts.

Our thoughts are very powerful. God tells us to renew our mind, and this exercise has to be constant!

"Whatever is true, whatever is honorable, whatever is right, whatever is pure, whatever is lovely, whatever is of good repute, if there is any excellence and if anything worthy of praise, let your mind dwell on these things…. And the God of peace shall be with you." —Phil. 4:8-9

We choose peace…or not.
We choose what we do.
We make our own schedule.
You are choosing the life you lead.

The mind controls the body's responses according to our perceptions. The book *The Energy Prescription* states, "An undisciplined mind leaks vital energy in a continuous stream of thoughts, worries, and skewed perceptions, many of which trigger disturbing emotions and degenerative chemical processes in the body." When we understand how important our thoughts are to the way we feel, this awareness helps us to help ourselves! Our Creator knows our make up; our design is perfect. This is true prevention.

The Body Runs in Two Phases

According to German New Medicine® (GNM), the 2nd biological law states the body runs in two phases, and every condition we experience runs in two phases. In this section, we will only talk about our normal, everyday cycle. This everyday cycle is called Normatonia and coincides with the circadian rhythm of the earth. The sun rises, and the sun sets—daytime, nighttime. Our bodies run on the same cycle. We have our daytime phase and our nighttime phase:

Active, daytime phase = sympathicatonic
Healing, nighttime phase = vagatonic

I'll describe both the daytime phase and the nighttime phase and include suggestions to assist your body in both phases to prepare the body for optimal rest.

The Daytime Phase Is Our Active Phase

When we wake up in the morning, we should be alert and should feel energized and ready for the day. We should be productive and have energy throughout the day. Our body was designed to handle normal activity and everyday stress. Yes, the body was designed to handle stress!

The question is how much unnecessary stress do we put on ourselves? Our modern lifestyle keeps the body in an active state for much longer periods than intended—whether we eat food that is too stimulating or we put too much in our day and cannot calm down or we face an unexpected conflict.

Rest, cont.

1. **We all have everyday responsibilities that should have boundaries.**

2. **Be happy with your stage of life.** Every stage of our lives is a natural part of becoming who we were meant to be.

3. **Express your creativity**—whatever that means for you—decorating, painting, reading, writing, singing, dancing, cooking, building, creating, etc.

4. **Set your intentions**—or what you are working on for the day and for your next stage of life.

5. **Purpose to wake up happy!**

6. **Make a gratefulness list,** and read it every morning.

7. **Say to yourself everyday, "I love you, I forgive you, thank you."** We are so hard on ourselves. We have to love ourselves so that we can love others.

8. **Use positive affirmations** (see Louise Hay's books).

9. **Quote inspirational Scripture.**

10. **Set realistic goals for the day**—what you need to accomplish instead of what you want to accomplish.

11. **Reset priorities** so that you are not disappointed in what you didn't get done.

- As a woman, you may be a stay-at-home mom, a working mom, a single mom, single, married with children, married with no children, partner, daughter, sister, or friend.
- As a man, balancing the demands of work, home, and personal relationships can be a difficult endeavor.
- You should be able to make it through the day without having to take a nap, unless you are a mom with small children.
- The best time to exercise is in the morning. This will help set your energy clock. Most vigorous activity should be done by 6 p.m.

Every day we should be productive, creative, and have a purpose to be fulfilled. In *The Blue Zones* book, Dan Buettner interviewed a one-hundred-year-old Okinawa woman who was the village matriarch. She met with the women of the village every day to discuss village needs, to pray, to laugh, to talk about men! She had an amazing purpose.

During the day, I constantly have my vision before me. Each day is a step towards my vision and goal. Live it out! In the morning, I always think about the patient I'm going to visit with and how I want the visit to go. While on the treadmill, I write emails, read a book, study, listen to a motivational teaching, or prepare for my day.

While reading a patient's health history prior to the visit, I set my intent for what I want to say during our time together. This usually leads to thinking and praying for others. I think about any meetings I'm going to have and my intent and purpose for the entire day—all the things I want to accomplish.

The body is designed to support you—your every thought, feeling, belief, as well as what you put into your body and how you respond to your environment. In the book, *The Genie in Your Genes*, Dawson Church says the molecules of our emotions share intimate connections with, and are indeed inseparable from, our physiology…. Consciously, or more frequently, unconsciously, we choose how we feel at every single moment!

When we understand how powerfully our thoughts affect how we feel, we will realize how our thoughts control our day.

He also says to "imagine the healing arts of the future reformulated around the idea of thoughts, driven by the power of feelings, as shapers of our reality. When a cardiac patient visits a doctor, the first prescription the doctor might offer might not be a drug, but a precisely formulated sequence of thoughts and feelings designed to affect the genetic predisposition of people at risk for heart disease!" Everything that happens in the body is based on a subjective experience and how we perceive it!

This is German New Medicine® in a nutshell. In his 35 years of research, Dr. Hamer proved the mind/body connection. Behind every symptom there is a very significant biological cause. Understanding the emotional connection to every symptom leads us to the conflict resolution which leads us to recovery. The body's design always has a meaningful purpose. See the GNM section on page 248, and for more teaching join me in the GNM classes and visit www.learninggnm.com.

Our Nighttime Phase Is Rest.

Every day your body needs to heal from the day's activities and stressors. Around 5–6 p.m., the body makes a natural transition into rest. It doesn't mean that we have to stop everything after 6 p.m.; it just means our activity should start changing to support the body's natural function.

The parasympathetic nervous system is the branch of the autonomic nervous system responsible for the body's ability to recuperate and return to a balanced state, known as "homeostasis." Just as the sympathetic nervous system is responsible for the "fight or flight" response, the parasympathetic nervous system is responsible

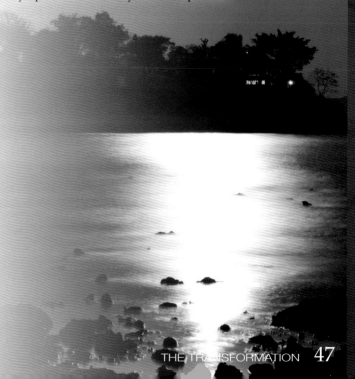

Rest, cont.

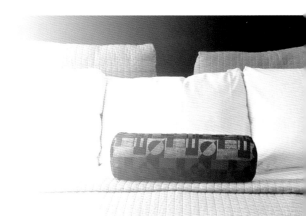

for the "relax and renew" process.

You can rest in little increments during the day by just sitting and relaxing at lunch or on a break or when the kids are taking a nap.

Avoid eating after 6 p.m., or at the latest, 7 p.m. Late, heavy meals interfere with the body's energy and the ability to rest and heal. You should wait to retire at least three hours after eating. When you sleep on an empty stomach, your body can rest, rebuild, and rejuvenate from the day. Many cultures eat their main meal at lunch or early afternoon.

In the evening, spend time with family and friends. This is a perfect activity to promote rest. When our kids were little, we used to play games. We made Friday night our movie night, which included homemade pizza. It became a family favorite!

Spend time outdoors in the evening. Most of us work and are closed-in all day. Take a walk an hour or so after eating, more leisurely than morning exercise. You can even do light rebounding for 5 to 10 minutes. Both will aid in digestion.

One of my personal favorite practices in the evening is enjoying a sauna for 30 minutes. It has a wonderful way of releasing the toxins from the day both physically and emotionally. Stretching or yoga is a wonderful practice to help relax the body. Find the things in the evening that promote relaxation and rest.

As it gets closer to bedtime:
- Take a short shower after a sauna.
- Soak 30 minutes in a magnesium crystal bath with essential oils.
- After a bath or shower, rub down with a towel.
- Apply one or more evening essential oils on the bottoms of your feet, the back of your neck, etc.

(See Daily Routine on page 80.)

The purpose of sleep is to relax and renew, to rejuvenate energy, and to heal the body from the day's activities and stressors. When it is time to get into bed, realize you

Every day your body needs to heal from the day's activities and stressors.

had enough time in the day to accomplish what needed to get done. Tomorrow is a new day, fresh, with no mistakes. We all have a programmed, preconceived idea that there is never enough time or enough resources. This is a lie. There is enough time and there is an abundance of resources.

One of the very important principles we can learn from GNM is the need to downgrade situations that cannot be resolved in the day they happen. We should surrender the day and every situation that was not resolved. This is not giving up; it is surrendering to the process of growth, learning, and progress.

Anything we fight or resist will not go away. We will keep on creating it! Don't be hard on yourself. You did all you could this day. Avoid negative self-talk, such as, "Ugh, I can never get anything done!" Think about all the things positive you did accomplish.

We operate out of one of two emotions: love or fear. Out of which are you operating? Remember, "Perfect love casts out fear."

Optimal Hours of Sleep

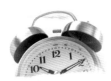

- We need 6–9 hours of uninterrupted sleep per night.
- Optimal hours—down by 10 p.m., up at 6 a.m.

Get into the habit of lying down at the same time every night. The body loves a schedule! It's on a time clock.

Prepare the bedroom for sleep. No electronic devices near the bed. Put your cell phone in another room to charge at night. Use Gia Wellness products to protect your room from electromagnetic radiation. Use a Home Harmonizer and cell chips. Do not use a night light. The pineal gland needs complete darkness to fully release melatonin to promote deep sleep.

If you need help falling asleep, try one of these ideas:

- reading
- listening to music
- yoga
- personal prayer
- meditation
- drink a glass of raw milk
- listening to relaxation CDs that guide you through personal healing. Experiment to find your favorite.

> "True silence
> is the rest
> of the mind;
> it is to the spirit
> what sleep is
> to the body,
> nourishment and
> refreshment."
> – William Penn

An old, new mode of prayer…

Did you ever wonder what the verse *"Pray without ceasing."* really means? How can we do that? As I learn about the wonderful design of the body, I understand it more and more. If at any moment our body is responding to how we feel, then at every single moment, we should have a prayerful thought of how we want to feel.

To feel as if your prayers were already answered, what would that feel like? Gregg Braden tells this story of a visit with his friend to pray for rain. The friend was praying for rain. Gregg went with him to a place that his ancestors went to pray. The man took off his shoes and acknowledged his ancestors and then was silent for a few seconds. Then he was done.

Gregg said, "I thought you were going to pray." He said, "I did. A prayer is a feeling. I felt what it would be like if it was raining, feeling the wet soil on my feet, and feeling deep within me of rain…."

Our feeling is our prayer. Our thoughts and feelings affect every part of us and speak to God. As Gregg would say, "Feel the prayer as if it had already happened." Create your day, as if it had already happened!

In his book, *Secrets of the Lost Mode of Prayer*, Gregg describes an ancient form of prayer that has no words or outward expressions. This little book is an absolute must read. It will comfort your soul and awaken the connection to the Divine Creator of the universe like never before.

Create a Home Environment that Promotes Rest and Wellness

This has been our goal for many years. Now we have a little home oasis. When you arrive home at night, you want to gather with family or friends and enjoy each other in a peaceful environment. Make your home a spa. We started out slow and added wellness features as we could afford them:

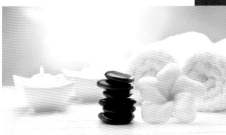

- soaker tub
- salt water pool
- exercise room
- ozone generated hot tub
- far infrared sauna

Use Natural Therapies to Assist in Achieving Rest

- SpectraVision™—correct disrupted energy patterns
- Far Infrared sauna
- Body Balance foot bath
- Natural sleep support supplements
  Bio-Identical Melatonin
  Deep Sleep
  Reset!

Understanding the importance of rest and good sleep is the foundation of our health. The body has to recuperate. Give yourself permission every night to rest. You will be refreshed and renewed for a new day.

PLEASE SEE THE SOURCE ACKNOWLEDGMENTS ON PAGE 272 FOR A LIST OF RESEARCH, BOOKS, AND WEBSITES USED FOR THIS SECTION.

Faith in God
& THE BODY'S DESIGN

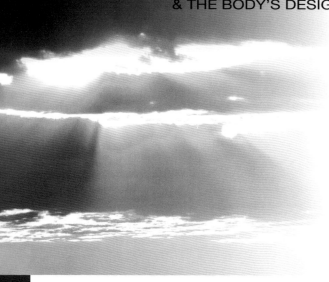

"Faith is the substance of things hoped for, the evidence of things not seen." Hebrews 11:1

Faith is an abstract concept, yet we have faith every day without thinking about it. We have faith that the sun will rise and set. We sleep, allowing our bodies to rest and rejuvenate. We wake up, ready to be nourished by food, not thinking about how the body digests it. We breathe in and out, not thinking about oxygen intake or the pumping of the blood by the heart. We live and love.

As I often have told my children, I cannot live your faith for you, nor can I tell you how to have faith or how to believe. But I do know that if we seek, we will find. God told us that His truth is written on our hearts. And because all living humans have the Spirit within them, part of our journey is discovering our faith and what we believe.

Acknowledging the Spirit and feeling the presence of God within us is a beautiful gift. It is our connection to all that is around us, created for our pleasure.

My purpose is to increase your faith by empowering you with transforming knowledge that may have been hidden by preconceived ideas of how we should live. Natural living fits the design of *nature* itself. Just as we have faith in the Divine, we can have faith in the natural function of the body. It's what I want you to walk away with when you read the 7 Laws of Wellness.

This part of our faith is often missing. We believe in God and the universe and the miraculous energy that holds everything together. We believe and have faith that the seasons will come and go. We seem to have faith in breathing, the heart pumping, going to sleep, waking up. Yet we have lost the faith in the body's design to heal.

The body has a wonderful, very intelligent design. We function as a whole. We don't have to tell the body to detox or breathe; these things are its nature. The faith I am describing is faith in the body's ability to heal as it was designed.

Symptoms & Causes

We often have a misconstrued view of our design. When we have a physical symptom, it is not unusual for us to become frightened. This fear is a learned response, based on our current belief that the body is malfunctioning, or something is attacking it. Our preconceived idea of health leads to fear and then resorts to harsh, invasive treatments, leaving our bodies weak and our hearts confused. It denies the power of God and His design of the body and nature itself.

Our spirit plays a huge role in understanding what is right and wrong. We can also trust the Holy Spirit to guide us as we learn how to take care of our bodies. We have to allow ourselves the opportunity to study and learn from the Spirit. The Spirit—the Divine—will not let us down. When I was seeking to know the truth about cancer, I read Dr. Hamer's work on the biological laws, and it resonated with me. The Spirit within me leaped, and I knew I had found truth. The information given in the Spirit is already there; we just have to seek to find the answers.

If you believe that illnesses, accidents, and disorders are relevant only to the physical self, you are refusing to acknowledge the majority of what makes you who you are! You have only to recall a situation where you've experienced instinctive reactions, such as your heart racing when you are afraid or that feeling in the pit of your stomach when you dread something. These automatic reactions are not from the physical body but are transferred to the body through thoughts or emotions.

A natural way to approach symptoms is to evaluate what has happened prior to the onset of symptoms. Since every condition is a result of what has taken place in our lives—toxic thoughts or emotions, toxic food, toxic lifestyle—we can understand that the body needs time to heal from those experiences.

Our symptoms help us understand ourselves and can become a wonderful part of the journey. *Accepting* symptoms as part of the healing process takes a huge step of faith since it is contrary to our current model. This is a paradigm shift that will take time to understand. Listen to your body because it is a reflection of who you are and want to be. **God has already given our bodies the capacity to heal.**

When we can forgive and love, we can resolve the turmoil within us and experience true healing. Healing in the physical body usually results in a stronger whole. This happens on all levels—body, mind, and spirit.

Science and Spirituality

There are many scientists today bridging the gap between science and spirituality. The *human genome project* was a perfect example that helped lead us in this direction. Billions of dollars were spent studying our DNA in hope of finding the answers to disease. What they discovered was that our genes have very little activity.

The working hypothesis was that there would be a gene that provided the blueprint for each of the 100,000 proteins, which are the building blocks of our cells, plus another 20,000 or so regulatory genes to orchestrate the complex dance of protein assembly. When the project was finished, they found just 23,688 genes.

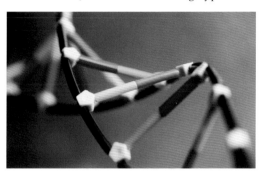
Genes account for 35% of longevity.

This developed the question: If all the information required to construct and maintain a human being is not contained in the genes, then where does it come from? And who is conducting the complex organ system?

This is just one aspect of science where our understanding is incomplete. Scientists are learning more about which factors influence the process that turns genes on and off. One factor that makes genes active is our experiences.

"Our experiences themselves are just part of the picture. We take facts and experiences and then assign meaning to them. What meaning we assign, mentally, emotionally, and spiritually, is often as important to genetic activation as the facts themselves. We are discovering that our genes dance with our awareness. Thoughts and feelings turn sets of genes on and off in complex relationships. Science is discovering that while we may have a fixed set of genes in our chromosomes, which of these genes is active has a great deal to do with our **subjective experiences**, and how we process them!" —*Dawson Church, PhD*

Genes only account for 35% of longevity. Good lifestyle, environmental factors, and support systems are the major reasons people live longer. The idea that our genes determine the way we are is very far from the truth. We are the *way* we are based on our beliefs about *who* we are. This is why it is so important that we study ourselves and rely on the Spirit to guide us.

Emotional perceptions play a large role in our health. Experts say that 99 percent of all illness is due to an emotional conflict or prolonged stress. Our bodies have significant biological responses designed with purpose to assist the body at all times. If our experiences and how we process them control what takes place in the body, then the responsibility is ours!

We have shifted our faith from creation to chemicals used to *"heal"* the body. We have too much faith in doctors and insurance companies to take care of us. There are many loving and caring doctors; they are just doing what they have been taught. But allopathic medicine views the body only as a chemical mechanism. It does not look at you as a whole person or ask you what has been going on in your life.

Faith in Natural Living

My heart's desire is to teach natural living so that you will trust the design and benefit from eating and living naturally. All of nature was created for us. We can grow our food and receive energy from the sun, earth, air, and water. Most of all, we need to maintain a clean thought life.

The tools of our consciousness—**our beliefs, prayers, thoughts, intentions, and faith**—often correlate much more strongly with our health, longevity, and happiness than our genes do! Studies show that a committed spiritual practice and faith can add many years to our lives, regardless of our genetic mix. The indigenous people groups that Dr. Price studied all had a strong spiritual belief system that contributed to their health.

Larry Dossey, MD, said, "Several studies show that what one *thinks* about one's health is one of the most accurate predictors of longevity ever discovered."

We talk to ourselves more than we talk to anyone else. If you would play those thoughts back, what would they say? Are they pleasant, joyful, encouraging, loving,

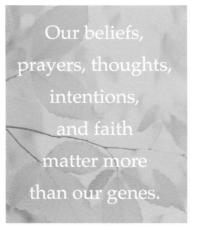

Our beliefs, prayers, thoughts, intentions, and faith matter more than our genes.

and thoughtful? Learning to see the good in everything takes time. When we realize that our perceptions are what control the body, we can truly help ourselves.

Jesus walked in love. Love has the highest vibration and is the highest level of consciousness. Walking in love is not always easy; it takes work on our part. Walking in love is where we will be happy and content and look at everything in life as a miracle.

Those who can forgive will do themselves a great service. Accepting God's forgiveness and forgiving others sometimes comes easier to us than forgiving ourselves. It took many years for me to forgive myself of mistakes made during young adulthood. We tend to be harder on ourselves and more critical of ourselves than anyone, even God. God's love is unconditional. He wants us to love ourselves, so that we can truly love others and give to others. Years ago, I learned a simple practice that enabled me to love and forgive myself. This allowed me to fully accept others' love, especially, and most importantly, God's love. This simple practice involves looking in the mirror everyday and reciting, "I love you, I forgive you and thank you." Although difficult at first, it made a profound difference in my life. I believe it will change the lives of those who learn to practice it.

Holding onto guilt and shame can destroy our self-image and result in symptoms to the physical body. This is reflected in any musculoskeletal condition. According to German New Medicine®, these conditions are considered a self-devaluation conflict, and in the healing phase, you may experience pain in your muscles and joints. We can't change the past, but we can change our perception of the past so that it doesn't continue to affect us.

When forgiving others, we must look at the situation and realize that we took part in creating it. This is sometimes called the mirror effect. When looking at the situation with the other person removed we can see why this situation is in our lives. This perspective allows us to process it with new eyes and possibly resolve the situation faster. We can then be thankful and forgive. The situation can be seen as benefiting our journey. We can forgive and not feel that others have taken advantage of us.

Lack of forgiveness—which often occurs as a result of hurt, humiliation, anger, fear, loss, guilt, or envy—can have profound effects on the way our bodies function:

- The body is in a state of stress or a prolonged active phase.
- Muscles tighten, causing imbalances or pain in the neck, back, and limbs.
- Blood flow to the joints is restricted, making it more difficult for the blood to remove wastes from the tissues and supply oxygen and nutrients to the cells.
- Normal processes of repair and recovery from injury or arthritis are impaired.
- Clenching the jaws contributes to problems with teeth and jaw joints.
- Headaches can become a problem.
- Chronic pain may get worse.

When we experience a symptom, the body is communicating to us that our way of thinking might be out of harmony with what is beneficial. Symptoms indicate an opportunity to change our belief system. It is truly a gift to bring back balance. According to German New Medicine®, repeated symptoms are called a "hanging healing," which means there has not been a complete resolution of the situation in your heart and mind.

"The physical body does not create illness," Lisa Bourbeau says, "because the physical body can do nothing by itself. What maintains its life is our soul, our inner self."

The genes only control 20–30 percent of the function of the body. The rest is controlled by who we are—our perceptions and belief system. Our body is controlled by our thoughts and emotions.

So, what is your outlook on life? How do you want to live? How do you want to age? All of this is within your control through your intention and thoughts. When my patients come in and say they want to be healthy and have vitality into old age, I say "Yes, and you can because you just said it." Believe it, and put faith into the steps to do it.

We Are Beings of Energy

This book is intended to remind us of the miraculous life that God has given us. It is our responsibility to take care of it. There is an energetic component to every biological process. The energy flows in, out, and around neurons, and genes interact constantly with the outside environment. Genes are the mechanism that organisms use to store information. Energy movement is how they communicate information.

In an appointment, I will help you recognize the true cause of your symptom—the conflict—and assist you in finding a creative solution. Then I'll suggest lifestyle changes and foods that will assist in the healing process. (See Therapies on page 242.)

When we understand how powerfully our thoughts affect how we feel, we will realize how what we think will control our day. All of these things would not be possible if we are not loving ourselves and thanking ourselves. Look in the mirror everyday and tell yourself, "I love you, I forgive you, and thank you."

"If someone wishes for good health, one must first ask oneself if he is ready to do away with the reasons for his illness. Only then is it possible to help him." —*Hippocrates*

PLEASE SEE THE SOURCE ACKNOWLEDGMENTS ON PAGE 272 FOR A LIST OF RESEARCH, BOOKS, AND WEBSITES USED FOR THIS SECTION.

As I understand the human body and all of what nature has to offer us, I am in awe of its wonder and magnificence.

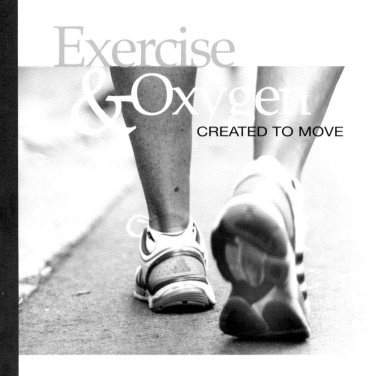

Exercise & Oxygen

CREATED TO MOVE

Our bodies were created to move!

Part of the natural care of the body is exercise.

Many natural functions of the body depend on it—

the heart, the lymphatic system, the immune system,

and especially our emotions. Walking, riding a bike,

hiking, swimming, dancing, playing a sport—all kinds

of physical activity can be fun and very beneficial.

Find a physical activity you enjoy, and just do it. If you get bored, try something new. You should exercise a minimum of 30 minutes every day for the rest of your life. **Here are a few important reasons to keep moving:**

• Physical activity stimulates brain chemicals that help you feel happier and more relaxed.

• You will feel better about your appearance when you exercise regularly, which will boost your confidence and improve your self-esteem.

• Exercise can help you maintain your ideal weight.

• Regular walking preserves bone density and increases bone mass.

• Exercise will help your cardiovascular system more efficiently deliver oxygen and nutrients to your tissues.

• Regular physical activity can deepen your sleep and help you fall asleep faster.

• Regular physical activity can lead to enhanced arousal for women.

• Men who exercise regularly are less likely to have problems with erectile dysfunction than are men who do not exercise.

• Exercise gives you a chance to unwind, enjoy the outdoors, and engage in activities that make you happy.

• Walking, taking a dance class, hitting the hiking trails, or joining a soccer team can help you connect with family or friends in a fun social setting.

Walking

The most natural form of exercise, I believe, is walking. It gets our body from where we are to where we want to be.

Remember your parents telling you how they walked miles to school in all sorts of weather? A hundred years

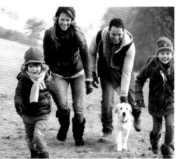

ago, exercise was not part of everyday vocabulary. Most people farmed or worked other physical jobs. Automobiles were a new invention, making them unaffordable for most people. There were only 8,000 cars on the road in the United States and the average person walked 3 to 6 miles a day. In modern America, we are fortunate if we walk one mile a day.

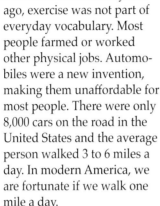

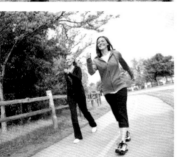

One of my textbooks, *Naturopathy for the 21st Century*, explains that a healthy young man should walk 6 to 12 miles a day; the convalescent, weak persons, and women should walk at least 3 to 5 miles a day. I believe we would be amazed how well we would feel if we followed this wonderful plan.

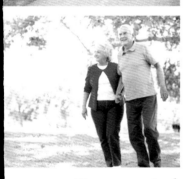

Consistency is key. A 30-minute walk at a good pace should take you about 1.5 miles. Start out slow, and work your way up to a 15-minute mile. Set a goal to walk at least three miles a day.

Vigorous exercise should be done before 6 p.m. so your body can prepare for rest and not be too energized to fall asleep. However, a leisurely walk after dinner can aid in digestion and be very relaxing.

Set a specific time each day to walk. I prefer first thing in the morning, and I am consistently walking three miles a day on weekdays and four miles on the weekends.

- When shopping, park far away and walk.
- Take the stairs whenever possible.
- Walk to a store instead of driving.
- Walk outside so you can be closer to nature. Choose a scenic route. This will boost your spirit!
- Invest in a good pair of walking shoes. Unfortunately, we usually walk on the pavement or a treadmill instead of soft ground.

Below is a great article someone gave me years ago. It was a photocopy so I don't know the author, but it is the best explanation of our unique design and the need to keep walking. What a beautiful design!

Two Feet / Two Hearts…

There is an especially valuable cardiac benefit from walking few people know about. It helps relieve an enormous pumping burden imposed on the heart by our upright posture and long legs.

The heart has to work against the force of gravity to pump "used" blood all the way back up from the feet for re-oxygenation and recirculation. That takes enormous pumping power! To help the heart with this extra load, the body has developed two "booster hearts"—one in each leg—which come into use as soon as you start walking.

When you're standing still, the heart pumps the blood all alone. But the instant you take a step, the booster hearts immediately spring into action and the calf muscles contract. This exerts a forceful upward "milking" action on a large vein through which blood returns from the feet to the heart! When the calf relaxes between steps, valves [in the vein] above it close to keep the blood from slipping back down. Each step repeats the process, pushing more blood up toward the heart. Thus, all the time you're walking, each leg serves as an assistant heart, helping the true heart pump blood.

Today walking is still the best way to condition or recondition your body. So get out and walk, walk, walk… for fun, for interest, for exercise!

Exercise & Oxygen, cont.

Rebounding

The rebounder—a mini trampoline—was originally invented back in 1938 by a man named Ed Russell. He wasn't a master at marketing. So it wasn't until the late 1970s that exercise expert Al Carter finally brought it into the spotlight.

Al Carter attended Oklahoma State University and the University of Utah with full scholarships in wrestling. He qualified twice for Olympic wrestling competition and won all-around gymnastic champion in the states of Montana, Texas, Louisiana, Oklahoma, and Arkansas.

He believed his exceptionally good health and superior strength were connected to his work on the trampoline, and he discovered the positive effects of rebounding on the human body. His research resulted in the book *Rebound to Better Health* and the development of the first home-sized rebounder "Dyna-Bound." His second book, *The Miracles of Rebound Exercise,* published in 1979, sold 1.3 million copies and became a national health and fitness bestseller.

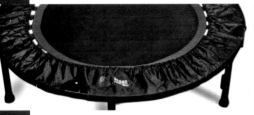 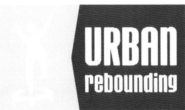

Rebounding is unlike other aerobic activities because it is a zero-impact exercise and places no strain on your joints. The aim of rebounding is not to bounce high but to perform a series of small, controlled movements.

A stabilizing bar fits to the rebounder which helps you feel steady. This attachment is especially helpful for the elderly, disabled, or handicapped and makes rebounding an exercise everyone can enjoy.

Rebounding stimulates the flow of lymph. "The lymphatic [flow] becomes very active during exercise but sluggish under resting conditions," states Arthur C. Guyton, MD, author of *Basic Human Physiology.* "During exercise, the rate of lymph flow can increase to 14 times normal because of the increased activity."

As you bounce on the trampoline, your body is subjected to gravitational pulls ranging from zero to three times the force of gravity. The change in gravitational forces gets your lymphatic system moving, which increases lymph flow by 14 to 30 times and increases the amount of waste products flushed from cells.

My husband Steven bought me my first rebounder 12 years ago. I have loved it ever since. It is such a fantastic overall workout, strengthening and detoxifying every cell and every organ in the body. It is the perfect exercise for women because it especially builds core strength.

You can easily rebound in your living room, your office, or your yard. Rebounding outside is a really wonderful experience.

There are many high quality rebounders available. I recommend the Urban Rebounder. It is great for home use and is very affordable. The rebounder comes with a stabilizing bar and an exercise DVD. The video explains different workout levels from which to choose. Other DVD workouts are available online.

Urban Rebounding was created by J.B. Berns while recovering from a knee injury. J.B. used his 20-plus years of martial arts, yoga, and personal/wellness training to develop the Urban Rebounder exercise system. It has sold millions and was listed by *Consumer Reports* in 2008 as one of their top 100 products. In 1999, *Fitness Magazine* named J.B. one of the top 10 personal trainers in the nation.

People who rebound find they are able to work longer, sleep better, and feel less tense and nervous. The effect is not just psychological, because the action of bouncing up and down against gravity effectively stimulates the lymphatic system without trauma to the musculoskeletal system. This unique discovery is central to why rebounding has become one of the most beneficial forms of exercise ever developed.

1. Provides an increased G-force (gravitational load), which benefits the body by strengthening the musculoskeletal system.

2. Protects the joints from the chronic fatigue and impact delivered by exercising on hard surfaces.

3. Helps manage body composition and improves muscle-to-fat ratio. Rebound exercise benefits you by giving you more control over these.

4. Benefits lymphatic circulation by stimulating the millions of one-way valves in the lymphatic system. This benefits the body's immune capacity for fighting current disease, destroying cancer cells, eliminating antigens, and preventing future illness.

5. Circulates more oxygen to the tissues.

6. Establishes a better equilibrium between the oxygen required by the tissues and the oxygen made available.

7. Increases capacity for respiration.

8. Tends to reduce the height to which the arterial pressures rise during exertion.

9. Lessens the time during which blood pressure remains abnormal after severe activity.

10. Assists in the rehabilitation of existing heart problems. Rebound exercise also benefits recovery from heart procedures, providing gentle, low-impact circulation.

11. Increases the functional activity of the red bone marrow in the production of red blood cells.

12. Gradually improves resting metabolic rate so that more calories are burned for hours after exercise. Related rebound exercise benefits the post-exercise "glycogen replenishment" process.

13. Causes core muscles and large muscle groups to contract, resulting in the rhythmic compression of the veins and arteries, which more effectively moves fluids, both blood and lymphatic, through the body and back to the heart, lowering peripheral blood pressure and lightening the heart's load.

14. Decreases the volume of blood pooling in the veins of the cardiovascular system, preventing chronic edema.

15. Encourages collateral circulation by increasing the capillary count in the muscles and decreasing the distance between the capillaries and the target cells.

16. Strengthens the heart and other muscles in the body so that they work more efficiently.

17. Gradually allows the resting heart to beat less often. Regular rebound exercise has been shown to benefit the heart rate, resulting in favorable decreases in resting heart rate.

18. Lowers circulating cholesterol and triglyceride levels.

19. Lowers low-density lipoprotein in the blood and increases high-density lipoprotein holding off the incidence of coronary artery disease.

20. Promotes tissue repair.

21. Rebounding for longer than 20 minutes at a moderate intensity at least 3 times per week increases the mitochondria count within the muscle cells, benefiting total endurance. Perhaps you will easily skip those naps.

22. Benefits the alkaline reserve of the body, which may be of significance in an emergency requiring prolonged effort.

23. Improves coordination between the propreoceptors in the joints, the transmission of nerve impulses to and from the brain, transmission of nerve impulses and responsiveness of the muscle fibers.

24. Improves the brain's responsiveness to the vestibular apparatus within the inner ear, thus improving balance.

25. Offers relief from neck and back pains, headaches, and other pain caused by lack of exercise. Rebound Exercise has been shown to benefit body alignment and posture.

26. Enhances digestion and elimination processes.

27. Allows for deeper and easier relaxation and sleep.

28. Results in better mental performance, with keener learning processes.

29. Curtails fatigue and menstrual discomfort for women.

30. Minimizes the number of colds, allergies, digestive disturbances, and abdominal problems.

31. Tends to slow down atrophy in the aging process.

32. Is an effective modality by which the user gains a sense of control and an improved self image.

33. Is enjoyable!

Exercise & Oxygen, cont.

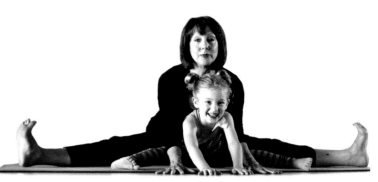

The Importance of a Strong Core

The center of our bodies is the *torso* or *core*. The muscles in the torso work together to stabilize all other movements. They not only include the abdominal muscles but also the side muscles and interior muscles. These core muscles support the spine when we sit, stand, bend over, twist, exercise, and more. It is very important that we develop strong core muscles to support our every move. Women especially should work on core strengthening exercises. We tend to lose muscle strength quicker as we age than men.

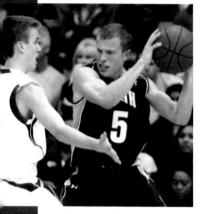

A strong core makes movement easier, creates balance and helps protect from injury. A weak core will lead to poor posture, lower back pain, and injuries. Many of these injuries are worse because the body lacks the strength to support itself and recover during falls and missteps. Sit-ups or crunches, rebounding, pilates, and yoga help strengthen the core.

Yoga

Yoga is an amazing full-body exercise, involving the body, mind, and spirit. I am by no means an expert on yoga, but I do believe yoga is an amazing, relaxing, strength-building discipline from which everyone can benefit.

Rachel Mor has been practicing yoga and teaching yoga since the 1970s. Here is what she says about the practice:

"I first began doing yoga in my teens because I had panic attacks which made living my daily life difficult. I was afraid all the time. The deep breathing and relaxation yoga brought to my mind and body was immediate. *Yoga* means to form a union of body, mind, and spirit. For me, it became a way for me to feel at home and safe within my body. Soon it became a way for me to experience my deeper or *soul* self and view life from the inside out. After practicing yoga, I am able to feel and experience myself and life from a deeper place of peace. This place within me feels eternal and infinite and loving.

Is this exercise? Yes. Does the practice make me healthy in my body? Yes; it makes me strong and flexible physically and mentally. Does it relieve stress and calm my emotions? Yes, always. When I practice yoga, I find a calmness and sense of joy and acceptance of this life, other people, and myself. This practice of yoga helps me through times of illness, suffering, and increases my sense of joy."

Personal Training, Resistance Exercise & Muscle Activation Techniques™

Some people desire to have a personal trainer to keep them accountable to an exercise routine. In my opinion, not all personal trainers are ranked the same. Find someone knowledgeable and who will teach exercises correctly. My friend, Daren, is just that person. I've asked him to write a few words for us on the subject.

"A professional personal fitness trainer is an individual trained to help coach, progress, motivate, and teach an individual in aspects that include learning new exercises all the way to learning valuable skills to live a more productive and healthy lifestyle.

Reasons to Hire a Personal Fitness Trainer:
• Create accountability
• Help to figure out your goals and build a plan
• Learn how to do an exercise properly
• Choose the right exercises for your body's design and shape

We also use a very unique approach to developing stability in the body called *Muscle Activation Techniques™ (MAT)*. The evaluation is based upon the understanding

that the body will protect itself when it recognizes instability; therefore, muscles tighten up as a protective measure when instability is recognized. When muscles are weak, then the joint that it supports becomes unstable and the natural protective mechanisms are diminished. The end result of MAT™ is that we not only increase joint *mobility*, but also increase *stability* through that range of motion."
—Daren Kosters, www.bodyrockfitness.com

Exercise & Emotional Wellbeing

According to German New Medicine®, the body functions according to significant biological programs driven by the psyche. Our perceptions and belief system have a great deal to do with physical symptoms. Therefore it is vital that we focus on our emotional wellbeing since it affects the entire body. (See GNM section, p. 248.)

If you are feeling down, exercise will lift you up. Your body's functions are made up of millions of chemical reactions as your nervous and endocrine systems facilitate everything from walking to digestion to your sense of wellbeing. Exercise releases the feel-good hormones that lift your mood and balance your emotions.

Serotonin, endorphins, and dopamine are hormones vital to feeling happy and calm. **Serotonin** is responsible for happiness, restful sleep, and a healthy appetite. Levels increase if you work out regularly. More serotonin means more energy and clearer thinking. **Endorphins** are released by your pituitary gland and make you feel exhilarated and happy. They also ease feelings of pain.

Exercise will also increase the release of **dopamine**, creating feelings of pleasure. Dopamine is one of the main neurotransmitters that your brain uses. It has a long-recognized connection with motivation and reward. That's one reason why people who exercise tend to lose weight, because they get a sense of satisfaction from the exercise. If you do not exercise, you might eat more food than you should because you are seeking pleasure from your food.

Exercise can reduce stress and improve your mood, stamina, and sex life. It is a great way to lift your mood and improve your emotions. When you exercise, your body feels more relaxed and calm. It is a great way to achieve balance.

Deep Breathing

The way you breathe affects your whole body. Deep breathing exercises will help you relax, release stress, and ease tension being held in the body. You can do breathing exercises at anytime during the day and especially first thing in the morning and right at bedtime. Yoga classes are a great place to learn and practice breathing.

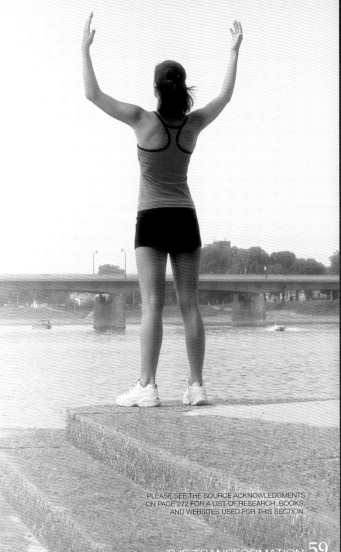

PLEASE SEE THE SOURCE ACKNOWLEDGMENTS ON PAGE 272 FOR A LIST OF RESEARCH, BOOKS, AND WEBSITES USED FOR THIS SECTION.

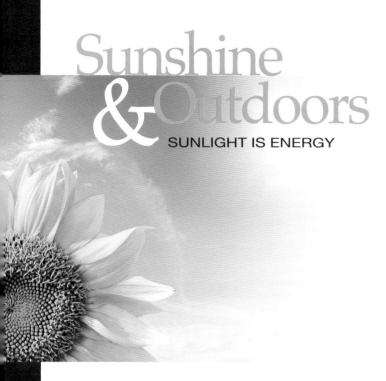

Sunshine & Outdoors
SUNLIGHT IS ENERGY

Sunlight is important for all living things!

The human body and all other living organisms need light to survive. Light is energy. We would not exist without the sun. Years ago, doctors sent people to the ocean for healing. The sun, the salt air, and salt water are all healing therapies given to us by our Creator— and they are free!

When I began this section, my thoughts turned to someone whom I value very highly. He is my teacher, mentor, and the inventor of the SpectraVision™—Lee Woolley. Lee has the best perspective on energy and light of anyone I know. Let's see what Lee has to say....

"Sunlight or photon energy acts as a source of information and regulation for all living systems. It can be seen as 'life-giving energy' as well, however, the requirement for the radiated energy from the sun sustains all life only because it is 'perfect' for us. It's amazing that the earth's distance from the sun and the angle of the earth's surface in relation to the sun's light creates the unique environment necessary for life itself.

"Any change in that angle or distance, and life as we know it wouldn't exist. The pineal gland, which is light sensitive, directs the light throughout the rest of the body. The photon energy it sends through the tissues has the ability to activate each and every cell in the body, creating the necessary biochemical and bioinformational processes to carry on metabolism and day-to-day living."
—Lee G. Woolley, CBP, BPA, BMD

The sun is so amazing and is literally our life source. It feels so magnificent, so calming, so relaxing! I could literally spend hours by the ocean or pool in the sunlight. The light and heat from the sun are indispensable to all nature. We are part of nature and need sunlight for health and wellbeing, for vitality and happiness.

The sun helps release our feel-good hormones. Exposure to light causes **endorphins** in the brain to be released. When released, they increase our body's threshold for pain and affect the way we feel emotionally. Before antibiotics, sunlight was successfully used to speed up the healing of wounds and injuries. Soldiers in World War II healed much better when their open wounds

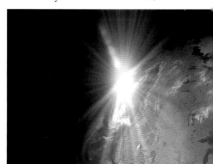

and broken bones were exposed to sunlight—and their survival rate increased. It's interesting that, chemically, endorphins are very much like morphine, but with no side effects!

Sunlight is also a very effective treatment for depression. Sunlight triggers the increased production of **serotonin**, the feel-good brain chemical that lifts your mood and helps alleviate depression. Too many days without sunlight can cause us to feel down or depressed. In addition, serotonin also affects our sleep patterns, body temperature, and sex drive. Daytime exposure to sunlight also increases **melatonin** production during the night—which helps regulate sleep and is a great antidote for insomnia.

Dr. Richard Hobday has many years experience with solar design in buildings and is a leading authority on the history of sunlight therapy. He states that sunlit houses can keep the body healthy, make us feel happier, and save energy.

The sun's rays support our body systems and assist the body in natural healing:

Sunlight strengthens the immune system and the cardiovascular system.

The body uses ultraviolet light to improve blood circulation, the pulse, and blood pressure.

Cholesterol levels can be balanced naturally.

Sunlight improves liver functions and is especially effective in treating jaundice.

They help the kidneys with part of their job—the elimination of waste products through the skin when we sweat.

The sun increases the body's metabolic rate by stimulating the thyroid gland, a weight-loss effect.

It also eases symptoms of premenstrual syndrome.

Sunlight exposure eases the healing of the swollen joints in cases of arthritis.

The thought of the sun healing our bodies is not new thinking. There are incredible healing powers of the sun that have been known for centuries. Cultures around the world have acknowledged the therapeutic qualities of the sun. From the pharaohs of Egypt to Greek, Roman, and Arabic physicians, countless wise and ancient scholars wrote stories and descriptions of the healing powers of sun therapies. Ancient records reveal how the sun was used to strengthen a person's health and treat a variety of illnesses and conditions.

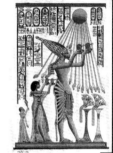

Understanding the therapeutic role that light can play in our lives today is vital as a preventative tool for overall health and wellness. It is natural healing at its best.

Today we have to get past the myth that sunlight is dangerous to our health. We have been told that unless we lather up with sunscreen, the sun has dangerous effects. How is this possible?

When we look at history, the sun was recommended to heal almost everything. For thousands of years, humans have lived in harmony with its heat and light. Yet we have lost this close contact with the sun and its healing powers. We have become afraid of it.

When we understand that the sun provides the foundation for all life-giving power on earth, and that the sun is the source of energy for all plants—and indirectly, for all animals—how can we believe it can harm us? If the sun causes cancer, I don't think we would be alive on the earth today.

"In recent years, we've all been trained to fear the sun due to the threat of skin cancer. Nothing could be further from the truth. Now there is a growing belief that exposure to the sun may not actually cause skin cancer. As a study published in the prestigious Cancer Journal indicates, exposure to sun actually decreases cancer rates."
—*The Vitamin D Council*

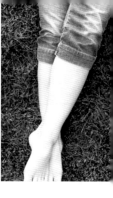

Your body is made to be in the sun, and when done properly, sun exposure is one of the best ways you can support your body's ability to protect you from cancer.

Sunlight & Vitamin D

Sunshine naturally triggers our skin to produce vitamin D. This vitamin supports cardiovascular health, promotes optimal cholesterol levels, enhances muscle strength, produces optimal blood pressure levels, helps maintain healthy immune systems, supports healthy kidney function, promotes healthy teeth, and keeps our bones strong and healthy.

Vitamin D deficiency has recently become an epidemic in the United States. How is this possible? During exposure to sunlight, the skin synthesizes vitamin D, which makes calcium absorption possible in the intestine, helping grow strong bones and healthy teeth. The sun helps prevent rickets (softening of the bones) in both children and adults and osteoporosis in the elderly. There is absolutely no reason in the world why anyone should suffer from a lack of vitamin D, when the remedy is as simple as spending a little time outdoors.

Since a lack of sunlight prevents the formation of vitamin D, it may be that high cholesterol levels are a result of a lack of sunlight. People who stay indoors and only go outside using industrial-strength sunblock might be subject to increased cholesterol levels for those reasons.

Sunlight-triggered vitamin D production also keeps your immune system healthy. Studies have shown that exposing the body to sunlight—or even ultraviolet (UV) light from an artificial source—increases the number of white blood cells or lymphocytes. These are the primary support for your body's ability to self-heal.

Vitamin D also increases the amount of oxygen your blood transports around the body. This boosts your energy levels, sharpens your mental faculties, and gives you an improved feeling of wellbeing.

The ideal way to get vitamin D is by exposing your skin to appropriate sunlight.

Healthy Sun Exposure Practices

The ideal way to get vitamin D is by exposing your skin to appropriate sunlight. Sun exposure (without sunscreen) for 10–15 minutes a day, with at least 40 percent of skin exposed, is a general guide. People with dark skin need to stay out significantly longer.

It is important to understand that in the summertime, when you put on your bathing suit and sunbathe for 30 minutes, your body produces about 20,000 IUs of vitamin D—as much as exists in 200 glasses of milk, or the equivalent of about 50 typical multivitamins!

The sun is a very powerful light source and overexposure that causes a burn can be harmful. We should have a healthy respect for the sun's rays, but should not completely eliminate it from our life. We will be missing out!

When you provide your body with the right fats and foods high in antioxidants, your skin can tolerate more sun exposure and thus reap all of the healing benefits you need. Don't let anyone tell you different—the sun is good for you!

The tan that develops with sun exposure is nature's way of protecting against too much UV radiation. Moderately tanned skin is more resistant to infections and sun burns than untanned skin. In addition, many skin conditions can be controlled and even cured through exposure to the sun. The best way to prevent skin damage from the sun is to expose your body to the sun throughout the year. Then in the summer you can tolerate more time in direct sunlight.

Start early in the season and expose most of your body to the sun for 15 minutes a day and continue to lengthen that time as you build a healthy, glowing tan. If you are unable to get healthy doses of sun exposure, then a safe tanning bed is another option.

The human body cannot go without light. People who cannot get outside regularly should install full-spectrum light fixtures in their work areas. We have these installed at Energetic Wellness.

Early morning sunlight in cool temperatures is beneficial to the body and will also set the body clock for a natural day-night cycle.

Could the fear of being exposed to the sun be fueled by companies that want to sell sun lotion products? I personally use coconut oil and/or Climb On Crème on my skin for tanning, after sun exposure, and everyday use. Coconut oil has natural sun protection—and although it will not completely prevent sunburn, it has an amazing ability to heal the skin. One of the primary reasons it is so effective in protecting the skin is its antioxidant properties, which help prevent burning and oxidative damage. You can apply coconut oil liberally. Re-apply the oil after swimming or sweating.

Avoid commercial sunscreen products at all costs. They are loaded with chemicals and prevent the absorption of light to produce vitamin D in the body. There are numerous studies that now show the dangers of sunscreen products. It is not a natural way to live!

Natural Life

It seems that modern medicine interprets the natural stage of a person's life as a condition instead of a very natural part of life and growth. The 7 Laws of Wellness will naturally assist us through all stages—Birth, Life, and Death.

Natural Conception & Birth

Our society has lost the understanding of how to care for young married couples preparing to have children. Couples of child-bearing years must nourish their bodies with nutrient-dense foods to give the next generation a solid foundation of health. Unfortunately, we use medicine to treat everything from infertility to delivery. A woman's body was designed to naturally bear children, but it needs the proper nutrients and care. We have forgotten that women have been giving birth since the beginning of time—our bodies instinctively know what to do.

Modern technology and emergency care is critical in life-threatening situations, but the majority of women do not even try natural childbirth. Surgery is automatically scheduled if there were previous problems. There is a significant health and biological purpose for the mother and the child to experience birth (GNM). When my daughter was first pregnant, I learned that only 2% of obstetricians have even seen a natural birth.

Natural Life

Men and women are being medicated through the natural stages of their lives—from puberty and menopause to emotional issues. These stages are natural and part of our design. We have replaced natural living practices with surgery and medication. The normal changes that occur should be handled in a delicate and natural way.

Natural Death

People want to spend their older years with energy and vitality. And most want a peaceful death. This is possible, but our current medical system does not have a good track record in this area. We can look to our Creator to receive wisdom and understanding regarding our body's natural design. Following the Laws of Nature and Nature's God will lead us through all the stages of life.

Healthy Eating Provides Protection

When your diet is balanced with a good ratio of essential fatty acids and is full of nutrient-dense foods and antioxidants, you'll be less prone to burning. When you eat a diet that contains too many omega-6 fatty acids, your skin balance is thrown off, making you more prone to sunburn. For example, processed foods made with vegetable oils—such as corn oil, cottonseed oil, safflower oil, sesame oil, sunflower oil, and soybean oil— all contain large amounts of omega-6 fatty acids.

When our diet is nutrient-dense, as outlined in this book, we have the best preventative medicine! Food is the best natural protector of all. The human diet should be high in omega-3 fatty acids—cod liver oil, salmon oil, pastured eggs, grass-fed beef, and my personal favorite, butter! A diet high in saturated fats will protect the skin from burning. So eat your coconut oil, palm oil, butter, and beef! Hmmm…do you think we have drifted from eating the foods that protect our body's ability to be in the sun? I do!

Foods like tomatoes, watermelon, and red peppers are rich in lycopene and will also help protect your skin from sun damage. Notice how tomatoes, watermelon, and red peppers are harvested and eaten fresh in the summer? What perfect design and timing! The complex antioxidants in green tea help boost the skin's ability to protect itself. Drink a cup of green tea a day to decrease the risk of sunburn. Tropical green tea extract can be applied directly to the skin before sun exposure.

I recommend that you do *not* take vitamin D3 supplementation. Instead, I believe that we can accomplish a healthy increase of our vitamin D levels by exposing our body to the sun and consuming whole foods:

• Sockeye salmon, tuna, trout, oysters, cavier, herring, sardines, sole, flounder, and mackerel
• Shiitake & button mushrooms
• Pastured eggs
• Raw milk and raw milk cheeses
• It is extremely important to supplement with fermented cod liver oil or salmon oil, especially in the winter.

Although care must be taken to avoid overexposure to ultraviolet (UV) rays, sunlight is known as a natural remedy for various skin conditions. The UV light from the sun slows production of skin cells and reduces inflammation.

So get out in the sun regularly. Build up a nice base tan. Eat nutrient-dense foods that protect the body from sun damage. Have a good healthy respect for the awesome power of the sun, and be grateful for the sun's amazing health benefits.

Cleaning—As a side note, sunlight is also very cleansing and can be used as a cleaning tool. That's why it is important to set out in the sun any rugs, blankets, and comforters that cannot be washed regularly.

Sun Gazing

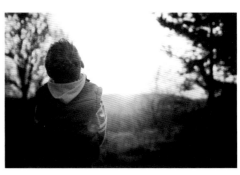

Sun gazing is also known as solar healing, solar gazing, sun staring, Sun Yoga, Surya Yoga, and Solar Yoga. All refer to the practice of staring directly at the sun to receive nourishment, physical healing, and spiritual enlightenment. The gazing is only done during the first hour after sunrise or the last hour before sunset, when the sun's rays are most gentle to your eyes.

Sun gazing was also practiced by ancient Egyptians, Aztecs, Greeks, and Mayans; in Tibetan Yoga and some traditions of Qigong, Tai Chi, and some Native American tribes. Here are some sun gazing benefits:

• Overall feeling of wellbeing
• A connection with nature
• Increased energy levels and decreased appetite
• Improved eyesight, including visual defects
• Alleviated mental disorders

Sun gazing is a beautiful practice, one in which I do often. Since there is much controversy over the risks and benefits, if you desire to practice sun gazing you will need further study than what is provided here. As with any practice, sun gazing must be done correctly and may not be appropriate for everyone.

Grounding/Earthing

The surface of the earth resonates with natural, subtle energies. Earthing refers to the process of connecting to the earth by walking barefoot outside.

Humans have practiced earthing throughout history—standing, sitting, working, or sleeping grounded indoors. Throughout most of history, humans walked barefoot and slept on the ground. They were directly connected to the earth almost 24/7. That's what the human body was accustomed to and the body knew exactly what to do with what the earth provides.

Our modern lifestyle involves wearing insulated shoes and sleeping in buildings that electrically isolate the body from the ground plane. While some people intuitively sense that they feel better when they walk or even sleep directly on the earth (as on a camping trip), most of the population is more or less permanently isolated from the earth's electrical influences.

For more than a decade, thousands of people around the world—men, women, children, and athletes—have incorporated earthing into their daily routines and report better sleep, less pain and stress, and faster recovery from trauma. Earthing immediately equalizes your body to the same energy level, or potential, as the earth.

The surface of the earth resonates with natural, subtle energies.

This results in:
- Synchronizing your internal biological clocks, hormonal cycles, and physiological rhythms.
- Suffusing your body with healing from negatively charged free electrons.

When we connect to the earth, the amount of the electrons we absorb is determined by the amount we need to balance the electrical charge of our body. It is always the perfect amount! In addition to restoring the body's natural electrical balance, contact with the earth reduces stress and inflammation. Earthing can have both short-term and long-term effects—sometimes quite dramatic and quick.

Women in particular are meant to be intimately tied to the earth, and there is no time in a woman's life where this becomes more obvious than during menopause. The earth is a woman's comfort, healing, and salvation as the natural change in a woman's life takes place. Without grounding, women can feel wired, frazzled, unsupported, depressed, and anxious. With the earth firmly anchoring our bodies—relieving the inflammation and stabilizing our hormones—the journey through this stage of life becomes deeper and more meaningful, filled with inspiration and power.

Grounding to the earth decreases hormone swings, lifts mood, increases the quality of sleep, and can comfort the soul like nothing else. Research and scientific data can explain the anti-aging, anti-inflammatory effects, the metabolism boost, blood sugar stabilization, and higher quality sleep. But earthing goes well beyond what we can measure.

When humans are barefoot and in direct contact with the earth, free electrons are conducted onto the skin's surface and into the body via the mucus membranes of the digestive and respiratory systems. The body gains the earth's electrical potential. This has been the natural bioelectrical environment of the human body and of other organisms throughout most of our history. Earthing is the most natural thing you can do!

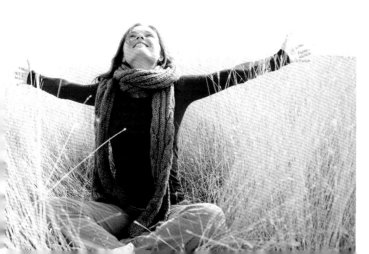

Fresh Air

The thought of going outside on a spring day, or most any day, is one of the most wonderful things. Taking time to be outdoors breathing in the fresh air is highly beneficial.

Ions are molecules that have gained or lost an electrical charge. They are created in nature as air molecules break apart due to sunlight, radiation, and moving air or water. If you have ever been to the beach, hiked a mountain, or walked beneath a waterfall, then you have experienced the power of negative ions.

Negative ions are odorless, tasteless, and invisible molecules that we inhale in abundance in certain environments. Once the negative ions reach our bloodstream, they are believed to produce biochemical reactions that increase levels of the mood chemical **serotonin**—helping to alleviate depression, relieve stress, and boost daytime energy.

While part of this euphoria is simply being around these wondrous settings and away from the normal pressures of home and work, the air circulating on the beach, for example, is said to contain tens of thousands of negative ions. This is much more than the average home or office building, which may only contain hundreds, dozens, or none at all.

How Negative Ions Affect
Your Brain & Renew Your Energy

Negative ions are said to increase the flow of oxygen to the brain, resulting in higher alertness, decreased drowsiness, and more mental energy. They clean the air, reducing irritants that could make you sneeze, cough, or have a sore throat. Negative ions can make us feel like we are walking on air. We are instantly refreshed when we open a window, step outside, or roll down the car window and breathe in fresh air.

Do you feel sleepy in air conditioning? Interestingly, air conditioning depletes the atmosphere of negative ions, but an ion generator releases ions into the room. People with winter depression experience relief with negative ion generators in their home or work setting. They can relieve depression the natural way.

Have you ever wondered why you always sleep more soundly after spending the day at the beach? The sea air is full of healthy negative ions. These charged particles, found abundantly in sea spray and concentrated in fresh air, improve our ability to absorb oxygen by neutralizing damaging free radicals (positive ions). These negative ions also help balance levels of serotonin, the body chemical associated with mood and stress. That is why a day at the beach leaves you feeling not only more alert and energized, but also deeply relaxed and able to rest more soundly. So next time you plan a vacation, try going to the beach. There is nothing like it!

Seawater

Outdoor beach activities give you the advantage of bathing in a natural therapeutic pool—the sea. Water is in great abundance on the earth, and about 97 percent of that is seawater. The beneficial healing qualities of seawater have been known to mankind for centuries.

Water has long been recognized for its healing properties.

Seawater contains many minerals needed by the body to help heal and detoxify. It helps heal wounds, reduces infection, and promotes pain relief. In recent years, studies regarding the benefits of ocean water have shown that many conditions—such as arthritis, psoriasis, and even depression—are improved by swimming in the ocean.

Beach Sand

Outdoor activities may also use the natural properties of beach sand to enhance your workout. It makes an excellent surface for exercising.

There is also nothing more relaxing than taking a walk on the beach. Growing up in New Jersey, we had the privilege of living near the Atlantic Ocean. Walking on the beach is my very favorite thing to do, as well as just sitting or laying on the beach, burying my feet in the sand.

The sand also acts as a natural exfoliant, helping the old skin to shed more quickly and improving its natural regeneration.

Hydrotherapy (Water Therapy)

Water molecules are composed of hydrogen and oxygen, which are essential for the survival of many known forms of life. Also known as nature's healer, water has favorable effects on the skin and muscles, calms the internal organs, stimulates nerve reflexes, and can calm the endocrine system.

The world's oldest medical literature makes numerous references to the beneficial use of the bath in treating various diseases. Hippocrates, a Greek physician who lived about five hundred years before Christ, was the first to write extensively on the healing of diseases with water.

He used water regularly, both internally and externally, in treating illness of all kinds.

Long before Hippocrates recorded his experiences with the healing properties of water, the Egyptians enjoyed bathing in their sacred river, the Nile. Pictures found in ancient Egyptian tombs show people preparing for a bath. The baby Moses was found in the rushes when Pharaoh's daughter went down to the river to bathe. Bathing held a prominent place in the instructions given by Moses, under divine guidance, for the government of the Hebrew nation. The relationship of bathing to the treatment of leprosy would, of course, lead us to believe that it was used for curative effects.

The ancient Persians, Greeks, and Romans erected stately and magnificent public buildings devoted to bathing. The baths of Darius I (about 558-486 B.C.), one of the earliest Persian kings, are said to be especially remarkable. The Greeks were probably the first nation to use the bath for personal cleanliness, as well as for health reasons. The Roman Empire integrated elaborate public bath houses into their city planning.

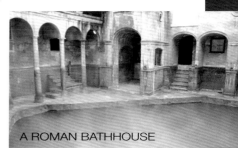
A ROMAN BATHHOUSE

During the early part of the eighteenth century, water was used medicinally. Baths were recommended for a variety of conditions. A book published by a minister, Mr. John Hancocke, in 1723 was called *Common Water, The Best Cure for Fevers*.

Sunshine & Outdoors, cont.

Water Therapies

Soaking in warm water will quiet and soothe your body. A nice 30-minute soak before bed is highly recommended. A soothing and relaxing bath can help counteract stress and its many effects on the body. It is the perfect way to heal from the day's activities and stressors.

A dip in cold water, in contrast, will stimulate and invigorate the body. Cold water therapy entails briefly and somewhat regularly exposing the body to natural stress that can enhance health. It can boost immune function, decrease inflammation and pain, and increase blood flow. Taking a cold shower will wake you up in the morning, but immersion is necessary for maximum benefit.

Exercising in water is very therapeutic and especially good for people with arthritis, those healing from a bone fracture, or overweight people. The buoyancy assists in supporting the body's weight. This decreases the load and reduces the stress placed on the joints, making it easier and less painful to perform exercises.

I do not recommend swimming or bathing in chemically treated chlorinated water. Salt-water pools are amazingly good for you and feel wonderful. I know…we have one!

> Clean water is key to our health.

Hot Tub—Good for Your Heart

A study at the Mayo Clinic found that soaking in hot water gives many of the health benefits of exercise with less strain on the heart. Immersion in hot water speeds up the heart to send blood to the surface and disperse extra body heat into the air. But after a few minutes, the warmed blood causes the blood vessels to dilate, which lessens resistance to blood flow and lowers the blood pressure.

Soaking in hot water is used for more than just relaxation—it has become known to cure a number of ills. Medical professionals around the globe use the natural hydrotherapy of warm water soaking to:

- ease anxiety and stress
- improve sleep and relieve insomnia
- relieve muscle and skeletal pain
- speed healing after injury and surgery
- protect the heart from rhythm disturbances
- improve the efficiency of the heart muscle
- have a positive effect on the regulatory mechanisms that control heart rate, blood pressure, and circulation

How to Enjoy Healthy Water at Home

Use a whole-house reverse osmosis water filter for your home or purchase one for drinking water and separate filters for each shower and tub in your home. Clean water is key to our health! It will be worth the investment.

PLEASE SEE THE SOURCE ACKNOWLEDGMENTS ON PAGE 272 FOR A LIST OF RESEARCH, BOOKS, AND WEBSITES USED FOR THIS SECTION.

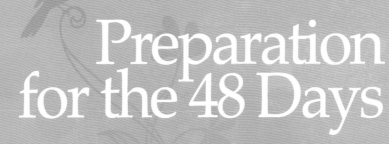

Preparation for the 48 Days

The Transformation

Let's Get Started

DATE

What You Will Need

☐ **Purchase food** from *Stage One: Foods for Life* list. Buy enough for a few days or plan for the week. *See page 132 for suggested menu ideas.*

☐ Purchase your **whole-food supplements** at the Oklahoma Energetic Wellness location or shop at www.energeticwellnessok.com. Plan to order at least a week before you want to start. *The products are optional, but if you want to get the most benefit from The Transformation, they are highly recommended.*

☐ Familiarize yourself with **this book**.

☐ **Schedule the conference calls** on your calendar if participating in the 48 Days group (offered several times a year). *Visit energeticwellnessok.com for more information.*

Purpose & Benefits of The Transformation

The purpose of the 48 Days is to take your body through a complete change. Change can sometimes be uncomfortable, but if you set your intention on experiencing the process, it can do an amazing thing for your body and your life.

Stage 1: Elimination, Days 1-15

The purpose of this stage is to stabilize insulin and blood sugar, reduce inflammation, reduce infection, enhance digestion, and help balance hormones in your body. The additional support and cleansing products gives you the tools to successfully make it through this most difficult stage.

Stage 2: Transformation, Days 16-30

The purpose of this stage is to maintain balance and continue to eliminate. When you have completed this stage, your body will have eliminated years of accumulated waste as well as rejuvenated your entire system!

Stage 3: Lifestyle, Days 31-48

Everyone waits for this stage to come as we add back potatoes and whole grains. The key to starting the Stage 3 food is to learn your body and how it responds to the additional foods. This is the stage that adds back your favorite foods so that you experience the most benefit from them. What do you need to maintain your desired weight? The keys to adding foods back are moderation and learning how to prepare them properly.

My purpose for guiding you through this amazing journey is to help you eliminate processed, denatured, refined foods and reeducate you as we add back only nutrient-dense, pure, whole foods that transform your health. Those of you who are patients are well on your way to this lifestyle of eating, and the program will only help you get there faster.

Starting the 48 Days will reset your metabolism and balance the body, but the main goal is to transform your way of eating for *life*. We will transform your body, your kitchen, and your lifestyle. You will have increased energy and vitality, adding years to your life.

This is a whole-body transformation! Diets don't work because they aren't a permanent lifestyle change—and they can seriously harm your body. Unless you lose weight by changing your habits, it will not be a long-term, healthy change and you will find yourself worse off than when you first started.

The body was perfectly designed. If given the right nutrients and lifestyle, your body will adjust to a balanced weight and support you through life. The perfect way to balance the natural design of the body is by applying the 7 Laws of Wellness. The 48 Days food plan, daily routine, and supplement plan help you get started and will assist your body in creating energy for balanced living. After the 48 Days, you can continue this way of eating and living—for life.

There are two reasons why the body has symptoms (including weight gain):
- We are what we eat and the way we live.
- We are what we think.

The Metabolism Craze

There is an abundance of contradictory information regarding metabolism and weight loss. It can be very confusing. If you have been frustrated with your body and blamed weight gain on your metabolism, I hope to help you begin loving your body—it is responding according to its design to take care of you!

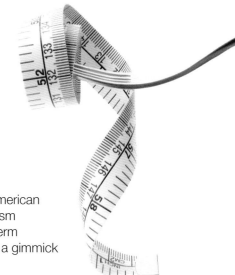

Metabolism is a popular buzzword created for our modern, diet-crazed American lifestyle. It is not unusual to hear people complain about a "slow" metabolism or wonder how to get their metabolism to speed up for weight loss. The term *metabolism* is not an actual medical term. It is overused by companies as a gimmick to sell diet plans and weight-loss products.

A hundred years ago, people did not need to talk about the latest diet or their slow metabolism. My parents are in their 80s, and they can't remember overweight people when they were young. We have a current epidemic of adult and childhood obesity. In June 2013, the American Medical Association (AMA) voted to declare obesity a *disease*. They say this will help America's leading physicians provide adults and children the medical assistance they need to lose weight. There is even testing being done for an obesity vaccine.

Declaring obesity a disease will most likely only benefit the pharmaceutical companies as they create more medication to treat symptoms. Creating a vaccine does not solve the root issues of chemically injected and processed food devoid of true nutrients. Our bodies are starving. Our food needs to be returned to its original design. We are what we eat.

My definition of metabolism is "the natural function of the body to create, store, and utilize energy." Food was created to be our medicine and medicine our food!

We Are What We Eat

Food gives the body the nutrients (fuel) to create, store, and utilize energy. It is used in every process of the body for the function of organs, tissues, and glands. Food sustains life, along with clean water, fresh air, sunshine, and rest—see the 7 Laws of Wellness on pages 23-68.

The food we eat is the fuel for energy in thinking, moving, and growing. Every function in the body needs energy. There are thousands of metabolic reactions happening at the same time. These processes are regulated by the body to keep our cells healthy and in proper, working order.

What we eat, how we move, and how much we rest determines how well our cells and tissues recover. Energy expenditure is continuous. The rate of energy varies during the day depending on what we do, what we did yesterday, and what we have eaten. Counting calories and following ridiculous weight-loss diets undermine the body's energy sources. We can balance the body by living and eating naturally, according to its design.

No Need to Count Calories
A calorie is not equal to a calorie. Most health care professionals recommend counting calories as a legitimate weight-loss approach. And most people do lose weight, but at great cost to their health. Eating whatever we want but limiting the amount of caloric intake—without thought of what we are putting in the body—is not wise. It does not lead to health and happiness. The foods we eat affect everything about us. **Real food supports the body's natural ability to function naturally—in body, mind, and spirit.**

The Transformation was designed for every body type, blood type, and addiction. It is the solution for balancing your metabolism and maintaining your perfect weight. The first step is to eliminate any addictive foods and beverages that are causing the problem.

In Stage 1, we eliminate key trigger foods, like refined white flour, white sugar, high-fructose corn syrup, artificial sweeteners, refined salt, and hydrogenated fats (trans-fats or vegetable oils)—all processed foods. This will give your body the ability to begin cleaning house and resetting/balancing your metabolism.

The foods recommended in *The Transformation* are organic and the most nutrient-dense foods available. If you cannot locate these foods, you can still apply these principles using the best whole foods that you can find. The key is eating "whole foods" instead of fake foods.

Fake, convenient, and devitalized food that accompanies a stressful lifestyle will weaken the body and leave it devoid of energy—the energy needed to heal. Eating pure, whole foods, living naturally, and giving the body every opportunity to function according to its biological design supports life the way it was intended.

Natural Balance
to Maintain Your Perfect Size

By eating and living naturally, I have weighed within a five-pound range for most of my adult life. It is not that my body can't gain weight, but I know how to control it through food, exercise, and proper rest. Many of my patients have achieved their balanced weight in the same way—it's a wonderful phenomenon!

Let's take a look at five incredible people! They are different ages, different body types, have different foundations, and started their transformation for different reasons.

JM, 37, came to EW two years ago—on medication, stuck in her weight (which was not too heavy but she just didn't feel herself), and with digestive problems (bloating, gas). Her exact words: "I always ate whatever I thought would help me lose weight. I wasn't connected to my body and only cared about what I looked like on the outside." She wanted to feel better, inside and out. After the 48 Days, she continues to eat the Foods for Life by maintaining a natural lifestyle. She is off medication, at her perfect weight, and feels better—inside and out.

Steven, 52, is my husband of 31 years. He has eaten pure, whole food over the years, but he works in the corporate world and travels a lot. He had accumulated weight, had a severe snoring issue and frequent back pain. After the 48 Days, he's been transformed—he lost 25 pounds, has less back pain, and as an added benefit to me, he no longer snores! He continues to limit his whole grain intake, and looks and feels great.

LH, 58, made her first wellness appointment in April 2010. She expressed feeling much older than she was and wanted to do something about it. She was overweight with a family history of obesity. During the 48 Days, LH did not add Stage 3 foods. She has learned how to maintain the 70 pounds she lost through eating the Foods for Life, and limiting potatoes and grains. She looks and feels amazing!

CJ, 65, came to me in July 2011. After not receiving the help she wanted from the medical community, she became interested in natural health. On several medications, discouraged, and not feeling well, she was ready to make a change to help her body heal itself. *The Transformation* has changed her life. CJ is off all medications—even one she had been on for 40 years. Although weight loss was not a priority, it came as a natural result. She has lost 24 pounds and is naturally maintaining her perfect weight.

RL, 74, came in November 2011. She was also on several medications, and I have to say, was the most curious of all my patients. She likes to research and was tired of taking medications and having to deal with the side effects. Having been through a divorce and the loss of a son, she was ready to start taking care of herself—body, mind, and spirit. After the 48 Days, RL remains on the Foods for Life and is doing great! On her 75th birthday she commented to me that she hadn't felt so good in 20 years. As a result of eating pure, whole foods and resolving conflicts, she naturally lost 25 pounds and is holding steady. Her children are following in her footsteps as a result of seeing the energy she has achieved.

During the 48 Days, **you** will discover how to balance your body for the purpose of maintaining **your** perfect weight for life!

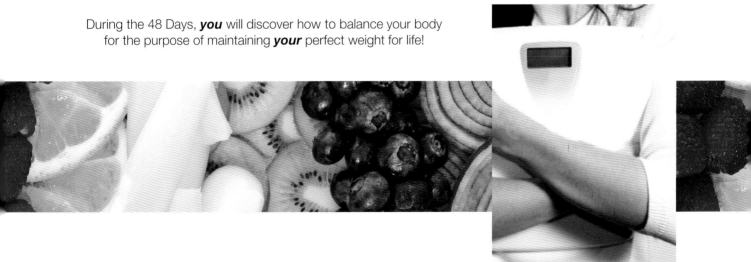

We Are What We Think

The body was designed to support your every thought, feeling and emotion.

According to the scientific evidence of Dr. Ryke Geerd Hamer, German New Medicine®, diseases are not errors of nature, but are created to support us during times of unexpected distress.

In light of Dr. Hamer's research, we know that a situation of abandonment and rejection can create a shock conflict in the kidney tubules, which increases water retention for extra fluid storage in the body. The feeling of rejection increases the size of the fat cells to protect you and to assist with "storage of fuel" during your time of need. A good analogy is feeling like a fish out of water. The biological response is to retain water. If the situation isn't resolved and you continue to feel abandoned or rejected, a life-long battle with weight may result. If you have experienced this type of conflict, please consider scheduling a GNM phone consultation for further discussion. (Call Energetic Wellness at 405-359-1245.)

Find a practical solution to downgrade and resolve your conflicts:

- Undergo natural therapies
- Seek professional counseling
- Talk to a friend
- Listen to Paraliminal CDs
- Prayer and meditation
- Recite positive affirmations
- Love and forgive yourself
- Forgive others
- Write in a journal

An ideal way to change old habits is by changing our perspective about life and about ourselves. The company Learning Strategies offers many Paraliminal CDs on various topics. A few helpful ones might be *Ideal Weight*, *Break the Habit*, and *Perfect Health*. I listen to one almost every night and often fall asleep while listening—they are powerful. See Resource Section (p. 265) for more information.

Louise Hay wrote a wonderful book called *Heal Your Body*. It lists numerous conditions with probable causes and new thought patterns to recite. Here is an example:

The Condition: Addictions

Probable Cause: Running from self. Fear—not knowing how to love the self.

New Thought Pattern: "I now discover how wonderful I am. I choose to love and enjoy myself."

The 48 Days & Weight Loss

The 48 Days will transform your health. Achieving your perfect weight will be a byproduct. If you intend to lose 20 pounds or more, then I suggest the following guidelines in addition to the Stages. The 48 Days will assist you in discovering the foods that are perfect to maintaining your perfect weight.

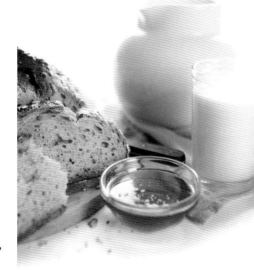

Stage — Eliminate the suggested dairy foods.

Stage — Continue to eliminate dairy and slowly add all the other Stage 2 foods. Pay attention to your body's response after each addition. *Do you like the way you feel? Do you have more or less energy?*

Stage — Continue to eliminate all dairy products and do not add grains until after the 48 Days.

If you are enjoying the momentum of losing weight (an average of 3 to 4 pounds a week), continue until you achieve your perfect weight.

After the 48 Days, begin adding dairy once a week, then twice a week, and see how you feel—and if it causes fluctuation in your weight. For the average person, raw goat milk and cheeses are very important and should not cause weight gain if eaten in moderation. Never eat processed dairy products.

You can also begin adding Stage 3 foods. Your body will let you know what it can tolerate. You may decide that you only want to eat (properly prepared) grains once or twice a week. This is a discovery that only you can make. Everyone's body, foundation, and body type is different and uses food energy in different ways.

As a side note: Those of you who are patients, continue to stay away from the foods that tested sensitive, even if they are on the "Foods for Life" list. Stay on all recommended supplements, even if they are not part of The Transformation *supplement list. If you have any questions, please call the office.*

What You Can Expect

Expect to learn a new, natural way of living!

By the end of the 48 Days, you will have transitioned into a natural way of eating and lifestyle!

Expect a possible reaction.

During the first two weeks, the restriction of certain foods that your body is addicted to—such as sugar, artificial sweeteners, caffeine, chemicals, preservatives, etc.—could cause your body to experience temporary withdrawal symptoms such as headaches, flu-like symptoms, increased carbohydrate cravings, fatigue, less energy, mood swings, and even changes in bowel habits. This may also happen due to increased cleansing of toxins from the body. This is the main purpose of consuming the suggested supplements, support supplements, and the cleansing supplements to help the body transition to this new way of eating with the least amount of discomfort. If you do experience any discomfort, remember that it is temporary, and your body needs extra rest and support. Make sure you are drinking the proper amount of water for your weight. These symptoms should only occur within the first two weeks, if at all.

Expect support from Energetic Wellness, especially me!

I want you to be successful. Expect our conference calls to provide you with continued information, motivation, and answers to questions. Please limit your questions on the call to those specifically pertaining to *The Transformation* and not your personal existing health condition. We can set up an individual wellness appointment so that all your personal concerns are heard and addressed.

Expect to be calm and not overwhelmed!

If for any reason you go off course while on the 48 Day plan, know that you can jump right back in and continue where you left off. The purpose of this process is to reduce stress by helping you make changes and guiding you into a natural lifestyle that usually has to be flexible. Plan on taking it one step at a time.

Expect a suggested daily routine.

This suggested daily routine reflects my 7 Laws of Wellness. Again, please take it one step at a time. Concentrate on changing your food and adopting everything else as you can. If you are comfortable starting everything, you will of course receive the most benefit. Any change you make is one step closer to a natural way of living, including more energy and vitality.

Expect to learn to love yourself.

I am so proud of you for making the decision to start this journey. This is a process, a journey of understanding who you are and how your body was designed. Take one day at a time. Learn a lot about yourself and your body. Learn to love yourself so that you can love others even more than you already do!

Expect an amazing transformation.

This will be an amazing transformation within your body and your life.

Once you complete the 48 Days, you can repeat it twice a year with my assistance or on your own. I have done different parts of this plan many times throughout each year and for years have lived on these wonderful foods for life, which includes all the pure, whole foods in the program.

Know that I will be praying for each one of you and making myself available to assist you through this wonderful journey!

God bless you!
The Transformation is for life!

Daily Routine

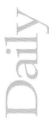

Daily

Use this routine and supplement plan throughout the 48 Days and as a guide to apply the 7 Laws of Wellness for life.

Hydration **Daily Water Intake**

- Drink spring or reverse-osmosis, purified and energized (iH2O) water with the recommended suggestions to increase energy in the water.
- Drink one half of your current weight in ounces every day.
- If possible, install a shower filter. Your skin is the largest organ of the body and can absorb harmful chemicals while showering.
- When out, buy FIJI, VOSS, or Mountain spring, non-sparkling bottled water.
- Save glass water bottles to refill at home. Buy a glass or stainless steel water bottle, and use it for home, work or travel.

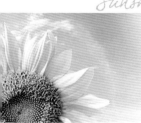

Sunshine/Outdoors **Fresh Air & Sun Exposure**

- First thing in the morning, get outside in the grass with your shoes off and connect with the earth! We walk on so much concrete that we are not receiving the energy we need on a daily basis from the earth.
- 20 minutes of sun exposure a day with most of the body exposed will increase your vitamin D.
- Take a break at work to get outside, every day!
- During fall and winter, take cod liver oil and/or use an ESB Tanning Systems indoor vitamin D lite tanning bed.
- Open windows to allow fresh air to cleanse indoor air at least 10 minutes a day, even in the winter.
- Wait as long as you can to turn on the air conditioning in summer and the heater in the winter.
- Use air filters.

Faith Strengthen Your Belief System / Renew Your Mind

These are just examples of exercising faith. Do what you like to strengthen and encourage yourself through this time of cleansing and changing your lifestyle.

- Practice morning prayer, devotion, or meditation.

- Make a list of things you are grateful for: people, things, something about yourself.
  Make a list of things you are grateful for about your spouse or loved one and share it with them.

- Look at yourself in the mirror every day and say, "I love you, I forgive you and thank you." So often we are so hard on ourselves. These statements are also powerful when spoken to your spouse, significant other, or children.

- Focus on your ability to obtain the perfect weight for you. Listen to *Ideal Weight* or *Perfect Health* by Paul Scheele daily if you have a hard time accepting yourself and especially your weight. Accept yourself, choose to eat properly and the weight will come off. Think: "Eat real food." Look in the *Recommended CDs & DVDs* section on pages 265–266 for web sites and ordering information.

- Listen to beautiful music; read inspirational material.

- Viewing the film "The Secret" is another wonderful way to transform your thinking by understanding the benefits of positive thinking and renewing your mind daily. Understand the law of attraction.

- Recommended book: *Everyday Miracles by God's Design* by Dr. David Jernigan. Look in the *Recommended Resources* section on page 265 under "Rest & Faith."

Detoxification Overview of Natural Therapies to Assist the Body in Its Natural Function

- Use the **Infrared Sauna** daily in winter, 3 times a week or more in the summer. You can purchase one for your home or buy a package of sessions at Energetic Wellness, a local gym or spa.

- **Body Balance Foot Bath** can be done daily or 3 times a week during the 48 Days and once a month for life. Purchase one for your home or buy a package of sessions at Energetic Wellness or a local spa.

- See the *Natural Therapies* section on page 252 for more information.

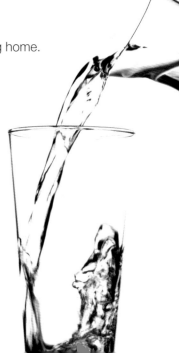

Morning

Nutrition and Detoxification **Morning Nourishment & Cleansing**

If you are taking my recommended supplements, then continue as directed per our appointment. Otherwise, start this daily supplement plan that will assist the body in natural detoxification and provide dense nutrition. For more information about the products, please refer to the Suggested Supplement Plan, starting on page 88. *An empty stomach is one half hour before a meal or two hours after.*

Morning Supplements—

Probiotics: 2 capsules or 1 scoop of powder in 8 oz. water or added to your green drink, on an empty stomach.

Cleansing green drink: If you are just starting out with a green drink, start out slowly!
  • Pure Synergy: start with 1 tsp. and work up to 1 Tbsp.
  • Mix together: Pure Synergy (1 Tbsp.) or Vitality Greens (2 scoops)
    • 6–8 oz. of pure clean water
    • 4 oz. of Inner Vitality or Energy Boost minerals
    • 1 tsp. of Master Cell Rejuvenator (MCR)
    • 1/2 tsp. vitamin C powder

Energy Water Bottle: Make water bottles for the day even if you are staying home. This will assure drinking one half your weight in ounces a day. Mix together:
  • 16 oz. pure clean water
And one of the following:
  • Fresh squeezed organic lemon or lime
  • 1 tsp. MCR (up to 4 tsp. daily)
  • 1–2 drops of Young Living Lemon Essential Oil
  • 1 Tbsp. Energy Boost minerals

Exercise/Oxygen **Get Moving!**

The body was created to move, and at least 30 minutes of exercise is a great way to start your day.

Caution: If you are on heart medication, diabetic, or haven't exercised in a long time, talk with your medical doctor and start out slowly (10–15 minutes) and work up to 30 minutes. If you are healthy, increase this to one hour or more.

Examples of exercises:
- Walk/run at intervals outside or on the treadmill, work up to 3–6 miles a day
- Rebounder used for 30 minutes with guided exercise (Urban Rebounding DVDs)
  This is by far one of the best ways to assist the lymphatic system and strengthen every organ. See Exercise & Oxygen in the 7 Laws of Wellness on page 54.
- Resistance exercises 3 times a week with a trainer or on your own
- Ab workout can be done every day
- Push-ups can be done every day
- Yoga at home or with a group in a studio
- Stretching at home or with a group can be done every day

Optional: While exercising listen to uplifting music or motivational CDs

Detoxification **Shower/Bath/Rubdown**

Taking proper care of the skin is vital to natural health.
- Always shower or bathe in filtered water.
- Rub down with towel, dry off.
- Apply virgin coconut oil from feet up to face. You can add a couple drops of an essential oil (lavender is my favorite) to the coconut oil before applying.
- For aromatherapy, choose your favorite essential oil—such as Young Living Company's Valor, Lavender, Thieves, or Frankincense. Apply 3 drops of oil on the palm of your hand, rub your hands together in circular motion three times, then cup your hands over your face, take several deep breaths, and then rub the remaining oil on top of your head, back of neck, and/or soles of feet. For women, apply Frankincense daily to your breasts.

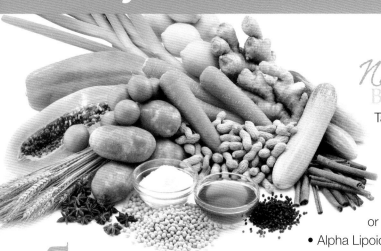

Nutrition
Breakfast / Lunch / Dinner

Take these mealtime supplements just prior to eating.

Breakfast
- Cod Liver Oil:
  2 capsules or
  1 tsp. per day,
  or Salmon Oil: 1 capsule
- Alpha Lipoic Acid: 1 capsule
- GI Restore: 1 capsule until bottle is gone (30 days)

See breakfast menu ideas or create your own breakfast from the appropriate food list.

Mid-Morning
- Syndrome K: 1 tsp. between breakfast and lunch until the bottle is gone (24 days)
- Lymph Care: 1 dropperful
- Reset!: 5 sprays in mouth

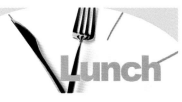

Lunch
- Cod Liver Oil: 2 capsules, or Salmon Oil: 1 capsule
- Alpha Lipoic Acid: 1 capsule

See lunch menu ideas or create your own meals
from the appropriate food list.

Mid-Afternoon
- Lymph Care: 1 dropperful
- Reset!: 5 sprays in mouth

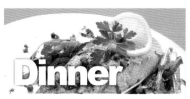

Dinner
- Cod Liver Oil: 2 capsules, or Salmon Oil: 1 capsule
- Alpha Lipoic Acid: 1 capsule
- GI Restore: 2 capsules
- Ultra GL: 2 tsp. until bottle is gone (24 days). ***Do not start until Day 25.***

See dinner menu ideas or create your own meals from the appropriate food list.

Try not to eat later than 6 or 7 p.m., or at least three hours prior to bedtime.

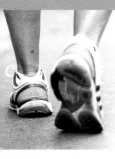

Exercise/Oxygen Gentle Movement

- Take a walk at least 1 to 2 hours after eating.
- Do breathing exercises.
- Rebound 10–15 minutes.
- Spend 30 minutes in the sauna—at least 2 hours after dinner, always after exercise.

Rest and Detoxification Evening Shower/Bath

These particular nighttime therapies assist you in releasing the tension and stressors from the day. The baths are very relaxing, yet purging.

- Take a short shower after the sauna, using warm water—just rinse.
- Soak 30 minutes in magnesium crystals with an essential oil.
- Rub down with a towel.
- Oil your body (same as morning).
- Aromatherapy (same as morning).
- Rub your choice of essential oils on soles of your feet, neck, etc.
- Apply Olbas oil on chest, neck, and under your nose.

Rest and Faith Prayer & Wind Down

The key to the evening wind down is very personal. Following are a few ideas to secure a restful sleep. Refer to "Rest" in the 7 Laws of Wellness on page 44 for more ideas.

- Read something inspirational.
- Use your own personal prayer… surrender all.
- Listen to music.
- Practice meditation/yoga.
- Listen to specific guided Paraliminal CDs by Learning Strategies:
  Ideal Weight, Relaxation, Anxiety-Free, Break the Habit, Deep Relaxation, Perfect Health, Positive Relationships, Personal Celebration
  See Recommended Resources, pp. 259 & 260.

Daily evening routine continued on next page.

Daily Routine, *cont.*

Get in bed before 10 p.m. This is key for the body's healing and rejuvenation. The best sleep is before midnight. Prepare the bedroom for restful sleep—remove cellphones and turn off all electronics.

At bedtime, wait one minute in between these homeopathics:

- Reset!: 5 sprays in mouth
- Lymph Care: 1 dropper, hold under tongue for 30 seconds
- Bio-Identical Melatonin: 1 dropper, hold under tongue for 30 seconds

You may also want to add these ideas to your daily routine.

Coconut Oil for *Brain Health and Weight Loss*

- Average person: 1–3 Tbsp. per day. This amount can be a combination of taken straight, in your food, and used in cooking.
  CAUTION: For some, taken straight can cause them to feel nauseated.
  Back down to a comfortable amount for you if it is too much, or use in cooking.
- Growing children could benefit from 2–4 tsp. per day.
- Breastfed babies consume natural lauric acid from mother's milk or, in homemade formulas, add 1/2 tsp. for every 5 lbs. of baby's weight per day.

The benefits of coconut oil for our overall health require a book of their own. Read Dr. Bruce Fife's books and Tropical Traditions™ Virgin Coconut Oil book or www.tropicaltraditions.com. See Recommended Resources, pp. 259 & 260.

Aromatherapy Essential Oils

Rub 3 times in circular motion in middle of the palm, cup, and inhale. Then rub remaining oil on top of head, back of neck, and soles of the feet.

- Lemon: brightening and cleansing
- Peppermint: energy and cooling
- Valor: morning, promotes courage
- Lavender: calms and relaxes, morning and/or night
- Thieves: antibacterial, morning and/or night
- Clove: highest value of antioxidants

To order Young Living Essential Oils, refer to the Resources section on page 268.

Oops!

If you go off of the 48 Days for a day, please don't beat yourself up! You might have to attend a business lunch at a Chinese restaurant that serves soybean oil. Try to choose your best option. Or you might have to stay up late because you have guests from out of town and miss your morning walk.

It's okay; things happen. But don't give up. It hasn't ruined your day. You have accomplished other things that are benefitting your wellbeing, such as drinking the amount of water you need or sitting out in the sun for half an hour.

Persevere . . .
you will see positive changes over time and how they benefit your life every day.

The Transformation is a significant change for most of you, and no one is perfect! Many of my patients have gone through the 48 Days several times, each time applying a new principle or adding a new element to their daily routine. **Wellness is a life journey**; a learning process.

The Transformation describes an ideal way of eating and living for life. The best of the best foods are listed for you to enjoy. If you cannot buy all organic fruits and vegetables, grass-fed meat, etc., then do the best you can. You will still be doing a wonderful service for your body, mind, and spirit by cutting out the processed food and eating whole foods. Always shop the perimeter of the grocery store where the fresh food is and not the center aisles where the processed foods are located.

If you have to attend a function where processed food is served, make the best choices possible. Also, it is better to consume **undesirable** foods in a short time frame rather than over several hours or the entire day. Consuming high carbohydrate foods within a one-hour time period will minimize the amount of extra insulin your body must produce. This will minimize the amount of fat the body stores and limit the overall effect that it may have.

Be kind to yourself. Things will happen, so just get right back on the road to wellness. You will soon realize that this way of living will become a part of you, and you won't even have to think about it; **you will just live it.**

Suggested Supplement Plan

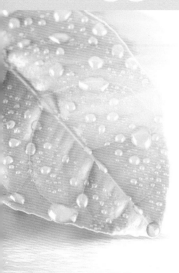

The Importance of Supplements

"There are two types of supplementation required in a wellness program. The first is *General Supplementation*—designed to give the body the basic building blocks for metabolic or detoxification functions. This provides the adequate vitamins, minerals, enzymes, and amino acids necessary for creating energy. Due to the many environmental poisons, toxins in food, and the challenge of eating a healthy diet, supplementation has become a necessity to maintaining a healthy lifestyle.

The second type of supplementation is known as *Supplemental Therapy*. It is outlined by the practitioner for you, **based on your own particular needs**. Supplemental Therapy is designed to naturally hone in on one of the many hundreds of functions needed to optimize health and increase healing responses in our body. For example, a product could key in on particular organs or glands, support lymphatic drainage, enhance pH regulation, provide the exact botanical blends for detoxification, or provide the cofactors needed for cellular nutrition and absorption.

Both types of supplementation are necessary and are important aids as the body regains its balance and begins working at optimal levels. The Supplemental Therapies may be periodically changed as the body heals."

Lee G. Woolley, CBP, BPA, BMD
Developer of the SpectraVision™ & Bionetic Technologies

The basic supplement package can be purchased to assist you through The Transformation and is recommended for life. These basics are my "Universal Supplements"—they can be used by everyone. Most of us grew up eating the standard American diet, and we need high-quality, whole-food supplements to support the natural function of the body. They will assist in natural detoxification and provide dense nutrition.

*I also recommend the support supplements and a cleansing package. The support supplements can be used throughout The Transformation and beyond, as needed. The support supplement, Reset!, will assist you through emotional stress and sugar cravings. Bio-Identical Melatonin will help with regulating sleep patterns and detoxifying the brain. The cleansing supplements will open the lymphatic system, cleanse the colon, kidneys, and liver/gallbladder. The cleansing products are safe for the average person and are recommended twice a year. **If you have an existing medical condition, please consider making an initial appointment or individual phone consultation through Energetic Wellness.***

Throughout the year, Energetic Wellness offers limited-time discounts on the supplements when purchased as a package. Purchase products by calling 405-359-1245 or shop online www.energeticwellnessok.com.

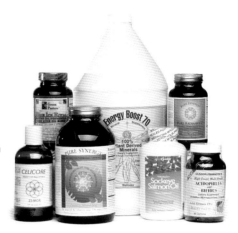

The Basic Supplement Package

- Probiotics: powder or capsules *(I recommend powder.)*
- Green Drink: Pure Synergy or Vitality Greens *(choose one)*
- Inner Vitality and/or Energy Boost 100% Organic Minerals: 1 gallon
- Cod Liver Oil or Sockeye Salmon Oil *(choose one)*
- Master Cell Rejuvenator: 8 oz.
- Pure Radiance C: powder or capsules *(I recommend powder.)*

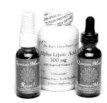

The Additional Support Package

- Reset!
- Bio-Identical Melatonin
- Alpha Lipoic Acid

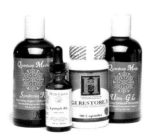

The Complete Cleansing Package

Only use these products during the 48 Days.

- Lymph Care: 2 bottles
- GI Restore: 1 bottle
- Syndrome K: 4 oz.
- Ultra GL: 8 oz.

Each package can be sold as an individual package or as part of a complete package.

The following section is a list of the supplements and ingredients Dr. Menzel recommends, and the reasons why she recommends them. The supplements are universal for everyone who comes to Energetic Wellness. After 15 years of self-study and 5+ years of education, Dr. Menzel compiled these supplements as the most needed. These supplements are of the highest quality available. Each supplement in the Basic package serves a specific purpose, assisting you during the 48 Days and *The Transformation* for life.

Use this supplement plan throughout the 48 Days and as a guide for life!

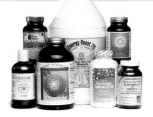

The Basic Package

Probiotics play an important role in human nutrition and health, and in naturally balancing the intestinal microflora. Health benefits attributed to the consumption of probiotics include: maintenance of the normal gut flora, alleviation of lactose (milk sugar) intolerance, improvement of digestive processes and absorption of nutrients, and stimulation of the body's immune system.

Dosage for Probiotic Capsules: Start with one capsule first thing in the morning and one at bedtime with one full glass of water, continue for 3 days. If you are not happy with the results, you can raise the dosage to two capsules first thing in the morning and two at bedtime for 3 days. Gradual increase in dosage is the best way to find this optimum personal level. The result you are looking for is a good, full bowel movement before noon each day. Every digestive system is unique. You need to find the dosage that yields the best results for you. It may be 1, 2, 4 or 6 capsules per day. Refrigerate.

Dosage for Probiotic Powder: Start with one scoop first thing in the morning on an empty stomach. Dissolve powder in a glass of clean non-chlorinated water and drink it. Do this once a day only. Stay at this dosage for 3-5 days. (1 scoop of powder is worth 4 capsules.) If you are not happy with the results you can raise the dosage to one scoop in the morning and one at night. Again, your body might do well on one, two, or three scoops a day. Refrigerate.

Green Drink *Start with either one of these green drinks. If you have been tested on the SpectraVision™ (SV), continue with the greens that tested well for you. If not, read the description of each green drink to select the one that best suits you. To find a SV practitioner in you area, see Therapies on page 247.*

PURE SYNERGY GREEN DRINK

My personal favorite! Pure Synergy is supported by over 30 years of research. Every bottle is fresh every month, and 100% organic. It was formulated to provide you with deep nourishment necessary to function optimally. Your body is able to then naturally detoxify, regenerate, and sustain abundant physical and mental energy throughout your busy days.

Pure Synergy is the most comprehensive and respected organic super food formula in the world—the standard by which all others are measured. Rediscover feeling healthy and energetic again—the palpable effect of this truly potent super food.

- Enhances vitality and vigor
- Provides sustained and steady energy
- Enhances mental clarity
- Assists purifying detoxification
- Supports healthy immune functions
- Enhances athletic endurance and recovery
- Greatly increases sense of wellbeing
- Provides essential support for healthy aging

Dosage for Pure Synergy Green Drink: *Start slowly to allow your body to comfortably acclimate to a deeper level of nutrition; work your way up to the recommended serving size. Begin with one tsp. of Pure Synergy and gradually increase to one heaping Tbsp. or more daily. Refrigerate.*

VITALITY SUPER GREENS

With a unique focus on nourishing the inner ecosystem, this very alkalizing formula, especially created by Donna Gates, will soothe and help rebuild the lining of your intestines. It's an excellent source of complete, easily assimilated protein, enzymes, vitamins, minerals, lignans, essential fatty acids, nucleic acids, and beneficial microflora. This formula is great for people with severe digestive conditions, as well as for gas, bloating, constipation, and/or diarrhea.

Dosage for Vitality Super Greens: *Two scoops in 8 oz. filtered water. Refrigerate.*

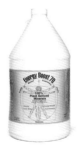

Energy Boost 70 is pure extracted Fulvic Acid from humate, which has been referred to as a "fountain of youth" because of its role in plant and animal nutrition. It contains the most easily digestible and bio-available organic mineral complexes and amino acids available. Leading natural health experts believe fulvic acid is one of the most important "missing links" in the modern food chain. Medical agricultural research continues to conclusively point to one conclusion: fulvic acid directly or indirectly holds the keys and solutions to many of the world's health problems.

Energy Boost 70 fulvic acid mineral complexes are the world's finest electrolyte, which improves energy function, increases assimilation, stimulates metabolism, restores electrochemical balance, reduces high blood pressure, enhances nutrients, and helps rebuild the immune system.

Dosage for Energy Boost 70: *1–4 oz. a day in 8 oz. of filtered water. This can be added to the green drink. Refrigerate.*

Inner Vitality is an all-natural, completely organic dietary supplement, chelated from ancient plant matter rich in essential minerals, trace elements and amino acids in a pH balanced state. Inner Vitality is a 4:1 rich source blend of bio-available Fulvic Mineral® (FA) and Humic Mineral® (HA) which are completely organic micro and macro mineral nutrients. Research results suggest that Humic and Fulvic Minerals complexes enhance mineral and trace element uptake, supporting the maintenance of mineral and trace element balances without harmful buildup in the body's cells. Following dissociation of the minerals and trace elements delivered by the Humic/Fulvic Mineral complex, the residual HA/FA complex can chelate heavy metals along the intestinal tract, in turn reducing heavy metal burdens in the digestive system. Inner Vitality reduces viral loads and toxins, while helping to rebuild cellular structure and speed healing. Plant derived, Inner Vitality's bio-available liquid minerals which ensure superior absorption into the bloodstream and allows the body to absorb more nutrients.

Dosage for Inner Vitality: *1–4 oz. a day in 8 oz. of filtered water. This can be added to the green drink. Refrigerate.*

Fish Oil

Choose one of the fish oils based on the description that most fits your need. Those without a gallbladder consistently do much better on the fermented oil because there is little digestion that needs to take place.

BLUE ICE COD LIVER OIL

Many of the great historical cultures had one sacred food which they relied on to ensure strong mind, body, and spirit: fermented fish or fish liver oil. The mighty Roman soldier was given a daily ration of fermented fish oil. The stoic Scandinavian Viking had a drum of fermenting cod livers outside the door of his home. Grandma always had a bottle of cod liver oil in the back cupboard.

Cod liver oil is high in EPA/DHA (omega-3 fatty acids) that supports the immune system, but it also promotes healthy blood lipids since omega-3 fatty acids can lower blood triglyceride levels. It also supports neurological and brain function. High in vitamins A & D, cod liver oil is great for the eyes! Higher doses of fish oil will greatly reduce inflammation and assist weight loss, but must be closely monitored. If you are currently taking a higher dose, please lower the amount. The omega-3 fatty acids must be carefully balanced with other foods when taking more than the recommended amount. For a complete evaluation of your omega-3 fatty acid needs, please make an office appointment, phone consult with Dr. Menzel or your local practitioner.

Dosage for Blue Ice Cod Liver Oil: *Take 1 tsp. per day or 6 capsules per day in divided doses with a meal. Refrigerate.*

BLUE ICE ROYAL COD LIVER OIL

Royal Cod Liver Oil is a combination of high-vitamin cod liver oil and high-vitamin butter oil in one.

Dr. Weston A. Price discovered High Vitamin Butter Oil in the 1930s. The pinnacle of his X-Factor discovery was the extreme synergistic effect between High Vitamin Butter Oil and traditional cod liver oil. "One without the other did not do his patients justice, but the two together worked like magic."

The high vitamin butter oil in Blue Ice Royal Cod Liver Oil is made from dairy oil extracted without heat from cows that eat 100 percent rapidly growing grass. The speed of the grass growth, timing of the grazing, species of grass, climate, and extraction method are all important to make real High Vitamin Butter Oil.

Dosage for Blue Ice Royal Cod Liver Oil: *6 capsules per day in divided doses with a meal. Refrigerate.*

SALMON OIL

Alaskan Sockeye Salmon are among the purest of all ocean fish, consistently testing free of hazardous levels of contaminants. In addition to ample omega-3s and vitamins A and D, whole, unrefined Vital Choice Sockeye Salmon Oil provides the full matrix of fatty acids, phospholipids, and antioxidants absent from standard, refined fish oils.

Dosage for Sockeye Salmon Oil: *3 capsules per day in divided doses with a meal. Refrigerate.*

Master Cell Rejuvenator

MCR is unlike any other product on the market due to its many benefits particularly for anti-aging, hormonal balance, and providing the necessary cofactors of metabolism. It is based on two ancient formulas—one from India and the other from the Orient. Both of these formulas have been tried and true for centuries and have functioned as the cornerstone for an all-around health regimen for the most royal and elite people in these countries. MCR is a uniquely modern adaptation of ancient knowledge blended from dozens of herbs containing vital ingredients that have been synergistically combined and uniquely designed to help maintain youthfulness, aid in metabolism, and counteract low energy at the cellular level. Because the ancients knew of the specific ways of preserving health and vitality, you can now take advantage of their knowledge.

Ayurvedic wisdom provides the base foundation to this formula, due to a unique combination of over 20 herbs working in synergy as a restorative to the body. Additionally this formula—containing a high percentage of Indian Gooseberry, which has a very strong rejuvenation effect—combined with the other constituents, strengthens the body, provides energy, and supports vitality. MCR also includes an additional ancient formula from Korea, which their ancient medical text has stated that those who take this formula daily for 27 years could live to be 360 years old. It includes over 29 of the most important botanicals, providing many of the plant-based nutrients necessary to help support virtually every aspect of male and female reproductive/endocrine systems, circulation, and the brain.

This is a breakthrough formula, which is based on micro-tincture blends of these uniquely formulated herbal extracts-designed to increase absorbability in the body by using the oral tissues rather than digestion for faster distribution. By using liquid oral therapies, our unique delivery system bypasses digestion and liver functions, so that the nutrients enter into the bloodstream more quickly. This process allows the nutrients to become more biologically available sooner. This is the ideal delivery system that supports and nourishes the body directly without the huge loss in biochemical conversion in the liver. In many cases, nutrients delivered by oral liquids, once they are consumed, can be found in the bloodstream in as few as 20 minutes!

Dosage for MCR: 1 tsp. in 8 oz. of water daily. It can be added to Green Drink. Use up to 4 tsp. a day if needed, 1 tsp. to every 8 oz. water. Do not refrigerate.

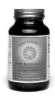

Pure Radiance C

Support your healthy immune system and overall wellbeing with this unique vitamin C. This organic whole food blend of vitamin C sources and flavonoids from around the world is as pure and potent as it gets.

Instead of being an unnaturally bright white like synthetic crystals of vitamin C, Pure Radiance C is a radiant mixture of tans, pinks, and golds. What you're seeing is a vibrant, living blend of wildcrafted camu camu, and organic amla, acerola, blueberries, raspberries, lemons, cranberries, cherries, rose hips, and sprouts—100% natural sources of vitamin C. And unlike isolated ascorbic acid powders, which have been chemically synthesized in a laboratory, Pure Radiance C provides all the well-researched, immune-supporting phytonutrients that only accompany genuine, 100% natural vitamin C.

Dosage for Pure Radiance C: *1/2 tsp. or 2 capsules daily. You may also do more if and when needed. The powder can go in Green Drink.*

The Support Package

Each supplement in the support package serves a specific purpose for assisting you during the 48 Days and can later be used as needed.

Reset!

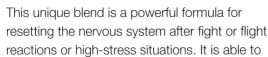

This unique blend is a powerful formula for resetting the nervous system after fight or flight reactions or high-stress situations. It is able to turn off the gnawing edge of distress or anxiety, and when taken regularly, it helps overcome the effects of long-term trauma. This unique formula is based on a synergistic blend of several relaxant herbs that won't make you drowsy, but will relieve the angst of stress and raw frayed nerve reactions in a calming way.

Excess stress results in lingering headaches, appetite loss or increase, and eventually a depressed immune system. Managing stress on a day-to-day basis can prevent many long-term effects such as high blood pressure, cholesterol, and heart disease. Stress can greatly affect our daily activities, preventing us from being fully attentive to our work and enjoying relationships and recreational activities.

For *The Transformation*, Reset! can be used to help balance blood sugar.

Dosage for Reset!: *5 sprays in mouth 3 times a day, especially at night and for sugar cravings. Take this supplement as needed throughout the 48 Days and as needed after The Transformation.*

Bio-Identical Melatonin

Melatonin occurs naturally in your body. It is produced by a small gland in the middle of your brain called the pineal gland. For most of us, the pineal gland is totally inactive during the day. But at night, when it gets dark, the pineal gland begins producing melatonin to be released into your blood. Melatonin makes you feel sleepy, less alert, and promotes and maintains sleep. Typically, in a normal night's sleep, your melatonin levels stay elevated for about 12 hours (generally between 9 p.m. and 9 a.m.). Then, as the sun rises and your day begins, your pineal gland turns "off" and the melatonin levels in your blood decrease until they are barely measurable at all.

The amount of melatonin you create and release every night varies depending on your age. Children usually have much higher levels of melatonin than adults. And as you grow older, your levels typically decrease. Researchers believe this may explain why many older adults occasionally experience disrupted sleep patterns. With less melatonin in their blood, the ability to fall asleep, stay asleep, and wake feeling rested can potentially be compromised. Indeed, that's just one of the reasons why we believe Bio-Identical Melatonin is very promising as a superior sleep supplement for people with occasional disrupted sleep patterns (e.g., the elderly, those with jet lag, and night-shift workers).

Melatonin & Detox

Bio-Identical Melatonin is nature's strongest antioxidant, offering protection against hydroxl free radicals that cause cell damage and cancer. Research shows melatonin to be 5.9 times more effective than glutathione and 11.3 times more effective than mannitol in defending against free radicals. Another study shows melatonin to be twice as good of a scavenger of the peroxyl radical than vitamin E.

The harmful effects of stress might include the development of irritable bowel syndrome, gastroesophageal reflux disease (GERD), or chronic constipation. If you already have one of these conditions, stress can make it worse. These conditions might also be exacerbated by poor eating habits that are typical during stressful times. People in challenging situations have a tendency to gain weight as well, since they don't stick to a healthy lifestyle or a daily exercise regimen as well as they should. It is not unusual for people in difficult circumstances to experience chronic pain, headaches, or difficulty sleeping.

Dosage for Bio-Identical Melatonin:
1 dropperful at bedtime. Hold under your tongue 30 seconds. Stay on this supplement the entire 48 Days and as needed after The Transformation.

Alpha Lipoic Acid

Alpha Lipoic Acid is one of the most potent antioxidants available today. It is required for the reduction of many enzyme functions for detoxification, and it is a potent free-radical scavenger itself. Without this critical substance, the body cannot produce cellular energy. Without cellular energy, natural detoxification is not possible. Alpha lipoic acid helps build a healthy liver and eliminate toxic heavy metals.

It is now known that Alpha Lipoic Acid is the only substance able to allow a cell to uptake glucose without the presence of insulin. How does this affect you? Smoother blood sugar, fewer cravings, and greater weight loss!

Dosage for Alpha Lipoic Acid: *3 capsules daily, 1 with each meal. Take this supplement through the entire 48 Days and as needed after* The Transformation.

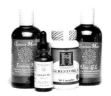

The Complete Cleansing Package

Each supplement in the cleansing package serves a specific purpose for maximizing your results during the 48 Days. You do not need to stay on these products or use them in the same way unless otherwise suggested through a wellness visit.

Lymph Care

Profound lymphatic drainage; lymphatic repair and immune boosting homeopathic.

The lymphatic system and the cardiovascular system are closely related structures and are joined by a capillary system. The lymphatic system filters out organisms that cause disease, produces certain white blood cells, and generates antibodies. It is also important for the distribution of fluids and nutrients in the body because it drains excess fluids and protein so that tissues do not swell. "Lymph" is a milky body fluid that contains a type of white blood cells, called "lymphocytes," along with proteins and fats. Lymph seeps outside the blood vessels in spaces of body tissues and is stored in the "lymphatic" system to flow back into the bloodstream.

As blood flows through arteries and into the veins or through the lymphatic system, the body eliminates the products of cellular breakdown and bacterial invasion. Lymph Care has been formulated to properly regulate lymphatic drainage while providing core nutrient support to get your body's immune system back on track!

Dosage for Lymph Care: *1 dropper 3 times a day, stay on throughout the 48 Days.*
For maximum effectiveness: Take remedy 15 minutes apart from food or anything strong in the mouth like peppermint or garlic. Hold liquid under the tongue for 30 seconds.

GI Restore X

Cleanses the bowel; releases stored acid.

GI Restore X provides results within 12 to 24 hours, helping rid the intestinal tract of excess waste, reduce bloating, increase energy, and may provide several pounds of weight loss within a few days. Included in the formula are effective natural laxatives, fiber, herbs to help soothe the intestinal lining, and acidophilus to help promote healthy bacteria levels in the intestinal tract. Added to this blend is bentonite clay, which has been used for centuries to bind and pull bacteria, metals, radiation, and harmful byproducts from the colon.

This unique formulation is designed to cleanse, nourish, and repair the colon for optimum nutrient absorption and vibrant health.

Dosage for GI Restore X: *Start on day 1. 3 capsules a day—1 with breakfast, 2 with dinner—until the bottle is finished in 30 days.*

Syndrome K

Deep kidney cleanse and emotional balance, including fear.

By increasing the potassium balance in the body and by aiding the neurogenetic regulation of the nervous system, Syndrome K balances the four main components of kidney health: the brain stem, mid-brain, neocortex, and the emotional abandonment stressors that created the strain in the kidney function leading to what is known as kidney syndrome.

This nourishing formula promotes vitality and longevity for men and women and should be used when the overall vitality is low. It reduces signs of aging and helps balance blood pressure. It includes Chinese herbs that have been used for thousands of years to heal and nurture the kidneys. Repairing the kidney function is a complicated and layered process. It must be approached using ingredients in a "multidimensional" array.

Dosage for Syndrome K: *1 tsp. daily on an empty stomach between breakfast and lunch until bottle is finished (24 days). Start on Day 1.*

Ultra GL

Deep liver and gallbladder cleanse.
Assists the liver through the 5-stage detox.

Ultra GL is guaranteed to be the most potent gallbladder/liver conditioner and detoxifier available. Ultra GL is especially useful for conditions where the liver gets stressed due to the toxicity of certain chemicals. Ultra GL also has antioxidant properties that preserve liver cell integrity when dealing with many overwhelming challenges. The liver is the largest internal organ, and it needs to function well since it is responsible for performing more than 500 different functions!

Various nutrients are required for liver detoxification to be successful. An adequate supply of key antioxidants is essential to prevent further liver damage. Milk thistle, vitamin C, selenium, beta carotene, vitamin E, and N-acetyl-cysteine (NAC) are powerful antioxidants that promote liver detoxification. Amino acids such as SAM-E, Arginine HCL, and many others play an important role in liver health. The B vitamins, including riboflavin and niacin, also aid in liver detoxification.

Dosage for Ultra GL: *Start on day 25! 2 tsp. with dinner until bottle is finished in 24 days.*

Additional Supplements

These additional products will assist you through The Transformation *and for life.*
I use many of them daily and have found great benefit from them.

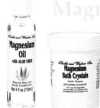

Magnesium Crystals and/or Oil

I highly recommend magnesium baths. They are an excellent way to supply the body with magnesium. They relieve back pain, muscle pain, arthritic pain, and stiffness. The Magnesium Bath Crystals are a highly concentrated, dry form of Magnesium Oil. Bathtub soaking, done 6 days a week, for 3–4 weeks, significantly raises the magnesium levels in the cells.

Anti-Stress
NATURAL VITALITY® NATURAL CALM®

A relaxing magnesium supplement The Anti-Stress Drink™

Natural Calm was developed by leading nutritional researcher Peter Gillham. Natural Calm is the only water-soluble magnesium blend utilizing Mr. Gillham's exclusive delivery formula and balanced pH, which provides superior magnesium absorption and maximum benefit.

Magnesium deficiency can be caused by a number of stresses on the body, including but not limited to: lack of adequate dietary magnesium, emotional stress, some drugs (diuretics, antibiotics, oral contraceptives, insulin, cortisone), heavy exercise, diabetes, gastrointestinal disorders and too much calcium in the diet.

Natural Calm is the solution both to restoring a healthy magnesium level and balancing your calcium intake, the result of which is natural stress relief. There are several reasons I recommend Natural Calm to patients. As a general use with *The Transformation* and for life, take 1–3 tsp. a day preferably in divided doses, especially when you have eaten out and in the evening to relax before bed.

Enzymes
FORMULA 30-P

Powdered Multiple Food Enzymes

I highly recommend taking digestive enzymes when you have to eat out and while traveling. Formula 30-P aids assimilation when enzyme-deficient food is consumed. It is also a powder formula. I recommend it in smoothies when you are using pasteurized yogurt or kefir to aid in the absorption of minerals. A powder is also a great option for children.

ASSIST FULL SPECTRUM ENZYMES

Assist Full Spectrum is a powerful, fast-acting, high potency enzyme formula. It is specially formulated to provide the widest range of useful digestive enzymes to help break down food, absorb nutrients, and prevent gas and bloating.

Olbas Oil

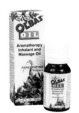

My earliest health discovery was Olbas Oil. I have been using this product and their cough syrup since my children were little. I still apply Olbas Oil to my chest, neck, and under my nose almost every night. This oil helps keep the lungs open. It is also great to use with children—but first must be mixed with a carrier oil (like coconut oil). Apply a drop or two to their nose, chest, and bottoms of feet.

Olbas Oil originated in Basel, Switzerland, over 100 years ago and continues to be a European and world-wide favorite. The essential oils are extracted from six medicinal herbs, which have for centuries been the basis of healing around the world. These oils are care-fully blended by Swiss herbalists, making the Olbas formula truly unique. The synergistic combination of these six essential oils provides amazing sensations to your body at multiple levels. Essential oils of peppermint, eucalyptus, cajeput, wintergreen, juniper, and clove.

Essential Oils

The numerous benefits of essential oils exceed the purpose of this book. They are a wonderful addition to *The Transformation*. (see Daily Routine, page 86) There are many helpful oils, but I have found Young Living Oils to be the most pure and beneficial. I have listed some of my favorites. *(Please note that I do not recommend any supplements from Young Living, but their oils are fine.)*

 LEMON OIL *(Citrus limon)* has a strong, purifying, citrus scent that is revitalizing and uplift-ing. Lemon consists of 68 percent d'limonene, a powerful antioxidant. It is delightfully refreshing in water and may be beneficial for the skin. Lemon may also be used to enhance the flavor of foods.

 PEPPERMINT OIL *(Mentha piperita)* has a strong, clean, fresh, minty aroma. It is one of the oldest and most highly regarded herbs for sooth-ing digestion, and helping restore digestive efficiency. Doctors and scientists have studied peppermint's sup-portive effect on the liver and respiratory systems and its ability to improve taste, smell, concentration, and mental sharpness. Another great benefit is peppermint's ability to directly affect the brain's satiety center—which triggers a sensation of fullness after meals. This power-ful essential oil is often diluted before topical application. Peppermint may also be used to enhance the flavor of food and water.

 VALOR® OIL is an empowering combination of therapeutic-grade essential oils that works with both the physical and spiritual aspects of the body to increase feelings of strength, courage, and self-esteem in the face of adversity. Renowned for its strengthening qualities, Valor enhances an individual's internal resources. It has also been found to help energy alignment in the body.

LAVENDER OIL *(Lavandula angustifolia)* has a fresh, sweet, floral, herbaceous aroma that is soothing and refreshing. Because it is the most versatile of all essential oils, no home should be without it. Lavender is an adaptogen, and therefore can assist the body when adapting to stress or imbalances. It is a great aid for relaxing and winding down before bed-time, yet has balancing properties that can also boost stamina and energy. Lavender is also highly regarded for skin and beauty. It may be used to soothe and cleanse common cuts, bruises, and skin irritations. Lavender may also be used to enhance the flavor of foods.

THIEVES' OIL was created based on research about four thieves in France who covered themselves with cloves, rosemary, and other aromatics while robbing plague victims. This proprietary essential oil blend was university tested for its cleansing abilities. It is highly effective in supporting the immune system and good health.

CLOVE OIL *(Syzygium aromaticum)* has a sweet, spicy fragrance that is stimulating and revitalizing. An important ingredient in our Thieves blend due to its wonderful immune-enhancing properties, its principal constituent is eugenol, which is used in the dental industry to numb the gums. Clove is the highest-scoring single ingredient ever tested for its antioxidant capacity. Always dilute for topical use. Clove may also be used to enhance the flavor of foods.

SACRED FRANKINCENSE OIL comes from the Boswellia sacra frankincense tree and is distilled at the Young Living distillery in Oman. Sacred Frankincense is ideal for those who wish to take their spiritual journey and meditation experiences to a higher level.

TRANSFORMATION™ OIL is now reformulated to include Idaho blue spruce, palo santo, and ocotea. These powerful essential oils empower you to replace negative beliefs with uplifting thoughts, which changes your overall attitude, emotions, and behavior.

Caution when using any essential oil:

Be sure to read the directions on each bottle. Some essential oils can cause skin sensitivity. If pregnant or under a doctor's care, be sure to consult your physician. Dilution is recommended for both topical and internal use. Do not apply directly to a fresh wound or burn. Dilute before using on sensitive areas such as the face, neck, genital area, etc. Keep out of reach of children. Avoid using on infants and very small children unless suggested by your healthcare provider.

I am often asked what I use on my skin. Our skin is our largest organ and must be nourished and protected. Any products we use quickly penetrate into our body. We do not want to put anything on the skin that we wouldn't be willing to eat. This eliminates almost all skin care and personal care products, even those in health-food stores.

Quickly after the start of my journey to eating and living naturally, I no longer had to wear a foundation on my face. After applying these principles, you will see an amazing improvement in your skin as well. The personal care products I have listed below are the ones I have faithfully used for many years.

You can purchase most of these products through the Energetic Wellness store. We can ship all items except the coconut oil. If you are not local to EW, you can purchase Tropical Traditions Coconut oil from www.tropicaltraditions.com.

Makeup & Nail Polish

Searching for organic makeup has been a challenge. Through the years, I have tried many different brands of eye makeup and lipstick. Most recently I have found a wonderful mascara called Mineral Fusion, a volumizing mascara that really works, a lip liner by Gabriel Cosmetics, and lipstick by Honeybee Gardens.

The key to finding truly natural cosmetics is looking for products free of paraben, FD&C colors and petrochemicals. This would include non-petroleum, nontoxic, chemical-free (such as formaldehyde) products. Most natural cosmetic companies offer nontoxic nail polish. I bring my nail polish with me if I go to a salon. Most health-food stores have a good selection. Do your research first before purchasing—it will save you time and money.

Nature's Plus Natural Beauty Cleansing Bar

The natural beauty bar works for my face, body, and hair—yes, I use it as my shampoo! Natural Beauty Cleansing Bar is absolutely free of soap and the harsh, irritating ingredients found in soap, such as caustic soda, lye, tallow, hexachlorophene, and alkalis. It is a unique cleanser made from natural, organic ingredients. Humectants and emollients are used to help maintain the skin's delicate moisture balance and to soothe irritated skin. They are combined with 500 IU of vitamin E and the special astringent and healing qualities of allantoin. This specially formulated cleanser is in a mildly acidic base (4.5 pH) to help maintain the body's normal acid mantle.

Coconut Oils

According to Dr. Bruce Fife of the Coconut Research Center, "One of the oldest uses for coconut oil is as a sunscreen/suntan lotion. Islanders have been using coconut oil for this purpose for thousands of years. In the tropics where the climate is hot, islanders traditionally wore little clothing so that they could keep themselves cool. To protect themselves from the burning rays of the hot tropical sun, they applied a thin layer of coconut oil over their entire body. This would protect them from sunburn, improve skin tone, and help keep annoying insects away. Coconut oil was applied on the skin daily. When a mother gave birth, one of the first things she would do is to rub coconut oil all over her newborn. Every day coconut oil would be used on the skin. As the children got older, they applied the oil themselves. They would continue this practice throughout their lifetime up until the day they died. Many islanders, even today, carry on this practice."

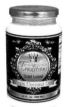

Tropical Traditions
Gold Label® Virgin Coconut Oil

Not only can you use virgin coconut oil for cooking, but it is an amazing lotion. I apply it from head to toe after a shower and use it as my daytime face moisturizer. If you apply it lightly, it will absorb into the skin and not appear greasy. It is also what I use to sunbathe (see Sunshine section, page 60).

Tropical Traditions Gold Label™ Virgin Coconut Oil is an unrefined coconut oil. Organic coconuts are used within 24–48 hours of harvest. They originate from small, family farms on Mt. Banahaw and other rural places in Quezon Province, the coconut capital of the Philippines. Only the highest quality coconuts are hand-picked from each harvest. The volcanic soil of Mt. Banahaw makes these organic coconuts some of the most nutritionally rich coconuts in the world.

Expeller-Pressed Coconut Oils

I apply the Tropical Traditions virgin coconut oil to my skin and use the expeller-pressed coconut oil in my cooking when I don't want the dish to have a coconut flavor. Tropical Traditions Expeller-Pressed Coconut Oil is a high-quality refined coconut oil. This oil is processed the *old* way by physical refining. The modern way of processing coconut oil is chemical extraction—using solvent extracts, which produces higher yields and is quicker and less expensive. Tropical Traditions Expeller-Pressed Coconut Oil *does not* use solvent extracts. It is made the *old* way by an expeller-pressed mechanical extraction. This oil is also *not* hydrogenated and contains *no* trans fatty acids. It is a very good quality food-grade coconut oil.

Tropical Traditions Organic Expeller-Pressed Coconut Oil is made from certified organic coconuts that have *not* been treated with chemicals or fertilizers. It is certified organic according to European and USDA standards. It is high in the medium-chain fatty acids, such as lauric acid. Organic Expeller-Pressed Coconut Oil goes through a steam deodorizing process which makes the taste very bland, unlike Virgin Coconut Oil which retains the odor and taste of fresh coconuts. Some people prefer a bland, tasteless oil. This coconut oil is solid below 76°F, and liquid above that.

Tropical Traditions Expeller-Pressed Coconut Oil, non-certified, is a 100% pure coconut oil made from high quality coconuts in the Philippines. This is the *common* type of oil that millions of people in Asia consume on a daily basis. The Expeller-Pressed Coconut Oil, non-certified, is shipped in from unpolluted areas of the Philippines where pesticides and fertilizers for coconut palms are virtually unknown. The coconuts typically come from very rural areas in the Philippines, far away from major urban centers.

Tropical Traditions Lavender Moisturizing Lotion & Baby Silk Moisturizing Lotion

My husband uses these lotions—they are fabulous! Tropical Traditions Moisturizing Lotions soothe the skin without harming the body.

Tropical Traditions Coconut Oil Deodorants

We use this deodorant and have been very happy with it. Tropical Traditions Coconut Oil Deodorants are chemical-free, paraben-free, and aluminum-free deodorant roll-ons made from the organic Gold Label Virgin Coconut Oil as their base. Your underarms are one of the most sensitive and absorbent areas of your body, so don't put harmful chemicals into your body through antiperspirants or harmful deodorants!

Climb On! Creme

This creme is my favorite nighttime moisturizer. Each night after I take my makeup off, I rinse my face with a warm wash cloth and liberally apply Climb On! to my chest, neck, and face. We say, "If you can't eat it, don't put it on your skin." Climb On! Creme is 100% pure and free from any fillers or synthetics. Only food-grade base ingredients and therapeutic-grade essential oils are used. Climb On! Creme is one of the most fabulous, multipurpose products on this planet. It is a deep moisturizer and acts like food for your skin.

Climb On! Lip Tube

This minty balm is made from peppermint essential oil which cools and soothes your lips. The aromatherapeutic value is one that stimulates the mind and focuses concentration. It can be used to moisturize skin after sun exposure, for wind-burned cheeks, dry cuticles, or tissue nose. And it is great for mosquito bites—just a dab and the itchiness seems to disappear. *(Of course, this statement has not been evaluated by the FDA.)* Use it under lipstick to prolong your color. Rub it on your temples if you have a headache. The smell of peppermint essential oil is said to stimulate and refresh.

SPF 30 Mineral Sunscreen

ClimbOn! sunscreen is good enough for humans, the environment, and animals. The FDA-approved sunscreen agent in this product is the non-nano zinc oxide. However, every ingredient used in this formulation is considered a sunscreen. One ingredient, Red Raspberry Seed oil (Rubus idaeus) is known to contain a high level of EFAs (essential fatty acids) which research shows to be connected with reduction of the effects of oxidative stress in the body. It also exhibits anti-inflammatory properties. It may also act as a broad-spectrum UVA and UVB shield.

If you are going to be out in the sun all day and feel the need to use sunscreen, this is the only one that I personally recommend. You can also use a combination of coconut oil and Climb On! Crème to give you an SPF of about 6–8.

Alba Botanica™ Un-Petroleum Multi-Purpose Jelly

The Un-Petroleum Jelly was a wonderful find when I was looking to replace Vaseline to remove eye makeup. Beeswax, moisture-rich coconut oil, and soothing, protective vitamin E, makes this natural, non-petroleum jelly perfect as an all-over body moisturizer to soothe skin and protect against irritation.

Body Brush

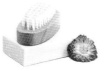

A body brush is an awesome tool for taking care of your skin and assisting the lymph to move impurities out of your body. Blood circulates through your body by the heart's pumping. As impurities are purged, they are deposited into the lymph; the layer just under your skin. The lymph, itself, has no internal pump to move waste out of your system (as perspiration) and is only stimulated by exercise and brushing. Lumps and hard knots in your groin or underarm areas are sometimes just

impurities that have not made their way out of your system. Daily skin brushing also helps rejuvenate the nervous system, combat cellulite by visibly improving the skin's texture, and sweep away dead skin cells. The gentle sweeping of the brush actually renews your cells! Find a good quality brush—many health-food stores sell them. Brush upwards from the soles of your feet to your groin and inward from your palms to your underarms. Avoid sensitive areas.

Cleaning Products

In my quest for natural cleaning products, there are two companies that have stood the test of time and have products that really work. Happy cleaning!

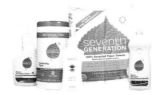

Seventh Generation

I use the Seventh Generation laundry detergent and many of their cleaning products in my home. Established in 1988, this company offers a complete line of natural household products designed to work as well as their traditional counterparts, but use renewable, nontoxic, phosphate-free, and biodegradable ingredients as often as possible, and are never tested on animals.

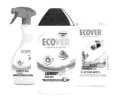

Ecover

Ecover is also a great company; I use several of their cleaning products, including a great liquid, non-abrasive scrub for sinks and tubs. The company is over 30 years old, which means they have had time to refine their products to produce refreshingly safe and effective cleaners for every corner of your home.

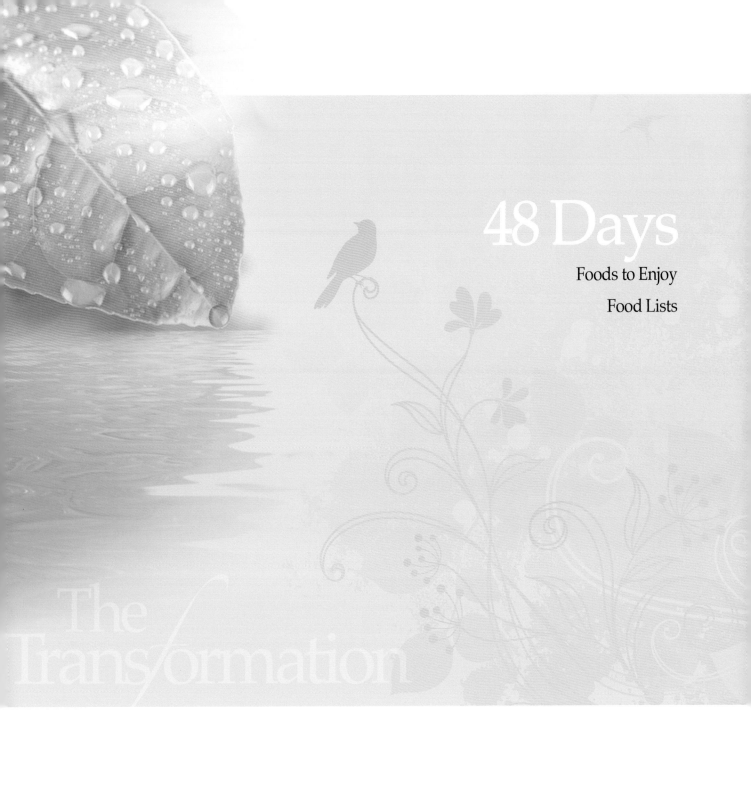

48 Days

Foods to Enjoy

Food Lists

The Transformation

Watch Portion Sizes

A good rule of thumb, one serving equals:

- Palm-sized portion of meat, fish, or poultry
- 1 1/2 ounces of cheddar cheese
- 1 cup yogurt or milk
- 1/2 cup berries
- 1/2 grapefruit or mango
- One small baked potato

- 1/2 cup of mashed potatoes
- 1/2 cup of cooked rice or pasta
- One slice of whole-grain bread
- One small pancake
- Two medium-sized cookies
- As many raw and cooked vegetables as desired with lots of butter!

At Home

- Use smaller dishes at meals.
- Try not to eat after 6 p.m. Eat your bigger protein meal at lunchtime or midafternoon.
- Serve food in the appropriate portion amounts, and don't go back for seconds.
- Put away leftovers in a separate container for tomorrow.
- Don't keep platters of food on the table. You are more likely to "pick" or have seconds.
- Periodic fasting—you don't always have to eat three meals a day.

At Restaurants

- Ask for half or smaller portions.
- Choose wild fish, brown rice, and a salad or vegetable side.
- Choose to go vegetarian if you know the meat is not grass-fed or the chicken is not free-range, and free of hormones and antibiotics.
- Avoid soy and canola oils and olive oil blends. Ask for pure olive oil or butter.
- Avoid sauces with sugar, and avoid food high in salt.
- See The Benefits of Nutrient-Dense Foods section on page 184 for an extended list of eating-out tips.

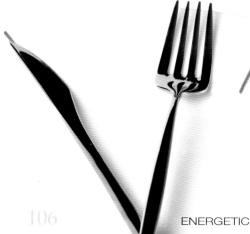

The Transformation

God created many diverse foods for us to enjoy—and we'll eventually get to all of them. But for now, we need to help our bodies overcome some of the effects of our previous diet and lifestyle. I recommend that the 48 Days be completed twice a year. Living on the Foods for Life will help you maintain optimum health.

In Stage 1, , we help the body undergo detoxification during days 1–15. The particular foods eaten and supplements taken help a healthy cleansing to occur. Though more limited than what we may be accustomed to, there are many foods to enjoy in this stage, and we provide menu suggestions and recipes to help you make the adjustment. This stage is very important.

For Stage 2, Transformation, days 16–30, remain on Stage 1 foods and introduce the Stage 2 foods to enjoy. These two weeks are when the body really responds to the healthy choices you're making. Pay attention, listen, and learn. Enjoy the process!

During Stage 3, Lifestyle, days 31–48, you learn to eat in a way that nourishes the body with whole foods. Your new way of eating includes the right fats, raw milk, grass-fed meats, organic fruits and vegetables, and sprouted grains. The pathway to a lifetime of nutritious eating lies ahead of you.

Let's begin to enjoy foods the way nature intended.

Foods for Life

Food Category

Eat from this column on Days 1–15.

Meat
Grass-fed, organic, fresh or frozen

Parentheses (...) indicate
a recommended brand.

Bacon
Beef
Beef or buffalo
  sausage—
   no sugar
Bone broth
Bone marrow

Bratwurst
Buffalo
Elk
Goat
Hot dogs—
  nitrite/nitrate
  & sugar-free

Lamb
Liverwurst
Organ meat—
  liver, heart, etc.
Pork
Venison
Veal

Fish
Wild freshwater or ocean-caught,
fresh or frozen

Cod
Fish broth
Grouper
Haddock
Halibut
Herring
Mackerel
Mahi mahi
Orange roughy
Pompano

Salmon
Salmon—*canned*
  in spring water
Sardines—*canned in*
  water or olive oil
Scrod
Sea bass
Shellfish
Snapper
Sole

Tilapia
Trout
Tuna
Tuna—*canned in*
  spring water or
  olive oil;
  (Crown Prince
  or Tonnino)
Wahoo
Whitefish

Poultry
Pastured, free-range
organic/non-GMO, fresh or frozen

Chicken
Chicken or turkey bacon—
  nitrite/nitrate free
Chicken or turkey sausage
  or hot dogs—*nitrite/nitrate*
  & sugar-free

Cornish game hen
Duck
Guinea fowl
Liver & heart
Poultry bone broth
Turkey

Eggs
Farm fresh, free-range,
organic/non-GMO

Chicken eggs—
  whole with yolk
Duck eggs—
  whole with yolk

Fish roe or caviar—*fresh,*
  not preserved

Luncheon Meat
Organic, free-range,
nitrite- & preservative-free

STAGE
2 Transformation
Eat from Stage 1 & 2 on days 16–30.

STAGE
3 Lifestyle
Eat from all the stages on days 31–48.

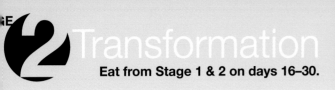
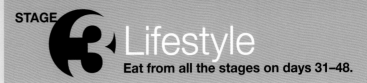

Why Grass-Fed Beef?

Have you ever taken a juicy bite of a freshly cooked piece of grass-fed beef? There is an incredible difference between grass-fed beef and beef that is fed grains and hormones. Not only is grass-fed beef the natural way to go, but it has reduced fat, more omega-3 fatty acids, no harmful additives, conjugated linoleic acid (which lowers the risk of cancer and clogged arteries), and it tastes so much better! Beef that is not grass-fed is higher in saturated fats and greases that become harmful. It can also lead to diseases such as arteriosclerosis (clogged arteries), diabetes, and so on. When cows live according to their design, their products are better for you. Make the healthy choice: Grass-fed beef is the way meat was intended!

Why No GMOs?

GMOs—or genetically modified organisms—are present in over 75% of all processed foods in stores across the country—94% of soy products and 75% of corn products. Genetically modified organisms have had specific changes introduced into their DNA by genetic engineering techniques. Many natural health-food brands are using GMOs in their so-called "natural" products.

Chicken
Roast Beef
Turkey

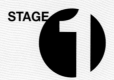

Dairy

Whole, raw, grass-fed, organic/non-GMO, no additions

When using pasteurized yogurt and kefir, I recommend you add enzyme powder to absorb minerals.

Cheese—*hard, goat milk*
Cheese—*hard, sheep milk*
Kefir—*goat milk*
  bought or homemade
  from grass-fed raw milk
Milk—*raw, goat*
Milk—*coconut*

Protein Powders—
  (Essential Living Whey)
Yogurt—*goat milk, plain,*
  bought or homemade
  from grass-fed raw milk
(Redwood Hill Farm goat
yogurt and kefir—only acceptable store-bought brand)

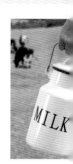

Vegetables

Organic, biodynamic, locally grown and in season, fresh or frozen

Artichokes
Asparagus
Beets
Broccoli rabe
Brussel sprouts*
Cabbage*
Carrots
Cauliflower*
Celery
Cucumber
Eggplant
Garlic

Leafy greens—*cooked*
  kale*, collard, endive,
  mustard greens, escarole
Leafy greens—*raw*
  radicchio, arugula,
  frisse, etc.
Lettuce leaf—*all kinds*
Mushrooms
Okra
Onion
Peas
Peppers

Pumpkin
Spinach*
Sprouts–
  broccoli,
  sunflower,
  pea shoots,
  radish, etc.
Squash
String beans
Tomatoes

Sea vegetables—kelp, dulse, nori, kombu, hijiki
Raw, fermented vegetables**—*lacto-fermented only, no vinegar*

*These cruciferous vegetables have a high level of oxalic acid and should be sautéed lightly in butter or coconut oil to neutralize and bring out the best nutrients for absorption.

**Refer to Nourishing Traditions Cookbook *listed in "Recommended Books" for fermenting recipes, including carrots, cabbage, onions, cucumbers, garlic, beets, daikon radish, turnips, red peppers, etc.*

Fruits

Organic, locally grown, fresh or fozen
Limit to 2–3 servings a day.

Blackberries
Blueberries
Cherries
Coconut—*unsweetened*
Coconut wraps

Grapefruit
Lemon
Lime
Pineapple
Raspberries
Strawberries

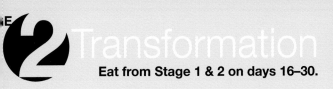

2 Transformation

Eat from Stage 1 & 2 on days 16–30.

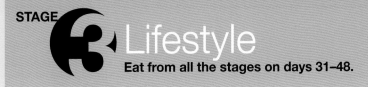

STAGE 3 Lifestyle

Eat from all the stages on days 31–48.

Goat milk feta cheese
Goat milk soft cheese

Milk—*raw, cow*

Products from cow milk
Cheeses—*hard, raw*
Cottage cheese
Cream
Feta cheese

Kefir—*cow milk, plain
bought or homemade
from grass-fed raw milk*
Ricotta cheese
Sour cream—*plain*
Yogurt—*cow milk, plain,
bought or homemade
from grass-fed raw milk*

Sweet potatoes
Yams

Corn—*organic only*
Corn tortillas—*sprouted, organic only*
Red potatoes

Why Organic Fruits & Vegetables?

Organic produce has higher levels of beneficial minerals like iron and zinc!

Organic fruits and vegetables contain up to 40% more antioxidants!

It is important to read the labels of all produce!
You do not want to buy genetically modified (GM) produce
with the 5-digit code "84011." Most GM food is not labeled.
Conventionally grown produce carries a 4-digit code: "4011"
and organic produce carries a 5-digit code: "94011."

Apples
Apricots
Grapes
Guava
Kiwi
Melon
Nectarines

Oranges
Passion fruit
Peaches
Pears
Plums
Pomegranates

Banana
Mango
Papaya—*organic only*
Canned fruit—*in its own juices, sparingly*
Dried fruit—*no sugar or sulfates: raisins, figs, dates, prunes
pineapple, papaya, peaches, and apples—sparingly*

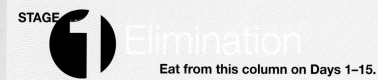

Foods for Life

Food Category

STAGE 1 Elimination

Eat from this column on Days 1–15.

Beans & Legumes
Organic, soaked or fermented

Miso—*fermented soybean paste, as a broth*
Lentils

Nuts & Seeds
Organic, raw, soaked & dried

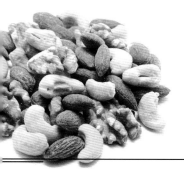

Raw Nuts & Seeds
Almonds
Coconut
Flaxseed—*ground*
Pumpkin seeds
Sunflower seeds

Raw Butters—
preferably sprouted
Almond butter
Pumpkin seed butter
Sunflower seed butter
Tahini / sesame seed butter

Fats & Oils
Organic & grass-fed

Avocado—*fresh, homemade guacamole;* (Wholly Guacamole)
Butter—*cow milk, raw, grass-fed, bought or homemade* (Kalona or Organic Valley)
Butter—*goat milk, raw bought or homemade*
Coconut milk or cream—*fresh or canned*

Coconut oil—*extra-virgin or expeller pressed*
Ghee
Lard
Olive oil—*extra virgin. Do not heat. Great for salad dressings.*
Palm oil—*virgin, red*
Sesame oil—*expeller cold-pressed*
Tallow

Condiments, Spices & Seasoning
Organic

Flavoring extracts— vanilla, almond, etc. *alcohol based, no sugar added*
Ginger—*pickled preservative- & color-free*
Guacamole—*homemade or bought* (Wholly Guacamole)
Herbamare seasoning
Herbs & spices—*no stabilizers*
Mayo (Wilderness Family)

Miso
Salad dressing & marinade— *raw & homemade*
Salsa—*fresh*
Salt (Celtic Sea Salt or Redmond Real Salt)
Umeboshi paste
Vinegar—*balsamic & apple cider*
Wasabi— *preservative- & color-free*

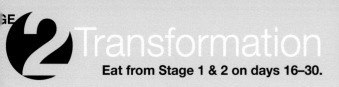

STAGE 2 Transformation

Eat from Stage 1 & 2 on days 16–30.

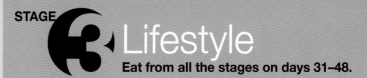

STAGE 3 Lifestyle

Eat from all the stages on days 31–48.

Black beans	Navy beans	Black-eyed peas	Garbanzo beans
Kidney beans	Tempeh	Broad beans	Lima beans
Mung beans	White beans	Edamame—	Pinto beans
		in small amounts,	Red beans
		only if non-GMO	Split peas

Brazil nuts	Use these commercial nuts sparingly
Cashews	if not prepared correctly by soaking and drying.
Hazelnuts	
Macadamia nuts	**Dry Roasted** / **Butters, Roasted**
Pecans	
Walnuts	

Dry Roasted
Almonds
Cashews
Macadamia nuts
Peanuts—*organic only*
Pecans
Pumpkin seeds
Sunflower seeds
Walnuts

Butters, Roasted
Almond butter
Cashew butter
Peanut butter—*organic, no sugar added*
Pumpkin seed butter
Sunflower butter
Tahini

Peanut oil—*expeller-pressed, in small amounts*

Cold-pressed, in small amounts
Flaxseed oil—*do not heat.* Sesame oil
Macadamia oil Sunflower oil
Safflower oil

Fat does not cause us to be fat.

In fact, fat enhances our ability to lose weight by balancing our metabolism.

Ketchup—*no sugar*
Salad dressings—*all natural, no sugar, no preservatives**
Marinades—*all natural, no preservatives**

*Be aware that so-called "all natural" salad dressings and marinades most likely contain soybean or canola oil which, if not organic, will be GMO.

Mustard
Soy sauce—*wheat-free, Tamari*
Tomato sauce—*no added sugar*

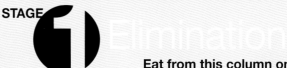

Beverages
Raw, organic, mineral-rich

Almond milk—*homemade*
Coconut water
Coffee—*Organic only. Freeze whole beans. Grind.*
  Flavor with acceptable dairy & sweetener for stages 1–3.
Green tea
Herbal teas—*unsweetened or with a little honey*
  or with acceptable sweeteners for stages 1–3
Kombucha—*homemade with acceptable natural sweeteners*
  or store-bought (Synergy)
Lacto-fermented beverages
Lemonade—*homemade*
Water—*natural spring water, reverse osmosis, nonchlorinated, no carbona*

Sweeteners
Organic, natural, local

Honey—*unheated, raw, 1 Tbsp./day*

Grains
Organic whole grain
Soaked, sprouted, or naturally fermented

Breads, Cereals & Pasta
Sprouted, naturally fermented, or sourdough

Why Sprouted Grains?

Why should you use sprouted grains?

Sprouting breaks down the starches in grains into simple sugars so your body can digest them like a vegetable (like a tomato, not a potato).

Not only does the sprouting process break down the starches, but it also produces vitamin C, increases the vitamin B content (B2, B5, and B6), and increases carotene up to eight times. Enzymes are also produced during sprouting, and sprouting neutralizes enzyme inhibitors and phytic acid.

Snacks
Limit desserts to a couple of times a week.

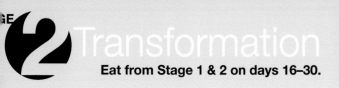
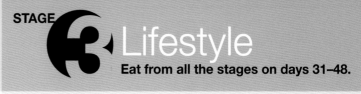
Beer—*organic*
Black tea—*organic*
Wine—*organic, preferably red*

Coconut sugar or nectar	Maple sugar or syrup
Date sugar	Whole cane sugar (Rapunzel)

Amaranth	Millet	Rye
Barley	Oats	Spelt
Einkorn	Quinoa	Teff
Kamut	Rice—*brown*	

(Phytic acid inhibits absorption of calcium, magnesium, iron, copper, and zinc.) Stay away from flours that break down into sugars and are heavy with starch. Take the sprouted route and keep those arteries clean!

Breads—*using acceptable grains from list above, sprouted, whole-grain sourdough or naturally fermented, bought or homemade*	Cereal—*sprouted or soaked* Granola—*sprouted or soaked* Pasta—whole grain einkorn, spelt, millet, quinoa or brown rice Tortillas—*sprouted*

Cacao—*raw powder* Cocoa & carob powders Desserts—*homemade*	Ice Cream—*homemade* Trail mix—*homemade* Zesty popcorn

Look for more snack options under "Occasional Healthy Foods" for after the 48 Days, page 122.

Pantry Transformation

This is by no means an exhaustive list.

When stocking your kitchen, think pure, whole food.
I have no boxed or prepared food or canned vegetables.
The only canned goods I recommend are organic
tomatoes—although an even better choice is to jar
your own garden tomatoes.

Refrigerator/Freezer Transformation

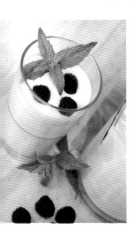

Refrigerated Produce
Fresh, in-season vegetables
Fresh, in-season fruit
Raw dairy products
Eggs
Raw beverages
Condiments

Freezer
Grass-fed meat
Pastured pork
Organ meats
Pastured, organic chickens
Freshwater and wild-caught fish
Homemade bone broths
Bones and feet for stock

Pantry Transformation

Fresh Pantry Produce
Garlic
Red potatoes
Sweet potatoes
Onions—*white, red*

Oils
Organic extra virgin olive oil
Virgin coconut oil
Expeller-pressed coconut oil
Assorted nut and seed oils

Dry Goods
*Tip: Always buy organic beans, grains, & nuts,
and store in glass jars.*
Dry beans
Grains & sprouted grains
Popcorn
Nuts—*raw*

Canned and Jar Goods
Capers
Coconut milk
Coconut cream
Black olives (non-GMO)
Tomatoes—*canned, homemade, or bought*
Tuna—*canned*
Salmon—*canned*
Whey protein (Essential Living)
Whole food supplements

Baking Cabinet

Flavor Extracts & Essential Oils
Anise
Lemon
Orange
Vanilla

Young Living Essential Oils
Oregano
Thyme
Orange
Lavender
Lemon

Natural Sugars

Coconut sugar
Coconut nectar
Date sugar
Honey—*raw, local*
Maple sugar
Maple syrup
Whole cane sugar (Rapunzel)

Baking Powders

Organic cacao powder
Organic cocoa powder
Organic carob powder
Organic maca powder
Rumford Aluminum-Free Baking Powder

Spice Cabinet

Tip: Buy organic herbs in bulk and store in mason jars, or grow your own.

Basil
Celery seed
Chili powder
Cinnamon
Chicken grilling seasoning (Simply Organic)
Cloves
Coriander
Cumin
Curry
Dill
Fennel
Garlic—*granulated*
Ginger
Herbamare
Italian seasoning
Marjoram
Nutmeg
Oregano
Parsley
Paprika

Peppercorns—*black, white*
Poultry seasoning
Salt (Redmond Real)
Red pepper—*crushed*
Rosemary
Sage
Thyme
Turmeric

Kitchen Equipment

Whisks
Spatulas
Large mixing spoons
Measuring cups
Measuring spoons
Knives—*serrated, straight edge*
Knife sharpener
Meat thermometer
Hand juicer
Hand mixer
Mixing bowls—*glass, stainless steel*
Strainer
Sifter
Colander
Lettuce spinner
Food processor
Blender (Vitamix)
Chopper
Dehydrator (Excalibur)
George Foreman Grill
Grain mill
Bread mixer
Pans and stock pots—*stainless steel*
Storage containers—*glass*
Cooling racks
Muffin papers—*regular, mini*
Muffin pans—*stainless steel*
Cookie sheets—*stainless steel*
Cake pans—*stainless steel*

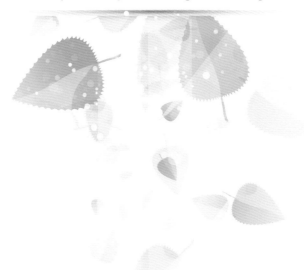

Congratulations!

You made it through the 48 Days!

You are well on your way to eating and living naturally for life!

On the following pages are the lists of
- **Foods for Life,**
- **Occasional Healthy Foods,** and the
- **Foods to Avoid for Life.**

They are your food guides as you continue your wellness journey.

. . . .

Nourish your body with the Foods for Life, moderate your consumption of the Occasional Healthy Foods, and stay away from Foods to Avoid for Life!

Foods for Life

*The following food list includes all of the foods from Stage and — the most nutrient-dense foods available — **organic, grass-fed, non-GMO and prepared correctly.** Parentheses (...) indicates a recommended brand. Enjoy these foods on a daily basis to support the body for life.*

Meat

Grass-fed & organic, fresh or frozen

Bacon
Beef
Beef or buffalo sausage—
  no sugar
Bone broth
Bone marrow
Bratwurst
Buffalo
Elk
Goat
Hot Dogs—*nitrite-, nitrate- & sugar-free*
Lamb
Liverwurst
Organ meats—*liver, heart, etc.*
Pork
Venison
Veal

Fish

Wild freshwater or ocean-caught, fresh or frozen

Cod
Fish bone broth
Grouper
Haddock
Halibut
Herring
Mackerel
Mahi mahi

Orange roughy
Pompano
Salmon
Salmon—*canned in spring water*
Sardines—*canned in water or olive oil*
Scrod
Sea bass
Shellfish
Snapper
Sole
Tilapia
Trout
Tuna
Tuna—*canned in spring water or olive oil* (Crown Prince & Tonnino)
Wahoo
Whitefish

Poultry

Pastured, free-range, organic/non-GMO, fresh or frozen

Chicken
Chicken or turkey bacon—*nitrite-, nitrate- & sugar-free*
Chicken or turkey sausage or hot dogs—*nitrite-, nitrate- & sugar-free*
Cornish game hen
Duck
Guinea fowl

Liver & heart
Poultry bone broth
Turkey

Luncheon Meat

Organic, free-range Nitrite- & preservative-free

Chicken
Roast beef
Turkey

Fats & Oils

Organic, grass-fed, unrefined

Butter—*goat milk, raw or bought*
Butter—*cow milk, raw or bought* (Kalona or Organic Valley)
Coconut milk/cream—*fresh or canned*
Coconut oil—*extra-virgin or expeller-pressed*
Ghee
Lard
Olive oil—*extra-virgin*
Palm oil—*virgin, red*
Tallow

Eggs

Farm fresh, free-range, organic/non-GMO

Chicken eggs—*whole with yolk*
Duck eggs—*whole with yolk*
Fish roe or caviar—*fresh, not preserved*

Dairy

Whole, raw, grass-fed, organic/non-GMO, no additions

Coconut milk

Cow milk products:
- cheese—*hard*
- cottage cheese
- cream
- feta cheese
- kefir—*plain, homemade or bought**
- milk
- ricotta cheese
- sour cream
- yogurt—*plain, whole milk homemade or bought**

Goat milk products:
- cheese—*hard*
- cheese—*soft*
- feta cheese
- kefir—*plain homemade or bought** (Redwood Hill Farm)

- milk
- yogurt—*plain homemade or bought** (Redwood Hill Farm)

Protein Powders— *grass-fed* (Essential Living Whey)

Sheep milk hard cheese

When using pasteurized yogurt or kefir, add enzyme powder to help your body absorb minerals.

Vegetables
Organic, biodynamic, local and in season, fresh or frozen

Artichokes
Asparagus
Avocado
Beets
Broccoli rabe
Brussel sprouts
Cabbage
Carrots
Cauliflower
Celery
Corn—*only organic*
Cucumber
Eggplant
Garlic
Leafy greens—*cooked* kale, collard, endive, mustard greens, escarole
Leafy greens—*raw* radicchio, arugula, frisse, etc.
Lettuce leaf—*all kinds*

Mushrooms
Okra
Onion
Peas
Peppers
Potatoes, red
Pumpkin
Raw, lacto-fermented vegetables
Sea vegetables— kelp, dulse, nori, kombu, hijiki
Spinach
Sprouts—broccoli, sunflower, pea shoots, radish, etc.
Squash
String beans
Sweet potatoes
Tomatoes
Yams

Fruits
Organic and/or locally grown— fresh or fozen
Limit to 2–3 servings/day

Apples
Apricots
Banana
Blackberries
Blueberries
Cherries
Coconut—*unsweetened*
Coconut wraps
Grapefruit
Grapes
Guava
Kiwi

Lemon
Lime
Mango
Melon
Nectarines
Oranges
Papaya—*only organic*
Passion Fruit
Peaches
Pears
Pineapple
Plums
Pomegranates
Raspberries
Strawberries

Beans & Legumes
Organic, soaked or fermented

Black beans
Black-eyed peas
Broad beans
Edamame— *in small amounts, only if non-GMO*
Garbanzo beans
Kidney beans
Lentils
Lima beans
Miso
Navy beans
Pinto beans
Red beans
Split peas
Tempeh
White beans

Nuts & Seeds
Organic, raw, soaked & dried

Almonds
Brazil nuts
Cashews
Coconut
Flaxseed (ground)
Hazelnuts
Macadamia nuts
Pecans
Pumpkin seeds
Sunflower seeds
Walnuts

Almond butter
Pumpkin seed butter
Sunflower seed butter
Tahini / sesame seed

Condiments, Spices & Seasoning

Organic, unrefined, non-irradiated

Flavoring extracts—
vanilla, almond, etc.
organic, alcohol-based, no sugar added
Ginger, pickled—*color- and preservative-free*
Guacamole—*homemade or bought*
(Wholly Guacamole)
Herbamare seasoning
Herbs & spices—
no added stabilizers
Ketchup—*homemade or bought, no sugar*
Mayonnaise—*homemade or bought, no sugar*
(Wilderness Family)
Miso
Mustard
Salad dressings
& marinades—*raw, homemade*
Salsa—*fresh, homemade or bought, no sugar*
Salt (Celtic Sea Salt & Redmond Real Salt)
Soy sauce—*wheat-free*
Tamari
Tomato sauce—*no sugar*
Umeboshi paste
Vinegar—*balsamic & apple cider*
Wasabi—*color- and preservative-free*

Beverages

Raw, organic, mineral-rich

Water— *natural spring water, reverse-osmosis, nonchlorinated, no carbonation*
Almond milk—*homemade*
Beer—*organic only*
Beet Kvass
Black tea
Coconut water
Coffee—*organic only*
Green tea
Herbal teas—*sweeten with acceptable sweeteners*
Kombucha (Synergy)
Lacto-fermented beverages
Lemonade—*homemade*
Wine—*organic only, preferably red*

Sweeteners

Organic, natural, local

Coconut nectar
Coconut sugar
Date sugar
Green stevia leaves
Green stevia powder
Honey—*unheated, raw*
Maple sugar
Maple syrup
Palm sugar
Sorghum syrup
Whole cane sugar
(Rapunzel)

Grains

Organic whole grain, soaked, sprouted, or naturally fermented

Amaranth
Barley
Einkorn
Kamut
Millet
Oats
Quinoa
Rice—*brown, wild*
Rye
Spelt
Teff

Bread & Baked Goods

Use acceptable grains from grain list.

Bread—*sprouted, sourdough or naturally fermented, homemade or bought*
Cereal/Granola—
sprouted or soaked, homemade or bought
Pasta—*whole grain*
Brown rice
Einkorn
Millet
Quinoa
Spelt
Tortillas—*sprouted*
corn, spelt

Snacks

Organic and prepared correctly using acceptable flours, nuts, and sweeteners. Limit desserts to a couple of times per week.

Cacao—*raw or raw powder*
Cocoa & carob powder
Crispy nuts
Desserts—*homemade*
Ice Cream—*homemade*
Popcorn—*organic only, no microwave*
Trail mix—*homemade*

Occasional Healthy Foods

*After the 48 Days, these are healthy, **non-organic** "whole" conventional food options. When consuming these foods, use digestive enzymes and take probiotics. These foods should be consumed in moderation. Remember, non-organic foods carry a toxic load of pesticides, herbicides, hormones, antibiotics, and are possibly genetically modified (GMO).*

Meats & Proteins
Organic or naturally raised

Canned broth or stock—
  without additives
  (Amy's soups, except
  chicken noodle)
Deli meats—*organic
  free-range, antibiotic-
  and hormone-free
  with no nitrates,*
  (Applegate Farms)
Eggs—*cage-free,
  non-organic*
Meat & deli meat—
  conventional
Salmon—*canned
  in spring water*
Tofu
Tuna—*low-sodium,
  canned in spring water
  or olive oil*

Dairy
*Whole, full-fat pasteurized,
non-homogenized*

Cheese—*hard
  goat milk;
  cheddar, Swiss,
  havarty, colby*
Cottage cheese—
  *dry-curd, goat milk
  or cow milk*
Cow milk—*vat-pasteurized*
  (Kalona Supernatural)
Cow milk - *pasteurized,
  non-homogenized*
  (Organic Valley
  Grass-fed/whole)
Cream—*cow milk*
Cream cheese
Sour cream
Yogurt or kefir—
  *pasteurized, cultured,
  from whole goat milk*
Yogurt or kefir—*plain,
  pasteurized, cultured,
  from cow milk*

Vegetables
*Fresh, in season, use
fruit and vegetable wash,
or frozen*

Lacto-fermented
  vegetables
Tomato products—
  *canned in BPA-free
  container*
All vegetables—
  *organic, canned in
  BPA-free containers*

Fruits
*Fresh, in season, use
fruit and vegetable wash,
or frozen*

All fresh fruits
Canned fruit—*sparingly,
  in their own juices,
  no added sugar*
Dried fruit—*no sugar
  or sulfates*
  raisins, figs, dates,
  prunes, pineapple,
  papaya, peaches,
  apples *(sparingly)*

Beans & Legumes
*Use sparingly when not
prepared correctly, one or
two times a month*

Beans—*dried, canned
  & plain*

Nuts & Seeds
*Use commercial nuts
sparingly if they are not
soaked & dried.*

Dry Roasted
Almonds
Cashews
Macadamia nuts
Peanuts—*organic only*
Pecans
Pumpkin seeds
Sunflower seeds
Walnuts

Butters, Roasted
Almond butter
Cashew butter
Peanut butter—*organic,
  no sugar added*
Pumpkin seed butter
Sunflower butter
Tahini

Sweeteners
Evaporated cane juice

Fats & Oils

Avocado oil—*unrefined*
Butter—*pasteurized
cow or goat milk*
Flaxseed Oil—*expeller-
pressed, do not heat*
Olive oil—*virgin,
conventional, or
expeller-pressed*
Palm oil, palm kernel oil,
& avocado oil—*unrefined*
Peanut oil—
*expeller-pressed,
unrefined, organic*
Safflower oil—
expeller-pressed
Sesame oil—
*expeller-pressed,
unrefined, organic*
Sunflower oil—
expeller-pressed
Walnut oil—
*expeller-pressed,
unrefined, organic*

Cold-pressed oils—
in small amounts
Macadamia oil
Safflower oil
Sesame oil
Sunflower oil

Condiments & Seasonings

Condiments—*wheat-free*
Fish sauce
Jams & jellies—*homemade
or bought, sweetened
with acceptable sugar*
Mayonnaise—*no sugar*
(Hain Safflower)
Salad dressings
& marinades—*bought,
all natural, sugar-free,
no preservatives**
Salsa
Soy sauce (tamari)
Tomato sauce
Wasabi

*Be aware that some "all-
natural" salad dressings and
marinades contain soybean oil
and/or canola oil, which are
GMO.*

Beverages

Almond milk—*homemade
or bought, unsweetened
and non-fortified*
Herbal teas—
*sweeten with
acceptable sweeteners*
Mineral waters—
naturally carbonated
Wines—*red & white*

Grains

Crackers—
(Mary's Be Gone,
DeLand Bakery
Millet Crackers)
Flours—*whole grain*
Pastas—*whole grain*
Whole grains—
not soaked or sprouted

Snacks

*Limit: a couple of times
per week*

Chocolate spreads—
organic, only with
acceptable sweeteners
Snack Bars*
(Thunderbird Energy Bars:
*Almond Cookie Pow Wow
Cashew Fig Carrot,
Cacao Hemp Walnut*)

(Essential Living Foods Bars:
*Raw Decadence Dark
Chocolate, Yoga Bar
White Chocolate*)

(Clif Kit's Organic Fruit &
Nut Bars: *Cashew,
Chocolate Almond
Coconut, Peanut Butter,
Berry Almond*)

*Although these bars are
organic, they should be
limited because the nuts
are not prepared correctly.*

*These foods are **fake foods, highly processed,** and should be **avoided** at all times. If these foods are eaten, it is vital to consume extra digestive enzymes. Also, increase your consumption of probiotics for three days after the food is eaten. 75% of food in the grocery store and in restaurants is genetically modified (GMO). Most of it is found in processed packaged foods and also in the feed of animals fed corn and soy. For a complete list of GM foods, refer to the Non-GMO shopping guide available at Energetic Wellness or through www.nongmoshoppingguide.com.*

Meats & Proteins
Bouillon cubes
Canned & dehydrated
  soups
Commercial eggs
Commercially grown
  beef, turkey, chicken,
  pork (including ham &
  bacon), etc.
Commercial hot dogs
  & sausages
Cured meats
Farm-raised fish,
  shellfish, etc.
Imitation eggs
Soy protein products—
  soybeans, soy protein
  isolate powders, textured
  vegetable protein (TVP),
  soy burgers, soy dogs,
  etc.

Dairy
Commercial ice cream—
  cow, soy or rice
Non-dairy creamer
Pasteurized, homogenized,
  low fat, skim milk,
  cheese & yogurt
Powdered milk
Processed imitation milk
  —*soy, rice, oats,
  hemp, etc.*

Vegetables
All pasteurized or heated
  pickled vegetables
Canned vegetables
Corn that is genetically
  engineered
Vegetable protein
  isolate powders

Fruits
Canned fruits
Fruit juices
Most Hawaiian papaya
  that is genetically
  engineered

Nuts & Seeds
Honey-roasted nuts
  & seeds
Non-organic peanut
  products
Nuts & seeds roasted
  in vegetable oil
Soy nut butter
Soy nuts

Fats & Oils
Hydrogenated oil and/or
  partially hydrogenated
All refined vegetable oils

Canola oil
Cottonseed oil
Grapeseed oil
Hemp oil
Margarine/spreads
Shortening
Soybean oil

Condiments, Spices & Seasoning
Jams with sugar added
Table salt—*iodized
  or regular*

Beverages
Bottled & frozen juices
Carbonated drinks
Distilled water
Protein powder drinks
Sodas
Stimulants such as
  coffee, energy drinks &
  mixed alcoholic drinks
Tap water or
  unpurified water

Sweeteners

Agave nectar
All artificial sweeteners
 (aspartame, NutraSweet®,
 Equal®, Splenda®,
 saccharin, sucralose)
Cane sugar—*refined white*
Corn syrup
Dextrose
(Florida Crystals)
Fructose
Fruit juices
Glucose
Heated honey
High-fructose corn syrup
Malt, barley malt
Rice syrup
Sucrose
Sugar alcohols—
 xylitol, sorbitol, etc.
Turbinado

Grains

White bread and any
 white flour products

Snacks

Candy, cakes & pies
Crackers
All snack food made with
 hydrogenated oil and
 high-fructose corn syrup
All snack food such as
 chips, pretzels, etc.

Misc.

All food preservatives
Anything you can't
 pronounce on a label
Breaded & deep-fried
 foods
Canned food
Flavor enhancers—
 like MSG
Food colorings
Foods cooked in aluminum
 cookware or with
 aluminum utensils
Microwaveable foods
Protein bars

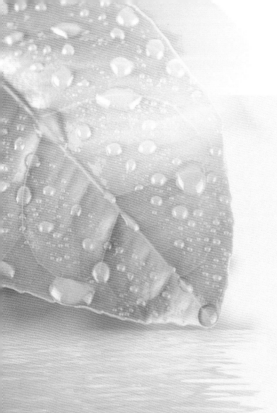

Menu Ideas & Recipes

Tips for a Healthy Lifestyle

Menu Ideas for Stages 1, 2 & 3

The Transformation

The following menu ideas and recipes will help you begin eating traditional, nutrient-dense foods. Pure, whole foods are full of flavor and more satisfying— the junk food cravings will decrease!

Tips for Making it Work

Years ago, I made the decision to eat only pure, whole food. Many people wrongly believe that this way of eating is too expensive. Our family of five lived on one income for more than 20 years and purchased organic, whole food as outlined in this book. It can be done. It might mean adjusting priorities, but the results are worth it.

Generally speaking, Americans consume way too much food. The food industry has created fake food that bypasses the body's "full" signals. Food that the body is not able to assimilate is not processed well and therefore gets stored as fat. The hidden sugar, salt, and fat in commercially processed food and served at restaurants causes problems. When you prepare your own food, you know how it is made and the origin of the ingredients. Most of all, it tastes better!

However, fitting in planning and food preparation can be a challenge. For many years I worked from home, took care of our family, homeschooled our children, and pre-pared our meals. I had a lot on my plate, but I was able to manage because I saw how important it was to my health and the health of my family. I made it a priority.

My husband and I are now empty-nesters and we both work full-time. Initially, finding the time for meal preparation was very difficult. However, we changed our methods and have made it work in our new stage of life. I eat small meals throughout the day, and when I get home (usually no earlier than 6 p.m.), Steven and I meet in the kitchen and prepare our meal together. We still make our meals from scratch, but it doesn't take long and we both enjoy it. As a general rule, we have one big meal a day—usually in the evening. On Saturday or Sunday, after our long morning walk, our big meal is usually brunch around 10 a.m.

Preparation is key for us. On the weekend, we chop up vegetables for salads and prep for meals that we can enjoy throughout the week. In the winter, crockpot meals are fabulous. I throw together a meal in the morning (which only takes 15–20 minutes), turn it on, and enjoy home-cooked food that evening. Soups can be prepared on the weekend and enjoyed throughout the week.

Since I have been trying to finish this book while running my practice, my weekends have become too full to prepare meals and plan for the week. We recently hired a cook. We do the grocery shopping and she marinates the meat we want to have during the week and chops up our vegetables. She prepares the meals according to our needs—whether the Food for Life or the stages of the

48 Days. This has saved us a lot of time, but still allows us to cook from scratch every night. You may think it is expensive, but if you compare the cost of picking up fast food, you are actually saving money (not to mention the cost to your health of eating out).

So whether we work at home, from home, or outside the home, we all work. Each stage of life poses challenges, but there is always an answer—because we have to eat. We were created to be busy, creative, and productive. If we want to be healthy, we have to make changes to our lifestyle and daily routine to make this natural way of life possible.

Food is our medicine, and if we don't get the right medicine on a daily basis, we will not function properly, the way God intended. We should have enough energy to accomplish the tasks we set for ourselves and the ones that are set before us—creating balance. What we consume, how we think, and how we live will determine how successful we are.

What's Your Lifestyle?

Here are some suggestions:

• **If you stay at home,** incorporate food prep into your daily schedule.

• **If you have kids at home,** include them in the food prep and grocery shopping. I adjusted our homeschooling schedule around daily living. This taught my children

important life skills. I am proud as I see my children—even my boys—cooking their meals. Most kids (and many adults) do not know how to cook. I involved my children in cooking and hospitality at an early age.

In our day and age, we have all but lost the art of hospitality. People want to get together at restaurants instead of taking the time to prepare a meal. Meal preparation is an investment of time—I get it! Going to a restaurant is very enjoyable and easy. But unfortunately, 75% of restaurant food is genetically engineered, uses the wrong fats, and has too much refined salt, hidden white sugar and fructose. Even the higher-end restaurants are making these mistakes.

• **If you work outside the home** and don't have time for meal prep on the weekends, consider hiring a cook or teen to help you. They can grocery shop, marinate meat, and prepare the vegetables for your meals for the week.

• **If you do eat out a lot,** make the best choices to the best of your ability. Familiarize yourself with the foods in each stage and only order from that list. Ask for your eggs to be cooked in butter, choose wild-caught fish prepared with 100% olive oil, and order vegetables over potato, rice, or pasta, and—skip the bread! This is what I do when I travel and have to eat out.

Menu Ideas

The following sample menu plans give you an idea of how to incorporate the foods from each stage into your diet. If you enjoy cooking and creating your own meals, feel free to make your own plan—just follow the list of foods for each stage. Be creative!

Once you have finished the 48 Days, purpose to eat the Foods for Life. Our nutritional needs differ based on age, activity levels, foundations, and weight. However, we have been given the guide and the rest is up to us. Whole foods for life works!

All Year Round—Throughout the 48 Days and for life, consume a probiotic or fermented food or beverage with every meal. This will aid in digestion and the absorption of nutrients. You can also drink a cup of bone broth with breakfast, lunch, or dinner. As a general rule, do not drink other liquids including water with your meals.

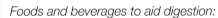

Foods and beverages to aid digestion:
- Bone broth
- Fermented vegetables of any kind
- Raw milk
- Yogurt
- Kefir
- Beet Kvass
- Kombucha
- Cocobiotic

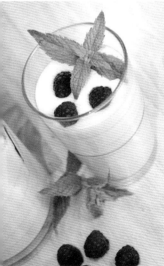

Meals—You do not need to eat three big meals a day! If you are eating pure, whole foods, your body needs less. Enjoy a nice breakfast with good fats and a moderate amount of protein. If dinner is your large meal, lunch can consist of a small portion of leftovers from the night before or a big salad. (I recommend a large salad every day.) I usually eat one light meal, one small meal, and one large meal. If this type of schedule causes you to snack frequently, you are not eating enough food at each meal, most likely not enough of the good fats. You should be full until the next meal. If you are not used to pure, whole foods, it may take time for you to figure out how much food your body actually needs—listen to your body's signals.

Periodic Fasts—Your body needs times of partial fasting to stimulate repair to its systems and maintain proper weight. I practice this sometimes several times a week. You may recall from my story that in years past, I fasted for long periods of time on just water and at that time in my life it was not beneficial to my body. I no longer believe that long periods of fasting is beneficial for anyone. A partial fast is restricting your meals for the day. This may mean, one or two meals to give the body a break. There are times when I drink broth for the day or have several glasses of raw milk and then have a normal dinner. The occasional skipping of a meal is beneficial to the body. Bone broth or raw milk fasts are very beneficial for the body and do not allow the breakdown of muscle or other vital tissue that can happen when you fast on water alone. Partial fasting is a great way to maintain your perfect weight. After you do it, you will come to enjoy how you feel and the benefits you will reap by this practice.

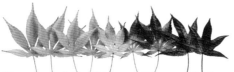

Spring/Summer & Fall/Winter Seasonal Menu Plans

Included are two sets of menu ideas for the different seasons of the year because it is beneficial to the body to eat according to the seasons. Some foods warm the body and some have a cooling effect. These relate to what is grown in season and help our body to function properly. Spring and summer is the best time to load up on the fresh, local, and cooling vegetables and fruits that are available. Fall and winter is a time to increase your intake of warming, mineral-rich bone broth and soups. See the list of seasonal produce in the Organic & Locally Grown section. There are also neutral foods that are good all year round—like green, leafy lettuces.

Stage 1:
Spring/Summer or Fall/Winter

Stage 2:
Spring/Summer or Fall/Winter

Stage 3: Lifestyle
Spring/Summer or Fall/Winter

Refer to the appropriate seasons' Menu Ideas when beginning the 48 Days.

Pure, whole foods are full of flavor and are much more satisfying, so the junk food cravings should dissipate. This way of eating includes a large variety of foods and food groups, so the possibilities are endless. These are just a few time-tested favorites. Enjoy! For additional recipes that support a traditional nutrient-dense way of eating, refer to *Nourishing Traditions* and *Sprouted Baking* and the websites listed in this book.

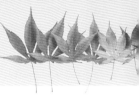

	Sample Day 1	Sample Day 2	Sample Day 3
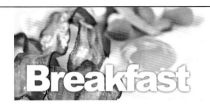**Breakfast**	Fried **eggs** any style (p. 138) **Stir-fried Veggies** (p. 139) 1/2–1 cup of raw milk	**Dr. Menzel's Pan Frittata** (p. 139) **Yogurt Cup** (p. 139) or 1/2–1 cup raw milk	**Anytime Energy Smoothie** (p. 139)
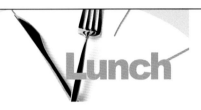**Lunch**	Cold Lentil Salad (p. 145)	Basic Green Salad with choice of protein (p. 144)	Hot Dog (p. 143) Choice of raw vegetables (anything seasonal in Stage 1)
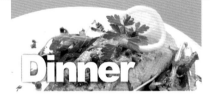**Dinner**	Beef Burgers (p. 164) Veggies on the Grill (p. 154) Basic Green Salad (p. 144)	Marinated Steak (p. 161) Cauliflower (p. 154) Basic Green Salad (p. 144)	Marinated Wild-Caught Salmon (p. 161) Cold Asparagus Salad (p. 146) Basic Green Salad (p. 144)

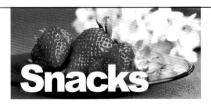
Snacks

1/2 cup berries with 1 oz. raw goat cheddar cheese

4–6 oz. plain or vanilla goat milk yogurt, 1/2 cup berries

Raw carrot and/or celery sticks with raw almond butter

1/2 cup **Crispy Almonds** (p. 172)

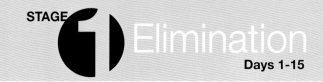
Sample Day 1	Sample Day 2	Sample Day 3
Fried Eggs (p. 138) Avocado **Stir-fried Veggies** (p. 139) 1 cup **bone broth** with 1 tsp–1Tbsp. coconut oil (pp. 148–149)	**Dr. Menzel's Breakfast Frittata** (p. 139) 1 cup **bone broth** with 1 tsp–1Tbsp. coconut oil (pp. 148–149)	**Breakfast Sausage** (p. 140) **Stir-fried Veggies** (p. 139) 1 cup **bone broth** with 1 tsp–1Tbsp. coconut oil (pp. 148–149)
Lentil Soup topped with seasoned yogurt (p. 150)	**Grilled Salmon** (p. 161) **Basic Green Salad** (p. 144)	**Roasted Butternut Squash Soup** (p. 151) **Basic Green Salad** (p. 144)
Greek Marinade for Beef (p. 161) **Broccoli Sauté** (p. 152) **Basic Green Salad** (p. 144)	**Oven Roasted Chicken with Vegetables** (p. 161) **Basic Green Salad** (p. 144)	**Acorn Squash Boats** (p. 154) **Bolognese Sauce** (p. 165) Shredded raw goat cheese **Basic Green Salad** (p. 144)

Suggested Preparation for the Week

• Make burger patties
and package according
to servings. Freeze.

• Make sausage patties
and package according
to servings. Freeze.

• Chop produce and
store in glass containers
in the refrigerator.

• Start a fermented
vegetable. (*Nourishing
Traditions* by Sally Fallon)

• Start a batch
of crispy nuts (p. 172).

1/2 cup berries with 1 oz. raw goat cheddar cheese

4–6 oz. plain or vanilla goat milk yogurt, 1/2 cup berries

Raw carrot and/or celery sticks with raw almond butter

1/2 cup **Crispy Almonds** (p. 172)

Menu Ideas for Spring & Summer

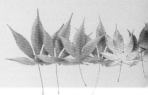

	Sample Day 1	Sample Day 2	Sample Day 3
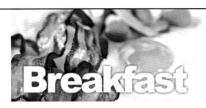 **Breakfast**	**Scrambled Eggs** (p. 138) Sliced peaches or melons (anything seasonal in Stage 2) Raw goat cheddar cheese	**Spinach & Feta Omelet** (p. 138) 1/2–1 cup raw milk	**Fried Eggs**, any style (p. 138) **Breakfast Sausage** (p. 140) 1/2–1 cup raw milk
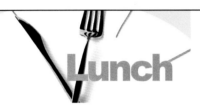 **Lunch**	**Tuna Salad** on a bed of romaine lettuce (p. 143) Baby carrots Cucumber slices	**Lunch Tray** (p. 143)	**Anytime Energy Smoothie** (p. 172)
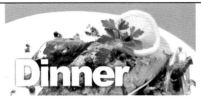 **Dinner**	**Coconut Chicken** (p. 162) **Sautéed Zucchini** (p. 153) **Basic Green Salad** (p. 144)	**Beef, Lamb or Turkey Burger** (p. 164) **Sweet Potato Rounds** (p. 155) **Basic Green Salad** (p. 144)	**Liver & Onions** (p. 166) **Sautéed Mixed Vegetables** (p. 152) **Basic Green Salad** (p. 144)

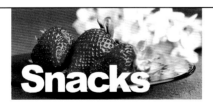

Snacks

1/2 cup berries with 1 oz. raw goat cheddar cheese

4–6 oz. plain or vanilla goat milk yogurt, 1/2 cup berries

Raw carrot and/or celery sticks with raw almond butter

1/2 cup **Crispy Almonds** (p. 172)

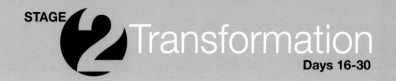
	Sample Day 1	Sample Day 2	Sample Day 3

Fried Eggs, any style
(p. 138)
Stir-fried Veggies
(p. 139)
1 cup **bone broth**
with 1 tsp–1Tbsp.
coconut oil
(pp. 148–149)

**Onion, Pepper &
Goat Cheese
Omelet** (p. 138)
Yogurt Cup (p. 139)
1 cup **bone broth**
with 1 tsp–1Tbsp.
coconut oil
(pp. 148–149)

Scrambled Eggs
(p. 138)
Breakfast Sausage
(p. 140)
1 cup **bone broth**
with 1 tsp–1Tbsp.
coconut oil
(pp. 148–149)

**Sautéed Cabbage
and Vegetables**
(p. 152)
Hot Dog
(p. 143)

**Roll Up Grilled Chicken
& Toppings
on Coconut Wrap**
(p. 143)

Basic Green Salad
(p. 144)

Lamb Burgers
(p. 164)
Sweet Potato Variation,
diced sweet potatoes
with peppers & onions
(p. 155)
Basic Green Salad
(p. 144)

Chicken Soup
(p. 148)
Basic Green Salad
(p. 144)

Easy Pan Chicken
(p. 162)
Sautéed Asparagus
(p. 153)

**Suggested
Preparation
for the Week**

• Make burger patties
and package according
to servings. Freeze.

• Make sausage patties
and package according
to servings. Freeze.

• Chop produce and
store in glass containers
in the refrigerator.

• Start a fermented
vegetable. (*Nourishing
Traditions* by Sally Fallon)

• Start a batch
of crispy nuts (p. 172).

1/2 cup berries with 1 oz. raw goat cheddar cheese

4–6 oz. plain or vanilla goat milk yogurt, 1/2 cup berries

Raw carrot and/or celery sticks with raw almond butter

1/2 cup **Crispy Almonds** (p. 172)

Menu Ideas for Spring & Summer

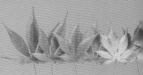

	Sample Day 1	Sample Day 2	Sample Day 3
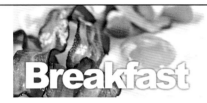 **Breakfast**	**Pancakes** (p. 140) **Fried Eggs**, any Style (p. 138) **Yogurt Cup** (p. 139)	**Dr. Menzel's Pan Frittata** (p. 139) 1/2–1 cup raw milk	**Anytime Energy Smoothie** with raw eggs (p. 139)
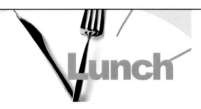 **Lunch**	**Ginger Carrots** (p. 153), prepare 3 days ahead **Lentil Burger** (p. 165) Avocado	**Roll-up or Sandwich** (p. 143) **Basic Green Salad** (p. 144)	**Basic Green Salad** (p. 144)
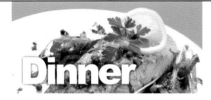 **Dinner**	**Easy Pan Chicken** (p. 162) **Sautéed Carrots** (p. 153) **Basic Green Salad** (p. 144)	**Asian Marinade for Fish** (p. 161) **Sautéed Chard, Kale** (p. 152) **Basic Green Salad** (p. 144)	**Grilled Garlic Butter Shrimp** (p. 166) **Sprouted Brown Rice** (p. 157) **Sautéed Spinach** (p. 152) **Basic Green Salad** (p. 144)

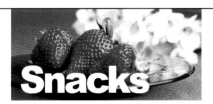 **Snacks**

1/2 cup berries with 1 oz. raw goat cheddar cheese

4–6 oz. plain or vanilla goat milk yogurt, 1/2 cup berries

Raw carrot and/or celery sticks with raw almond butter

1/2 cup **Crispy Almonds** (p. 172)

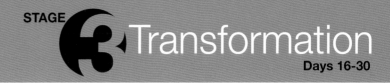
Sample Day 1	**Sample Day 2**	**Sample Day 3**

Basic Sprouted Oatmeal
with butter
(p. 142)
1 cup **bone broth**
with 1 tsp–1Tbsp.
coconut oil
(pp. 148–149)

Fried Eggs
(p. 138)
Breakfast Sausage
(p. 140)
1 cup **bone broth**
with 1 tsp–1Tbsp.
coconut oil
(pp. 148–149)

Ginger Basic Muffin
loaded with butter
(p. 141)
Fried Eggs, any style (p. 138)
1 cup **bone broth**
with 1 tsp–1Tbsp.
coconut oil
(pp. 148–149)

Suggested Preparation for the Week

Lamb Meatballs
(p. 163)
Shredded Carrot Salad
(p. 146)

Basic Green Salad
(p. 144)
with protein of choice

Basic Green Salad
(p. 144)
with protein of choice

• Make burger patties
and package according
to servings. Freeze.

• Make sausage patties
and package according
to servings. Freeze.

Minestrone Soup
(p. 151)
Basic Green Salad
(p. 144)

Spicy Meatloaf
(p. 164)
Mashed Potatoes
(p. 157)
Sautéed Green Beans
(p. 153)
Basic Green Salad
(p. 144)

Crockpot Beef Stew
(p. 166)
Basic Green Salad
(p. 144)

• Chop produce and
store in glass containers
in the refrigerator.

• Start a fermented
vegetable. (*Nourishing
Traditions* by Sally Fallon)

• Start a batch
of crispy nuts (p. 172).

1/2 cup berries with 1 oz. raw goat cheddar cheese

4–6 oz. plain or vanilla goat milk yogurt, 1/2 cup berries

Raw carrot and/or celery sticks with raw almond butter

1/2 cup **Crispy Almonds** (p. 172)

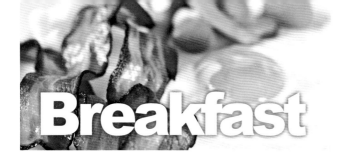

Breakfast

When using coconut oil, if you do not want food to taste "coconutty," use expeller-pressed coconut oil.

Fried Eggs

Prepare as desired: over easy, medium, or well done. Fry in virgin or expeller-pressed coconut oil or butter.

Soft and Hard-Boiled Eggs

Wash eggs and cover with water. Boil 4 minutes for soft-boiled eggs and 12 minutes for hard-boiled eggs. Plunge eggs in cold water for easy peeling. Refrigerate for a convenient addition to any meal or snack.

Scrambled Eggs

For results that have a more pleasant texture and superior taste, add cream instead of milk. The extra yolk makes a super scramble.

1 fresh egg	Pinch sea salt
1 egg yolk (optional)	2 tsp. butter
1 Tbsp. cream	

Beat egg, optional yolk, cream, and salt thoroughly with a wire whisk. Melt butter in a heavy skillet. Add beaten egg mixture and stir constantly with a wooden spoon until egg is scrambled. Serve immediately with a side of your choice.

Nourishing Traditions

Basic Omelet

4 eggs
3 Tbsp. water
Pinch sea salt
2 Tbsp. butter or extra-virgin coconut oil

Crack eggs into a bowl; add water and salt. Blend with a wire whisk. (Do not whisk for too long or the omelet will be tough.) Melt butter in a seasoned cast-iron skillet. When foam subsides, add egg mixture. Tip pan to allow egg to cover the entire pan. Cook several minutes over medium heat until underside is lightly browned. Lift up one side with a spatula and fold omelet in half. Reduce heat and cook another half minute or so—allowing the egg to cook on the inside. Slide omelet onto a heated platter and serve. *The Maker's Diet*

Variations:

Onion, Pepper & Goat Cheese Omelet—In 2 Tbsp. butter, sauté 1 small onion (thinly sliced) and 1/2 red pepper (cut into strips) until tender. Sprinkle evenly over the egg mixture as it begins to cook, along with 2 oz. of goat's milk cheddar or feta cheese.

Herb Omelet—Sprinkle 1 Tbsp. parsley, 1 Tbsp. chives, and 1 Tbsp. thyme or other garden herb (all finely chopped) over the omelet as it begins to cook.

Mushroom Omelet—Sauté 1/2 lb. fresh mushrooms (washed, dried, and thinly sliced) in 2 Tbsp. each of butter and olive oil. Scatter over the omelet as it begins to cook.

Sausage Omelet—Sauté 1/2 cup turkey sausage mixture in 2 Tbsp. butter until crumbly. Scatter over the omelet as it begins to cook.

Spinach & Feta Omelet—Add chopped onion to beaten eggs. Add more onions, spinach, tomatoes, and feta cheese as it begins to cook.

Tomato & Basil Omelet—Scatter 1/4 cup diced tomato and chopped fresh basil over omelet as it begins to cook.

Dr. Menzel's Pan Frittata

1/4 cup broccoli and/or spinach
1/4 small onion
1/4 red or green pepper
1 Tbsp. or less butter or coconut oil
2 eggs
Sea salt, pepper, Herbamare, or other spices
Grated raw goat cheddar cheese
   or grated pecorino romano

Sauté any combination of veggies listed or other leftover veggies in butter or coconut oil. Add a pinch of salt, pepper, and a little Herbamare. Crack 2 eggs over softened veggies. Cook until done. Top with goat cheddar or pecorino romano. Cover for 2 minutes for cheese to melt. Yummy! *You can double or triple this easy recipe for a great quick breakfast everyone will love!*

Stir-fried Veggies

Sautée vegetables of your choice in butter or coconut oil with a pinch of sea salt.

Sample veggies: onion, spinach, kale, broccoli, peppers, carrots, mushrooms or any combination you choose. Use leftover veggies from the night before.

Serve as a side or tossed in sprouted brown rice.

Green Breakfast Smoothie

1 cup pure, filtered water
1/2 cup frozen berries
1/2 of a frozen banana
1 tsp. honey
1 Tbsp. Pure Synergy

Mix in blender at high speed.

Pure Synergy

Anytime Energy Smoothie

6–8 oz. raw goat milk *or* yogurt *or* kefir
    or full-fat coconut milk (Thai brand)
    or raw cow milk
1 tsp.–1 Tbsp. virgin coconut oil (optional)
1–2 raw eggs
1 Tbsp. flax seed oil (optional)
1 tsp.–1 Tbsp. raw honey
2–3 Tbsp. Essential Living Whey protein powder
1/2 cup fresh or frozen fruit (berries are best)
1–2 scoops digestive enzyme powder (Formula 30-P)
1 tsp. vanilla extract (optional)

Blend all in a high-speed blender (Vita-Mix).

Yogurt Cup

6 oz. plain goat yogurt
1 tsp. honey
1/2 cup fruit (berries, apples, bananas, melons,
   oranges, peaches, etc.)
1/8 cup crispy nuts
Sprinkle of cinnamon, nutmeg, or cocoa
   (great for the fall and winter months)

Mix together yogurt and honey. Top with fruit, nuts, and spices.

Jessica Menzel Brown

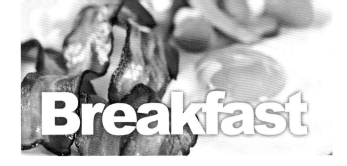

Breakfast

Turkey Breakfast Sausage

1 lb. ground turkey
1 small onion, peeled and finely chopped
1/2 tsp. each cumin, marjoram, pepper, nutmeg,
    oregano, cayenne pepper, ginger, dried basil,
    thyme, and sage
1 tsp. sea salt
2 Tbsp. whole-grain breadcrumbs
1 egg, lightly beaten
2 Tbsp. butter

Mix all ingredients and chill. Make into patties and
sauté in butter. To store, make into patties and store
in an airtight container, using parchment paper to line
the container and to separate the patties.

Breakfast Sausage

1 egg, slightly beaten
1/3 cup onion, finely chopped
1/2 cup red delicious apple, finely chopped
1/4 cup homemade breadcrumbs
2 Tbsp. fresh parsley, snipped

1/2 tsp. sea salt	1/4 tsp. black pepper
1/2 tsp. ground sage	1/8 tsp. cayenne pepper
1/4 tsp. ground nutmeg	1 lb. ground turkey,
	beef, or lamb

In medium size mixing bowl, combine egg, onion, apple,
bread crumbs, parsley, salt, sage, nutmeg, black pepper, and cayenne pepper. Add ground meat and mix
well. Shape mixture into nine 2" wide patties.
    Preheat indoor grill to 300° and cook 4 minutes or
until desired doneness.

Pancakes

1 egg	1 Tbsp. honey
1 cup sprouted spelt flour	2 Tbsp. coconut oil
(option: whole-grain flour)	3 tsp. baking powder
3/4 cup raw buttermilk or raw milk	1/4 tsp. sea salt

If coconut oil is solid, heat on very low until soft, almost
liquid. Mix all ingredients in a medium bowl. Heat skillet
or griddle. Grease with butter and ladle pancake batter
onto the surface. Cook 1-2 min. on each side. Serve hot
with butter and 100% pure maple syrup.

Gluten-Free Millet Pancakes

1 cup sprouted millet flour	2 Tbsp. applesauce
2 Tbsp. Rapunzel	3 Tbsp. coconut oil
whole cane sugar	1/2 cup water
1 tsp. baking powder	(or more if needed for
1/4 tsp. sea salt	desired consistency)

In a medium bowl, mix together dry ingredients. Add
wet ingredients; mix until just blended. Do not overmix
or pancakes will be tough. Pour 1/4 cup of batter onto
hot griddle or skillet. Cook until bubbles form, then flip
and brown on the other side. Serve alone or top with
butter and 100% pure maple syrup! These freeze well.

Jessica Menzel Brown

Fruit Topping

Butter
Apples (fresh), or blueberries, strawberries, or peaches
    (fresh or frozen)
Rapunzel whole cane sugar (or any Stage 3 sweetener)

Put fruit and butter in a frying pan and sprinkle with
whole cane sugar. Simmer until soft and warm. Pour
over favorite pancakes or waffles.

Basic Muffins 🌙

3 cups spelt flour
2 cups buttermilk, kefir,
    or yogurt
2 eggs, lightly beaten
1 tsp. sea salt

1/4 cup maple syrup
2 tsp. baking soda
1 tsp. vanilla extract
3 Tbsp. melted butter

Soak flour in buttermilk, kefir, or yogurt in a warm place for 12–24 hours. Muffins will rise better if soaked for 24 hours. (Those with milk allergies may use 2 cups filtered water plus 2 tablespoons whey, lemon juice, or vinegar.)
   Preheat oven to 325°. Blend in remaining ingredients. Pour into well-buttered muffin tins (preferably stoneware), filling about 3/4 full. Bake for 1 hour or until a toothpick comes out clean. Makes about 15.

Nourishing Traditions

Variations:

Raisin Muffins—Add 1/2 cup raisins and 1/2 tsp. cinnamon.

Blueberry Muffins—Add 1 cup blueberries, fresh or frozen. To prevent blueberries from falling to the bottom of the muffins, do not mix into batter. Place 5-7 blueberries on top of the batter in each muffin tin.

Dried Cherry Muffins—Add 4 oz. dried cherries and 1/2 cup chopped crispy pecans.

Fruit Spice Muffins—Add 2 ripe pears or peaches, peeled and cut into small pieces, 1/2 tsp. cinnamon, 1/8 tsp. cloves, and 1/8 tsp. nutmeg.

Lemon Muffins—Add grated rind of 2 lemons and 1/2 cup chopped crispy pecans.

Ginger Muffins—Add 1 Tbsp. freshly grated ginger and 1 tsp. ground ginger. Omit vanilla.

Basic Sprouted Muffins 🌙

2 Tbsp. raw apple cider vinegar or kombucha
1 cup raw cow or goat milk
2 eggs

1/2 cup Rapunzel whole cane sugar
    (If coarse, make into a powder in food processor.)
1 tsp. vanilla
1/2 cup coconut oil, expeller-pressed, melted
2 1/2 cups sprouted spelt flour
3/4 tsp. sea salt
2 tsp. aluminum-free baking powder
Spices of your choice: 2 tsp. cinnamon
                          1 tsp. ginger
                          1/4 tsp. nutmeg

Add-ins of your choice:

1/2 cup raisins
1/2 cup chopped crispy nuts (p. 172)
1/2 cup unsweetened, shredded coconut
1 cup zucchini, apple, or carrot, shredded
    (extra moisture may require longer cooking time)

Preheat oven to 375°. In mixing bowl, combine vinegar, milk, eggs, sugar, and vanilla. Whisk well. While whisking, add coconut oil.
   Combine flour, salt, spices, and baking powder in a separate bowl and fluff with fork. Add wet ingredients and mix until smooth. Do not overmix. Combine add-ins and fold in. Fill oiled or paper-lined muffin tin 3/4 full with batter. Bake for 20–25 minutes until toothpick comes out clean.   Wardeh Harmon, www.gnowfglins.com

Wild Blueberry Muffins 🌙

1 1/3 cups sprouted spelt flour
1 tsp. baking soda
2 tsp. aluminum-free baking powder
1/2 tsp. sea salt
3/4 cup Rapunzel whole cane sugar
1/2 cup expeller-pressed coconut oil
1 egg
1 cup yogurt
1 cup frozen wild blueberries

Preheat oven to 350°. Sift together flour, baking soda, baking powder, and salt. Set aside. Whisk together

CONTINUED ON NEXT PAGE

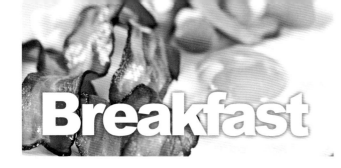

Breakfast

sugar, oil, egg, and yogurt. Add the dry ingredients, reserving 1 Tbsp. to toss with blueberries. Stir well by hand, but do not overmix. Mix in 1/2 cup wild blueberries. Spoon batter into muffin pan. Sprinkle the remaining blueberries on top, pressing down lightly. Place in oven and increase temperature to 400°. Bake for 20-25 minutes.

Breakfast Porridge

1 cup oats, rolled or cracked
1 cup warm filtered water
  plus 2 Tbsp. whey, yogurt, kefir, or buttermilk
1/2 tsp. sea salt
1 cup filtered water
1 Tbsp. flax seeds (optional)

For highest benefits and best assimilation, porridge should be soaked overnight or longer. Once soaked, oatmeal cooks in less than 5 minutes—truly a fast food. *(Those with severe milk allergies can use lemon juice or vinegar in place of whey, yogurt, kefir, or buttermilk.)*

Mix oats with warm water mixture, cover, and leave in a warm place for 7–24 hours. Bring an additional 1 cup of water to a boil with sea salt. Add soaked oats, reduce heat, cover, and simmer several minutes. Grind optional flax seeds in a mini grinder. Remove oats from heat, stir in optional flax seeds, and let stand for a few minutes. Serve with plenty of butter or cream and a natural sweetener like Rapadura, date sugar, maple syrup, maple sugar or raw honey. You may also wish to add apricot butter, chopped crispy nuts, or dried sweetened coconut meat.

Nourishing Traditions,
Revised by Michele Menzel

Baked Oatmeal

2 1/2 cups oats
1 3/4 cups raw milk
1/2 cup coconut oil
4 eggs
1/2 cup Rapunzel sugar, maple syrup, or honey
2 cups raisins
1 tsp. baking powder
1/2 tsp. sea salt
2 tsp. cinnamon
2 tsp. vanilla

Optional add-ins *(or sprinkle on each serving after baking)*:
  2 cups chopped nuts
  2 cups chopped apples or pears

Soak oats and raw milk overnight in a covered bowl on kitchen counter. In the morning, mix in oil, sugar, and eggs until glossy. Mix in baking powder, salt, cinnamon and vanilla. Stir in oats, raisins, and chopped apples (or pears). Pour into 9"×13" baking dish and bake at 350° for 20 minutes.

Soaked Baked Oatmeal

2 1/2 cups oats
2 1/2 cups warm filtered water
5 Tbsp. whey, yogurt, or kefir

Mix in a bowl. Soak overnight in a warm place 7–24 hours. In the morning, beat together:

1/2 cup coconut oil (virgin or expeller pressed)
4 eggs
1/2 cup Rapunzel whole cane sugar,
  maple syrup, or honey
Add: 1 tsp. aluminum-free baking powder
    1 tsp. sea salt
    2 tsp. cinnamon
    2 tsp. vanilla
Stir in the soaked oatmeal and pour into a greased (with coconut oil or butter) 9"×13" baking dish. Bake at 350° for 20 minutes or until solid.

Toppings: chopped apple, pears, berries, chopped crispy nuts, raisins, warm raw milk.

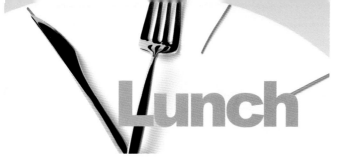

Lunch

Tuna Salad

1 5-oz. can water-packed tuna, drained
1 Tbsp. or more Wilderness Family mayonnaise,
  to your desired consistency
Onion, chopped
Celery, chopped
Pickles, chopped
Black olives, chopped

Mix all ingredients with a pinch of salt and pepper.
Serve tuna on a bed of lettuce, coconut wrap,
a sprouted bun or sliced, sprouted bread of your
choice, with raw veggies on the side. Can also
be served on the side of a small tossed salad with
homemade salad dressing.

Hot Dog & Kraut

1 or 2 grass-fed hot dogs
1–2 spoonfuls of sauerkraut
1 Tbsp. butter
Favorite mustard

Sauté hot dogs in a pan with butter, until heated. Top
with sauerkraut and mustard. If in stage 3, place on a
sprouted spelt bun with mustard. Serve with a tossed
salad and/or homemade sweet potato fries, homemade
French fries, or crispy potatoes.

Roll-ups or Sandwich

Turkey, grilled chicken or roast beef
Sliced goat or cow raw cheddar cheese
Mustard and/or mayonnaise
Lettuce   Sprouts
Tomato   Avocado
Coconut wrap, tortilla or bread of choice

As roll-ups, roll cheese in choice of meat. As sandwich,
use bread of choice or tortilla. Layer meat, cheese, lettuce,
tomato, sprouts, avocado and condiment of choice.

Lunch Tray

Crispy nuts, handful (p. 172)
1 sliced apple or other fruit
2–4 slices raw goat cheddar cheese
Hot dog, cut into bite-sized pieces

Arrange on plate and enjoy!

Einkorn Wheat Berry Salad

1 1/2 cups Einkorn wheat berries
4 fresh tomatoes, diced
1 cucumber, sliced
1 scallion, sliced
3 Tbsp. parsley, minced
3 oz. feta cheese
3 Tbsp. olive oil
1 Tbsp. apple cider vinegar

Cook Einkorn according to basic cooking instructions
on box. Set aside to cool. In a medium serving bowl,
whisk olive oil, vinegar, scallions and parsley together.
Add tomatoes, cucumbers and feta and mix well. Toss
with wheat berries and serve with salt and pepper to
taste.

Jovial Foods

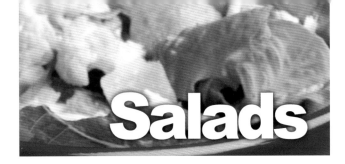

Salads

Basic Green Salad
Use organic ingredients.

1 head Romaine, Boston, red leaf, green leaf,
 or mixed greens, washed well and torn or
 chopped
1/2 cucumber, quartered
2 plum tomatoes, diced
    or several cherry or grape tomatoes
1/2 small red onion, chopped or sliced
2–3 oz. raw cheddar cheese, diced or grated (opt.)

Combine in a large bowl. Toss with your dressing of
choice.

Basic Variations:
Beets
Cabbage—green & purple, finely chopped
Carrots, chopped or shredded
Celery
Cucumbers
Mushrooms
Peppers—red, green, yellow
Red onion, finely chopped
Scallions
Sprouts
Zucchini, julienne sliced or diced
Hard-boiled eggs
Grilled chicken
Grilled salmon
Tuna
Ground sprouted flax seeds
Cheese
Crispy nuts & seeds

Basic Balsamic Dressing
1 tsp. Dijon-type mustard, smooth or grainy
2 Tbsp. plus 1 tsp. balsamic vinegar
1/2 cup extra virgin olive oil
1 Tbsp. expeller-pressed flax oil

Dip a fork into the jar of mustard to transfer about
1 teaspoon to a small bowl. Add vinegar and mix.
Add olive oil in a thin stream, stirring until oil is well-
mixed or emulsified. Add flax oil and use immediately.
Makes about 3/4 cup.

Nourishing Traditions

Variations:
Herb Dressing
3/4 cup Basic Balsamic Dressing
    1 tsp. finely chopped fresh herbs—
    parsley, tarragon, thyme, basil, oregano, etc.

Prepare basic dressing and add herbs. Makes 3/4 cup.

Garlic Dressing
3/4 cup Basic Balsamic Dressing
1 clove garlic, minced

Prepare basic dressing. Add garlic and stir. Let sit a few
minutes to allow amalgamation of garlic flavor. Makes
3/4 cup.

Creamy Dilled Vinaigrette
1/4 cup extra virgin olive oil
1/4 cup Wilderness Family mayo
1/4 cup lemon juice
1/8 tsp. sea salt
1/4 tsp. dill weed
2 cloves garlic, minced
Pinch of white pepper

Whisk together. Also good on baked potatoes.

Creamy Avocado Dressing

1 large avocado
1 Tbsp. plus 2 tsp. fresh lemon juice
1/2 cup plain yogurt
1/4 cup extra virgin olive oil or coconut oil
2 garlic cloves, minced
3/4 tsp. sea salt
1–3 tsp. maple syrup

Blend together all ingredients until smooth and creamy. Use immediately or store in the refrigerator.

Karen Williamson

Miso-Ginger Dressing

1 cup water
1/2 Tbsp. fresh ginger, peeled and chopped
1 1/2 Tbsp. mellow white miso
1 Tbsp. lemon juice
1 Tbsp. tahini
1/2 scallion, chopped
2 cloves garlic, minced
3 Tbsp. Barlean's organic flax oil

Combine all ingredients in blender or food processor until creamy. Makes 1 1/3 cups.

Cold Lentil Salad

Enjoy this protein- and fiber-packed recipe that's not only delicious, but great for your body, too!

1 cup lentils, soaked overnight, cooked, and cooled
1 Tbsp. extra virgin olive oil
2 Tbsp. lemon juice, freshly squeezed
1 clove garlic, minced
2 Tbsp. balsamic vinegar
2 green onions, chopped
2 Tbsp. Italian parsley, chopped
1/4 small, red onion, chopped
1 carrot, chopped
Sea salt and pepper to taste

To soak lentils:

In glass bowl, add enough warm, filtered water to fully cover lentils. Add 1 Tbsp. of whey or lemon juice. Let sit on counter for at least 7 hours. Drain and rinse. Cover and cook over medium-high heat for 30–45 minutes, or until tender (but not falling apart). Drain, rinse with cold water, and set aside.

In a small bowl, whisk together olive oil, lemon juice, garlic, and vinegar. Set aside.

In a medium bowl, combine cooked lentils, green onions, parsley, red onion, and carrot. Drizzle olive oil mixture over salad and toss well. Season to taste. Refrigerate, covered, for at least 30 minutes, preferably 2–3 hours.

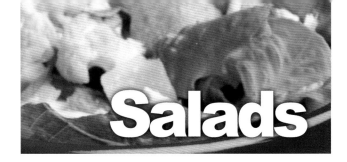

Salads

Cold Cucumber & Tomato Salad

1–2 cucumbers
6–8 cherry or grape tomatoes, cut in half
    (or two plum tomatoes, diced)
1/2 small red onion, diced

Combine and toss with favorite homemade salad dressing (p. 144).

Cold Asparagus Salad

1 bunch of asparagus, woody ends removed

Lemon vinaigrette dressing:
1/3 cup extra virgin olive oil
1/4 cup lemon juice
1/4 cup green onions, sliced
1 Tbsp. Dijon-style mustard
1 tsp. honey
1/2 tsp. sea salt

Blanch the asparagus by immersing into boiling water for 2 to 3 minutes and then immediately into ice water to stop the cooking. In a container with a tight lid, combine vinaigrette ingredients and shake to combine. Pour over asparagus and toss. Chill until ready to serve, cold or at room temperature.

Bean Salad

4 cups cooked black beans (p. 167)
2 tomatoes, diced
2 avocados, diced
2 bell peppers, diced (red, yellow, or orange)
1 poblano or 2 jalapeño peppers, seeded, diced small
1 small red onion, diced
1–2 cloves garlic, minced
Juice of 1/2–1 lime, to taste
1/4 cup olive oil, or more
Sea salt and pepper to taste

Prepare black beans according to the Basic Bean recipe (p. 167). Do not overcook. Chill. Toss together all the ingredients. Serve in a bowl as a salad, a side, or dip. Serve cold.

Tammi Foster

Shredded Carrot Salad

4–5 cups carrots, shredded raw
1/2 cup raisins
1 Tbsp. Dijon mustard (check ingredients)
2–3 Tbsp. maple syrup
2–3 Tbsp. orange juice, freshly squeezed

Mix all together. To enhance taste, refrigerate for at least 1–2 hours before serving.

Potato Salad or Pasta Salad

3 lb. red potatoes
    or 1/2 lb. whole spelt elbow noodles
1/2 small onion, finely chopped
1–2 celery sticks, finely chopped
4–6 hard-boiled eggs, finely chopped
Several heaping Tbsp. of Wilderness Family
  mayonnaise, Hain safflower mayonnaise
  or homemade mayonnaise
Sea salt and pepper
Paprika

For potatoes: Boil potatoes with the skin on until you can slide a fork in and out without resistance. Leave the skins on the potatoes and cut into bite-sized pieces.

For noodles: Boil noodles according to instructions on box, until tender. Drain. Rinse with cool, filtered water.

Put all ingredients in a bowl, mixing in the mayonnaise last. Use as much mayonnaise as you desire. Salt and pepper to taste. Garnish with paprika.

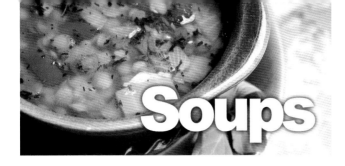

Chicken Stock (Bone Broth)

8-quart stockpot
1 whole free-range chicken (3 lbs.)
　　or bony chicken parts, such as necks,
　　backs, breastbones, and wings
Gizzards from one chicken (optional)
Feet from the chicken (optional)
4–6 quarts cold filtered water
2 Tbsp. vinegar
1 large onion, coarsely chopped
2 or more carrots, peeled and coarsely chopped
3 celery sticks with leaves, coarsely chopped
1 Tbsp. sea salt
1 bunch parsley

Place chicken or chicken pieces in a large stainless steel pot with water, vinegar, and all vegetables except parsley. Let stand 30 minutes to 1 hour. This allows minerals to begin releasing from the bones. Bring to a boil, and remove scum that rises to the top. Reduce heat, cover, and simmer for about 3 hours. Remove chicken and debone. Place chicken meat in a glass container and refrigerate for use in chicken soup recipe. Put all the bones, fat and everything else back into the broth and cook for an additional 21 hours. The longer you cook the stock, the richer and more flavorful it will be. About 10 minutes before finishing the stock, add parsley. This will impart additional mineral ions to the broth.

　　Strain the stock into a large bowl and refrigerate until the fat rises to the top and congeals. Skim off this fat and reserve the stock in covered containers in your refrigerator or freezer.

Variations: Use whole turkey or duck. Use carcass of chicken, turkey, or duck.

Carcass version: Debone leftover chicken, turkey, or duck. Put meat in a container and store in refrigerator or freezer for later use. Place all bones, fat, neck, and gizzards in pot with water and vegetables. Bring to a boil, reduce heat, and simmer overnight at least 12 to 24 hours. Keep the lid on so water does not evaporate.

These stocks will have a stronger flavor. Use several sprigs of fresh thyme, tied together during cooking.

Chicken Soup

4–6 quarts homemade chicken stock
　　(reserved from making homemade broth)
1–1½ cups each of finely diced vegetables
　　such as carrot, celery, string beans (fresh or frozen),
　　turnips, onions, spinach (fresh or frozen)
1/2–1 Tbsp. sea salt
1/2–1 Tbsp. Herbamare seasoning
Chicken meat, cooked & diced

Put stock, all vegetables, salt, and Herbamare in a 6-qt. stainless steel stockpot and cook until vegetables are tender (approximately one hour). Add diced cooked chicken about 10 minutes before soup is done.

Variation: You may also add cooked brown rice (p.157) or cooked whole grain pasta (follow instructions on box) right before serving.

Beef Stock (Bone Broth)

4 lbs. beef marrow and knuckle bones
1 calf's foot, cut into pieces (optional)
3 lbs. meaty rib or neck bones
4 qts. cold, filtered water
1/2 cup vinegar
3 onions, coarsely chopped
3 carrots, coarsely chopped
3 celery sticks, coarsely chopped
Several sprigs of fresh thyme, tied together
1 tsp. dried green peppercorns, crushed
1 bunch parsley

Good beef stock must be made with different bone parts: feet and knuckle bones impart large quantities of gelatin; marrow and knuckle bones impart flavor and nutrients; and meaty rib or neck bones add color and flavor.

Place the marrow and knuckle bones and foot in a very large pot with vinegar and cover with water. Let stand for 1 hour. Meanwhile, place the meaty bones in a roasting pan at 350° in the oven until well browned. Add bones and vegetables to the pot. Pour the fat out of the roasting pan, add cold water to the pan, and bring to a boil. Stir with a wooden spoon to loosen coagulated juices. Add this liquid to the pot. Add additional water, if necessary, to cover the bones; no higher than within 1" of the rim of the pot. Bring to a boil. Remove scum with a spoon. Reduce heat. Add thyme and peppercorns.

Simmer stock for at least 12, and as long as 72 hours. Add the parsley and simmer another 10 minutes.

You now have a pot of rather repulsive-looking brown liquid containing globs of gelatinous and fatty material. After straining, you will have a delicious and nourishing clear broth that forms the basis for many other recipes.

Remove bones and strain the stock into a large bowl. Let cool in the refrigerator and remove the congealed fat that rises to the top. Transfer to smaller containers and to the freezer for long-term storage.

Nourishing Traditions

Lamb Stock (Bone Broth)

Salt before roasting. Roast 1 lb. lamb soup bones at 500° for 20–25 minutes. Stir occasionally to prevent sticking.

Remove from oven and transfer bones to stock pot. Add 2 qt. water and 1/4 c. red wine (use something cheap but robust) to roasting pan and deglaze. Add all of the deglazed juices to the stock pot.

1 small onion or 1 leek, halved
1 med. carrot, halved lengthwise
1 sprig rosemary
1 tsp. thyme
2 cloves garlic, smashed and peeled
1 tsp. sea salt
5 peppercorns
1 Tbsp. sweet vermouth

Add to the stock pot and bring to a boil. Let it boil for 5 minutes, then cover the pot and simmer for 12–24 hours. Check periodically. If the water volume has dropped by more than half, add water back to a little over half and continue to simmer.

Strain through a cheesecloth-lined colander and chill overnight. Skim off the fat, package, and freeze.

Nancy Osborn, Cordero Farms

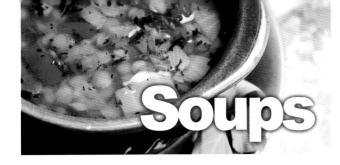

Soups

Red Meat Chile

3 lbs. ground beef or lamb
4 Tbsp. extra virgin olive oil or lard
1/4 cup red wine
2 cups beef stock
2 onions, finely chopped
2–4 small green chiles, seeded and chopped
2 cans tomatoes, briefly chopped in food processor
3 cloves garlic, peeled and mashed
1 Tbsp. ground cumin
2 Tbsp. dried oregano
2 Tbsp. dried basil
1/4–1/2 tsp. crushed red pepper
4 cups black or kidney beans, cooked
Garnish options: tortilla chips, organic & non-GMO
        chopped green onions
        piima cream or creme fraiche
        avocado slices
        chopped cilantro

In a heavy pot, brown meat in oil until crumbly. Add remaining ingredients, except garnishes, and simmer about 1 hour. Serve with garnishes.

Nourishing Traditions

Lentil Soup

4 cups lentils
Warm water
2 Tbsp. whey or lemon juice

4 Tbsp. butter, or 2 Tbsp. butter and 2 Tbsp. olive oil
1 small stalk celery, finely chopped
8 carrots, finely chopped
1 large onion, finely chopped
16–18 cups of water
2 heaping Tbsp. miso
1 Tbsp. Herbamare seasoning
Sea salt to taste
Parsley (fresh or dried)

Toppings:
    Grated Pecorino Romano cheese
    Plain yogurt
    Sour cream

Option: cooked whole grain pasta (follow instructions on box) or cooked brown rice (p. 113)

Cover lentils with warm water. Stir in 2 Tbsp. whey or lemon juice and leave in a warm place to soak for 7 hours. After soaking, drain water from lentils; set aside. Sauté vegetables in butter then add lentils, water, Herbamare, dried parsley, and salt. Bring to a soft boil, then simmer vegetables and lentils up to an hour, until lentils are soft. 15 minutes before done, ladle out 1/2 cup broth from soup, mix with miso until dissolved, then return back to soup. Serve in bowl with favorite topping. Sprinkle with fresh parsley.

During stage , add cooked spelt pasta or sprouted brown rice to each bowl before serving. This recipe makes a lot of soup and can be divided in half.

Vera Angeline (Dr. Menzel's mom)

Roasted Butternut Squash Soup

1/2 cup coconut oil
2 large butternut squash
1 onion, cut into large chunks
1 head garlic
1/2 tsp. rice bran oil or coconut oil

2 cups chicken stock
2 Tbsp. fresh lime juice
Sea salt & pepper to taste
Ground nutmeg, optional

Preheat oven to 350°. Pour oil into a roasting pan to coat the bottom. Cut the squash in half and remove the seeds. Place in pan, cut side down. Prick the skins with a sharp knife. Place onion around the edges. Cut the top of the garlic head off and drizzle with rice bran or coconut oil. Place in pan with the other vegetables. Bake for 45–60 minutes, or until tender. Remove from oven and cool slightly.

Scrape baked squash into a large stock pot. Add the roasted onion and garlic, squeezed out from the skins. Add chicken stock and lime juice and bring to a boil. Reduce heat and simmer for 15 minutes. Using a hand blender, purée the soup until smooth. Add nutmeg, salt, and pepper as desired.

The Eat-Clean Diet Favorites

Minestrone Soup

3–4 cloves garlic, minced
1 onion, chopped
4 Tbsp. olive oil/butter mixture
3 carrots, chopped
4 celery stalks, chopped

8–10 cups homemade vegetable, beef, or chicken stock
    or water with 2-3 Tbsp. miso
2 Tbsp. chopped fresh parsley, basil, and oregano
    (1 tsp. each if using dried herbs)
1 bay leaf
Sea salt & pepper to taste
1 28 oz. can crushed tomatoes
1/2 small head cabbage, shredded
1 zucchini, sliced
1 cup frozen spinach or 3 cups fresh
1 cup frozen green beans or fresh
4 oz. frozen organic corn (optional)
1 cup garbanzo beans, soaked & cooked
1 cup kidney beans, soaked & cooked
1 cup white canelli beans, soaked & cooked
Grated Pecorino Romano cheese
Fresh basil or parsley for garnish
Whole grain small pasta (einkorn, spelt, millet, or rice)

Follow the Basic Beans recipe (p. 167) for soaking and cooking beans. Sauté the first four ingredients in olive oil/butter mixture. Add remaining ingredients, except miso and cook until tender. About 15 minutes before serving take a cup of broth out of the soup and mix in the miso; add broth back to soup. Sprinkle grated cheese on top and garnish with fresh basil or parsley.

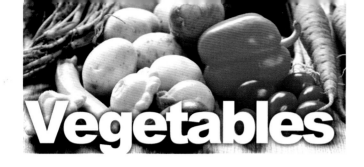

Vegetables

Sautéed Mixed Vegetables

4 cups spinach—trim, soak in cold water
     for 10 minutes and spin dry
2 cloves garlic, minced or pressed
2 Tbsp. cilantro, coarsely chopped
2 Tbsp. yellow onion, finely minced
2 Tbsp. butter or coconut oil
Sea salt & pepper

Heat butter or oil in a skillet on medium-high heat.
Sauté the onion and garlic for 2–3 minutes. Add the
spinach, cilantro, salt, and pepper and cook for about
2 minutes.

The Lazy Person's Whole Food Cookbook

Sautéed Garlic Spinach

Spinach or other greens
Butter or coconut oil
3 cloves garlic, pressed or finely chopped
Sea salt & pepper

Trim greens and wash. Melt butter or coconut oil in
skillet. Place leaves and garlic in the skillet. Sauté until
wilted, stirring occasionally. Season to taste.

Broccoli Sauté

2 Tbsp. butter
2 cloves garlic, minced
1/2 tsp. lemon zest
1 1/2 cups raw broccoli
1 Tbsp. lemon juice
1/2 tsp. sea salt
1/8 tsp. white pepper

Melt butter in a skillet. Add the garlic and lemon zest.
Add the broccoli and sauté for two minutes. Add
lemon juice, salt, and pepper. Toss and serve.

Sautéed Chard, Kale

*Don't be intimidated by chard. It's very tasty and loaded
with minerals. This recipe is one of my favorites.*

2 Tbsp. butter or 1 Tbsp. coconut oil
1/2 cup sliced onion
2 cloves garlic, pressed or finely chopped
1 bunch green chard, kale, or a mixture of any greens
1/4 tsp. sea salt

Heat butter or oil in a large skillet. Sauté the onion and
garlic together until they are translucent, 2–3 minutes.
Add the greens, stir, and cook on medium-high for
3–4 minutes.

Sautéed Cabbage & Vegetables

1 head green or Savoy cabbage,
     chopped into bite-sized pieces
1 bunch Swiss chard, collards or kale,
     chopped into bite size pieces
1 head broccoli, chopped into bite-sized pieces
1 medium onion, diced
2 cloves garlic, minced; or garlic powder to taste
1 stick organic butter
Sea salt and pepper to taste
Thyme to taste

Melt butter in large skillet. Add all vegetables to skillet.
Sprinkle thyme liberally on top and salt and pepper to
taste. Sauté until vegetables are tender.

Optional: To make a one-dish meal, add cooked
Italian beef sausage cut into bite-sized pieces.

Sautéed Vegetables

2 Tbsp. butter or coconut oil
1 medium onion, diced or sliced thin
2 gloves of garlic, minced
Sea salt and pepper to taste
Spice of choice
Vegetable of choice: Broccoli
                    Green beans
                    Peppers
                    Zucchini

Sauté butter, onions, and garlic. Add your favorite vegetable and sauté until tender. Use any vegetable or a combination of vegetables from the list. Thyme is one of my favorite herbs to add to green beans.

Sautéed Carrots

Carrots, julienne
Butter
Sea salt to taste
Cinnamon (optional)

Sauté carrots in butter until tender. Salt to taste. Yummy!

Sautéed Asparagus

3 Tbsp. butter
3 cloves garlic, minced
1 bunch of fresh asparagus spears
2 plum tomatoes (optional), diced
Sea salt and pepper to taste

Sauté butter, garlic, and asparagus for approximately 10 minutes or until tender. Add optional tomato and sauté an additional 5 minutes.

Honey-Lime Brussel Sprouts

1 lb. brussel sprouts
1 lime, for zest and juice
1 tsp. honey
2 Tbsp. butter
1 Tbsp. expeller-pressed coconut oil
Sea salt & pepper

Trim brussel sprouts; discard ends and remove outer leaves. Cut each in half lengthwise, then place on a cutting surface, cut-side down. Cut into thin slices.

Finely grate lime peel to make 1 tsp. zest. Cut lime in half and squeeze to make 1 1/2 to 2 Tbsp. juice. Mix lime zest, juice, and honey in a small bowl. Set aside.

Melt butter in a large skillet over medium-high heat. Add oil and tilt skillet to blend. Add sprouts and cook 3–4 minutes or until they begin to wilt and brown. Season to taste with salt and pepper. Stir in lime mixture and cook 1 more minute. Remove from heat and serve while hot.

Ginger Carrots

Prepare 3 days ahead.

4 cups grated carrots, loosely packed
1 Tbsp. fresh ginger, grated
1 tsp. sea salt
2 Tbsp. whey
   (if not available, add an additional 1 tsp. salt)
Canning jar

Mix all ingredients in a bowl and pound with a wooden pounder to release juices. Place in a quart-sized wide-mouth mason jar and press down firmly until juices cover the carrots. The top of the carrots should be at least 1" below the top of the jar. Cover tightly and leave at room temperature for 3 days before moving to cold storage.

Nourishing Traditions

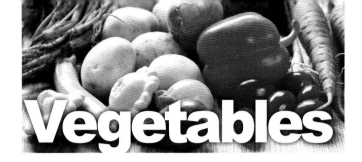

Vegetables

Veggies on the Grill

1 eggplant, thinly sliced
2 zucchinis, thinly sliced, lengthwise
5 plum tomatoes, sliced lengthwise
1 onion, thinly sliced
2 yellow squash, thinly sliced, lengthwise
3–5 baby bella or portabella mushrooms, sliced
Arugula leaves
Raw goat cheddar cheese (optional)
Sprouted whole grain buns

Marinade: 4 Tbsp. olive oil
                  2 Tbsp. balsamic vinegar
                  2 tsp. lemon juice
                  4 cloves garlic
Or use Greek Marinade (p. 161).

Marinate veggies for several hours or overnight. You can make more marinade if you wish and use it as you are grilling to keep the veggies moist.

Grill using a veggie basket for the grill or a George Foreman Indoor Grill, or roast in the oven, or pan sauté. Serve as a side dish or on a sprouted whole grain bun topped with melted raw goat cheddar and arugula leaves.

Spaghetti or Acorn Squash

1 squash
Water
Butter
Sea salt

Preheat oven to 350°. Cut squash in half, scrape out the seeds, and place face-down in a baking dish with 1 inch of water. Bake for 1 hour. For spaghetti squash, scoop out squash noodles onto plate and serve with butter and salt or serve topped with Bolognese sauce (p. 165). Acorn squash creates it own bowl; serve with butter, salt, or topped with Bolognese sauce.
Jessica Menzel Brown

Cauliflower

1 small onion, diced small
3 sticks celery, diced small
1 head cauliflower, diced small
4 Tbsp. butter
Sea salt to taste

Cut each of the vegetables very small and sauté in butter until tender. Salt to taste.
Jessica Menzel Brown

Beets

3–4 beets
Filtered water

Wash beets and cut off stems. Place in a sauce pan and fill with filtered water. Bring to a boil and cook until tender. Fork should slide out easily. Peel and slice. Store beets in glass container and use in salads, ferment, or sauté in butter and add a pinch of salt.

Sweet Potato Rounds

2 sweet potatoes, peeled and sliced thin
4 Tbsp. butter
Sea salt to taste

Melt butter in a large frying pan on medium-high heat.
Add potato slices and sprinkle with salt. Cook until
tender and crispy.

Variations:
Sweet Potatoes, diced
Onions, diced
Green Peppers, diced
Mushrooms, sliced
Mix-and-match variations
Cumin to taste
Coriander to taste

Rosalie Larkin,
Variations by Michele Menzel

Spinach Casserole

Absolutely my family's favorite Thanksgiving side dish!

2 pkgs. chopped spinach, thawed
1 stick butter, melted
2 eggs
4 oz. fresh mushrooms, chopped
1/4 cup Pecorino Romano cheese, grated
1 cup homemade breadcrumbs (p. 158)
1/2 tsp. sea salt
1 tsp. garlic powder
1/4 tsp. pepper

Preheat oven to 325°. Mix all ingredients together.
Bake covered for 25 minutes. Uncover and bake
10 more minutes.

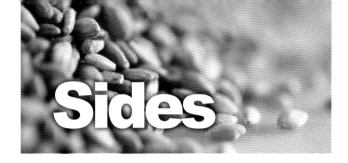

Sides

Grilled Pineapple

1 whole, fresh pineapple*
3 Tbsp. honey
1 Tbsp. lemon juice, lime juice, or orange juice
   (your choice), freshly squeezed
1/2 tsp. black pepper, freshly ground

Cut off the top of the pineapple, then peel it with a serrated knife. Remove any eyes with a paring knife. Cut into quarters from top to bottom. Slice out the core from each quarter. Cut each quarter slice into four pieces (two pieces lengthwise and two cross-wise). You should now have 16 wedges of pineapple (each about 3" x 1").

Heat grill to medium. In a small bowl, combine honey, juice, and black pepper. Thoroughly brush the glaze onto each slice of pineapple. Oil grill rack. Place pineapple wedges on the grill and cook approximately 4 minutes on each side until the pineapple becomes fragrant and starts to dry out on the surface. NOTE: Do not overcook the pineapple spears or they will turn mushy and burn. Remove from the grill and brush with any additional glaze. Serve and enjoy!

Note: The grilled pineapple can be kept at room temperature for up to 8 hours. Warm before serving.

*Smell the pineapple when purchasing. The stronger the smell, the riper the fruit. Turn the pineapple upside down in an empty container for a few hours before you grill it to distribute the sugar throughout the fruit.

www.whatscookingamerica.net

Deviled Eggs

12 eggs
Several Tbsp. Wilderness Family Naturals Mayonnaise
   or homemade mayonnaise
1/2 tsp. mustard
1/2–1 tsp. dried parsley
Sea salt and pepper to taste
Sprinkle with paprika for garnish

Put eggs in a pot to boil. When the water comes to a boil, set timer for 10 minutes. Remove from heat, drain, bathe with cold water. Peel and rinse. Slice each egg in half lengthwise, removing the yolks and putting them in bowl. Display whites on a serving dish. Mix yolks with all other ingredients until smooth. Spoon into holes of the egg whites and garnish with paprika. Makes 24 deviled eggs.

Stuffed Mushrooms

8 large mushrooms
2 Tbsp. butter
1 large garlic clove, crushed
3 Tbsp. homemade breadcrumbs (p. 158)
1/4 tsp. basil
1 tsp. lemon juice
Pepper to taste

Preheat oven to 375°. Remove and chop mushroom stems. Sauté chopped mushroom stems in butter. Add garlic and breadcrumbs. Stir in basil, lemon juice, and pepper. Sauté briefly. Fill the mushroom caps with the stuffing. Place stuffed mushrooms in a pan and cover with parchment paper. Bake for 20 minutes. Serve immediately.

Sue Lampman

Basic Soaked Brown Rice

2 cups brown rice
4 Tbsp. whey, yogurt, kefir or lemon juice
  added to 4 cups warm water
1 tsp. sea salt
2-4 Tbsp. butter

Place rice and warm water mixture in a flameproof casserole and leave in a warm place for at least 7 hours. Bring to a boil, skim, reduce heat, stir in salt and butter and cover tightly. Without removing lid, cook over lowest possible heat for about 45 minutes.

Nourishing Traditions

Sprouted Brown Rice

2 1/2 cups water   2 Tbsp. butter
1 cup rice   1/2 tsp. sea salt

Heat water until hot, add rice, butter and salt. Bring to a boil. Simmer for 50 minutes.

Steven Menzel

Brown Rice with Onions & Pecans

1 cup brown rice, sprouted
3 Tbsp. butter
1/2 cup red onion, chopped
1/2 cup green onion, chopped
2 garlic cloves, minced
1/2 cup crispy pecans, coarsely chopped
2 Tbsp. green onions, chopped

Prepare brown rice in medium saucepan. About 15 minutes before rice is done, melt butter in heavy skillet over medium-low heat. Add red onions and sauté, stirring frequently until softened, about 10 minutes. Stir in garlic, pecans, and green onions. Sauté, stirring constantly until the onions are golden and garlic is tender, about 5 minutes. Remove rice from heat into bowl; spoon the onions/nuts on top of rice and toss lightly. Garnish with green onions.

Mashed Potatoes

Mashed potatoes are an American favorite and can be a healthy part of a meal. We don't have them very often but they are a must with spicy meatloaf or Thanksgiving dinner!

3 lb. red potatoes
Filtered water
Sea salt and pepper
2 Tbsp. (or more) butter, melted
1/4 cup (or more) warm raw goat or cow milk

Optional: garlic powder
         sour cream

Wash and dice potatoes. In salted water, boil potatoes with the skin on until tender. Drain water and mash in pot. This will keep the potatoes hot. Put butter and milk in a saucepan on low until butter is melted. Pour butter and milk into the pot and mash. Salt and pepper to taste. Add garlic and/or sour cream if desired.

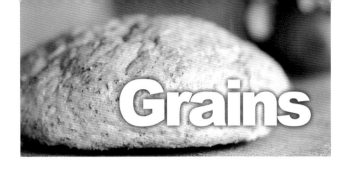

Grains

Sprouted Spelt Biscuits

Hearty but yummy! Great with soups.
Can be used for topping of Vegetable Pot Pie (p. 163).

2 cups sprouted spelt flour
2 tsp. aluminum-free baking powder
1/2 tsp. sea salt
4 Tbsp. coconut oil
3/4 cup raw cow or goat milk
    (or Kalona Supernatural whole milk
    or Organic Valley grass-fed whole milk)

Preheat oven to 400°. Sift the dry ingredients together. Combine oil and milk, then stir into dry mixture. Form dough (may need more flour or milk) and roll into balls. Drop onto greased cookie sheets and press down into biscuit form. Bake for 20 minutes.

Jessica Menzel Brown

Homemade Italian Breadcrumbs

1/2 loaf sprouted, sourdough or naturally fermented
    bread (approx. 9 slices)
1/2 tsp. Herbamare
1 tsp. sea salt
1 tsp. garlic
1 Tbsp. Italian seasoning or create your own
    (parsley, basil, oregano)
2 Tbsp. finely grated Pecorino Romano cheese
    (optional)

In a food processor, chop all ingredients into fine crumbs. Store in freezer. Use as breading for eggplant, chicken Parmesan, fish, in the stuffed mushrooms recipe, or any recipe that calls for breadcrumbs.

Sprouted Crackers

5 cups sprouted flour (your preference)
2 1/4 cups whole buttermilk or yogurt
1/2 cup unsalted butter, melted
1 Tbsp. aluminum-free baking powder
2 tsp. sea salt

Preheat oven to 300°. Place flour and buttermilk in bowl and mix until a slightly stiff dough forms. Add melted butter, baking powder, salt and flavoring (see Variations, below). Blend well.

Roll out 1/4 of the dough at a time onto a floured surface to about 1/8" thick. Cut into squares with knife or pizza wheel. Place close together on lightly buttered baking sheets. Lightly brush with extra melted butter. Bake for 30 minutes. Reduce heat to 200° and continue to bake for three more hours or until completely dried. Will be crispy and full of flavor.

Variations:

Rosemary/Walnut: Add 2 rounded Tbsp. of ground
    rosemary, 1 Tbsp. dried rosemary leaves, and
    1/4 tsp. of walnut oil
Sesame/Poppyseed: Add 2 Tbsp. each of the seeds
Cinnamon: Add 4 Tbsp. ground cinnamon, 1/2 tsp.
    cinnamon oil and 3/4 cup date or maple sugar
Cracked Pepper: Add 2 Tbsp. of cracked black, green,
    or pink peppercorns. Sprinkle tops with sea salt.
Herbed: Add 1 1/2 Tbsp. dried dill, 1 tsp. each basil,
    thyme, oregano, and tarragon

To Your Health Sprouted Flour Co.

Scottish Oatmeal Scones

1/2 cup butter, melted
1/3 cup raw cow or goat milk
1 egg
1 1/2 cups sprouted spelt flour
1 1/4 cups of sprouted oats
1/4 cup Rapunzel whole cane sugar
1 Tbsp. baking powder
1 tsp. cream of tartar
1/2 tsp. sea salt
1/2 cup raisins (or dried cherries)

Combine all dry ingredients and add all liquids. Mix until moistened. Stir in raisins. Knead dough a few times on floured surface and shape into two circles. Cut each circle into 6 or 8 wedges. Bake at 425° for 12–15 minutes or until lightly browned. Serve with butter and honey.

Sweet Potato Scones

1/2 cup raw cow or goat milk
2 cups sprouted spelt flour
1 Tbsp. baking powder
1/2 tsp. baking soda
1/2 tsp. sea salt
1/2 cup Rapunzel whole cane sugar or 1/3 cup honey
1/2 tsp. cinnamon
4 Tbsp. butter, melted
1 cup cooked sweet potato, mashed
1 egg, slightly beaten

Preheat oven to 400°. Whisk all dry ingredients together. Combine all wet ingredients. Mix together. Spoon onto greased cookie sheet and bake for 15 minutes.

Sweet Potato Rolls

2 1/4 tsp. yeast
1/2 cup lukewarm water
1/2 cup yogurt
3/4 cup sweet potato purée
1 Tbsp. butter, melted
1 1/4 tsp. sea salt
2 large egg yolks, lightly beaten
4 cups sprouted spelt flour
2 Tbsp. butter or olive oil, melted

In a large bowl, dissolve the yeast in warm water, and let stand 5 minutes. Fold in the yogurt. Whisk in sweet potato purée, 1 Tbsp. butter, salt, and egg yolks. Lightly spoon the flour into a dry measuring cup; level with a knife. Add 3 1/2 cups of flour and stir until a soft dough forms.

Turn the dough out onto a floured surface. Knead until smooth and elastic (about 8 minutes). Add enough of the remaining flour, 1 Tbsp. at a time, to prevent the dough from sticking to your hands (it will feel soft and tacky). Place the dough in a large bowl coated with olive oil, turning to coat the top. Cover and let rise in a warm place 45 minutes or until doubled in size. Punch down the dough, cover, and let rest 5 minutes.

Line two baking sheets with parchment paper. Divide the dough into 24 equal pieces. Cover to prevent drying. Shape each piece into a 9" rope and tie it into a knot, tucking the ends under the roll. Place rolls on the prepared sheet. Cover and let the rolls rise 30–45 minutes, or until doubled in size.

Preheat the oven to 400°. Bake for 8 minutes. Rotate the pans from top to bottom; bake an additional 6–8 minutes or until the rolls are golden-brown. Remove from pans and cool on wire racks. Brush rolls with melted butter or olive oil.

Essential Eating Sprouted Baking

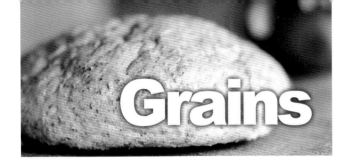

Grains

Sprouted Spelt Tortillas

2 cups sprouted spelt flour
1 tsp. sea salt
2 Tbsp. lard or coconut oil
Approximately 1 cup warm water

Mix flour and salt. Add oil and mix with hands or a
fork until crumbly. Slowly add water until dough forms
into a ball that is not too sticky but holds together
well. Knead for 3 minutes. Divide dough into 1" balls.
Put the balls in an oiled mixing bowl and cover with
a moist towel. Heat a cast iron skillet or tortilla maker
over medium heat and add a small amount of oil. Oil
a clean, flat work surface. With an oiled rolling pin,
roll out one ball of dough about 1/8" thick (or to your
desired thickness) and about 6–8" across. Place tortilla in the pan. Cook for 25 seconds or until bubbles
form. Flip with a spatula and cook for another 15–25
seconds, or until the bubbles are browned. Remove
tortilla from pan and place between moist towels in
low oven to keep warm and moist. Repeat until all of
the balls have been rolled out and cooked. Add oil
to pan and rolling pin as needed. Makes about 10
medium tortillas.

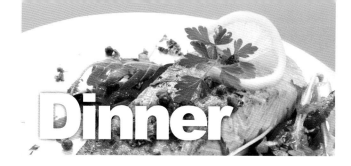

Dinner

Greek Marinade
for Fish, Chicken, or Beef

1/2 cup lemon juice
1/2 cup olive oil
3 Tbsp. fresh oregano, chopped
3 Tbsp. fresh mint, chopped
1 tsp. garlic, minced
1 tsp. lemon peel (zest), finely shredded
1/4 tsp. sea salt

Stir together lemon juice, olive oil, oregano, mint, garlic, lemon zest, and salt. Pour over meat of choice. Turn to coat with marinade. Marinate in refrigerator for at least 30 minutes. Drain meat, reserving marinade. Cook meat over medium heat for 8–15 minutes or until it reaches desired temperature: fish (145°), chicken (160°–175°), beef (125°–160°), turning once and brushing with marinade halfway through cooking. Discard any remaining marinade.
The Cooking Girl, Christa Carretero

Asian Marinade
for Fish, Chicken, or Beef

1/4 cup organic unpasturized soy sauce or tamari
2 Tbsp. dark sesame oil   1 Tbsp. minced garlic
2 Tbsp. rice vinegar   1 Tbsp. minced ginger
Ground black pepper to taste   1 scallion, sliced thin

See Greek Marinade for instructions.
The Cooking Girl, Christa Carretero

Latin Marinade
for Fish, Chicken, or Beef

1/2 cup fresh lime juice
1/2 cup fresh orange juice
1 garlic clove, minced
1/2 medium red onion, finely diced
4 jalapeño chilies, minced (seeds and ribs removed
    to control spiciness, if desired)
Sea salt and pepper to taste
1 cup extra-virgin olive oil
Cilantro leaves

See Greek Marinade for instructions.
The Cooking Girl, Christa Carretero

Crock Pot or Oven Roasted
Chicken & Vegetables

1 whole organic, free-range chicken, rinsed
6–7 med. red potatoes, chopped
3–4 stalks of celery, chopped   Sea salt & pepper
5 carrots, chopped   Water/chicken broth
1 onion, sliced   Optional spices:
1 1/2 tsp. garlic powder   parsley, sage, thyme

Preheat oven to 350°. Place chicken and chopped vegetables in a baking pan, drizzle with olive oil, and/or cover chicken with pats of butter. Pour water or chicken broth into pan until it covers the bottom at least 2" deep. Sprinkle with salt, pepper, and garlic powder. Top with optional spices. Place in oven. Cook for 1 1/2–2 hours. Check regularly to make sure there is liquid in the bottom. Spoon the liquid over the top of the chicken and veggies to keep them moist.

Serve immediately. Make broth from leftover chicken carcass—refer to chicken stock recipe (p. 148).

For crockpot: Follow same instructions for oven except place everything in crockpot and cook according to your crockpot directions for chicken. This is usually 8-10 hours on low or 4-5 hours on high.

Rena Menzel

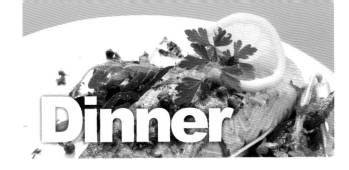

Dinner

Italian Sautéed Chicken

6 Tbsp. coconut oil
1 medium onion, chopped
4 garlic cloves, minced
7–8 pieces of chicken, bone-in or boneless
Sea salt & pepper
Basil, fresh or dried
1/2 cup wine
Homemade canned tomatoes or 28 oz. can
    crushed tomatoes or fresh diced tomatoes
    or 1 jar tomato sauce, no sugar
Bunch fresh spinach (optional)

Sauté onion about 3 minutes. Add garlic, then chicken. Brown. Add salt, pepper, and basil to taste. Add wine and tomatoes (or sauce). Cook until heated through. Ten minutes before serving, top with fresh spinach.

Coconut Chicken

1 quart chicken stock
1 1/2 cups whole coconut milk
    or 7 oz. creamed coconut
1/2 lb. chicken, cubed
    or leftover chicken already cooked
1/4 tsp. red pepper flakes,
    or fresh diced jalapeño chilies,
    or 1/4 tsp. dried cayenne pepper
1 tsp. fresh ginger, grated
Sea salt or fish sauce (optional)
Juice of 1 lemon
2–3 green onions, finely chopped (optional)
Chopped cilantro for garnish

Simmer all ingredients, except cilantro, until meat is cooked. Garnish with cilantro.

Nourishing Traditions

Easy Pan Chicken

6 pieces of chicken (bone-in or boneless)
6 Tbsp. expeller-pressed coconut oil, butter,
    extra virgin olive oil, or combination
1 medium onion, finely sliced
1 3.5-oz. jar organic capers
2–3 cloves of garlic
1/2 cup chicken broth, more as needed
1 tsp. sea salt
Simply Organic Chicken Seasoning

Melt oil in a large skillet over medium-high heat. Sprinkle seasoning and salt on both sides of the chicken. Put in pan and add onions, garlic, capers and chicken broth. Cover and let chicken cook on medium heat for 20 minutes (10 minutes if boneless). Cook until meat thermometer reads 180°. Add any variation of vegetables below, cover with lid, and cook an additional few minutes until vegetables are tender.

Vegetable Variations:

    Mushrooms, sliced
    Tomatoes, sliced
    Squash, sliced
    Spinach, kale, or chard, fresh or frozen
    Zucchini, sliced

Jessica Menzel Brown & Michele Menzel

Tuna Spaghetti

1 lb. whole-grain spaghetti
    from acceptable grain list
1 can water-packed tuna,
    undrained
6 Tbsp. olive oil
2 tsp. lemon juice
1/2 c. fresh parsley, chopped
1/2 tsp. garlic powder
1 tsp. sea salt
1/2 tsp. pepper
1/2 tsp. dill weed
1/4 cup Pecorino
    Romano cheese,
    grated

Cook pasta and drain well. Add all other ingredients into the pot of the cooked pasta and toss. Top with grated cheese. Serve immediately.

Sue Lampman

Chicken with Sweet & Sour Sauce

8 chicken breasts, skin on
1 cup fresh orange juice
1 cup fresh lemon juice
1 cup apple cider vinegar
2 Tbsp. fresh ginger, minced

2 Tbsp. garlic, minced
1/2 tsp. red pepper flakes
3 Tbsp. extra virgin olive oil
2 cups chicken stock

Trim chicken breasts and pound lightly with the small prong side of a meat hammer. In a saucepan, combine remaining ingredients except olive oil and chicken stock. Bring to a boil. Reduce heat and simmer for several minutes. Allow to cool and stir in olive oil. Marinate the chicken breasts in this mixture for several hours or overnight. Remove from marinade and broil about 7 minutes per side. Keep warm on a heated platter in the oven while making sauce.

Place marinade and stock in a saucepan and boil vigorously until sauce is reduced by half. To serve, slice the chicken breasts across the grain, arrange on individual plates and spoon sauce over it. Serve with steamed cabbage, sautéed red peppers, and sautéed mushroom slices.

Nourishing Traditions

Vegetable, Chicken, or Beef Pot Pie

4 cups chicken broth, vegetable stock, beef stock or
  water, with 1 Tbsp. miso
1 Tbsp. fresh parsley, chopped
  or 1 1/2 tsp. dried parsley
1 cup onion, chopped
2 cups carrots, sliced
1 cup potatoes, diced
1 cup green beans, fresh or frozen
1 cup peas
1 cup corn (non-GMO, organic)
2 cups cooked chicken or beef, diced
2/3 cup sprouted spelt flour
1/2 cup raw cow or goat milk, or cream

Preheat oven to 450°. Mix everything in large pot. Add peas, corn, and meat. Cook until veggies are tender. Blend flour and milk and add to pot. Stir until thickened, about 15 minutes. Pour into 3-quart casserole dish, and top with company pie crust (p. 170) or biscuits (p. 158). Bake for 15 minutes. Reduce heat to 350° and bake an additional 30 minutes.

Lamb Meatballs

1 medium onion, finely diced (optional)
1 Tbsp. olive oil
1 cup homemade Italian breadcrumbs (p. 158)
1/2 cup fresh cream or raw milk
2 lbs. ground lamb
2 tsp. dried thyme
2 eggs
1 tsp. sea salt
1 tsp. fresh ground pepper

Preheat oven to 350°. Sauté onion in olive oil. Soak breadcrumbs in cream and set aside. Combine meat, thyme, eggs, salt, and pepper. Mix in onion and bread-crumb mixture. Mix with hands thoroughly. Form into 1 1/2" balls and place on stainless steel baking sheets. Bake until cooked through, about 10–15 minutes.

Place the cooked meatballs in a crock pot with two quarts of warm lamb broth and serve.

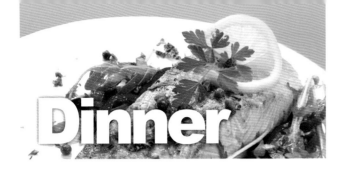

Dinner

Spicy Meatloaf

2 lbs. of ground beef or other meat (lamb, turkey, etc.)
1/2 lb. ground heart (optional)
1 medium onion, peeled and finely chopped
1 carrot, peeled and finely chopped
1 stalk celery, finely chopped
4 Tbsp. butter
1/2 tsp. red pepper flakes
1 tsp. dried thyme
1 tsp. cracked pepper
1 tsp. sea salt
1 1/2 cups homemade Italian breadcrumbs (p. 158)
1 cup raw goat milk or raw cream*
1 egg
1 Tbsp. fish sauce (optional)
4 Tbsp. tomato paste

Soak breadcrumbs in cream. Sauté onions, carrots, and celery in butter until soft. Mix in red pepper flakes, thyme, pepper and salt.

Have a 9"x13" pan ready. Using your hands, mix meat with sautéed vegetables, soaked breadcrumbs, egg, and optional fish sauce. Form into a loaf and set in the pan. Top with tomato paste. (I usually place a sliced onion on the top.) Add about 1 cup water to the pan. Bake at 350° for about 1 1/2 hours.

*Use raw milk or raw cream if available. If you don't have either, buy organic cream at the health-food store.

Original recipe from Nourishing Traditions
Revision by Michele Menzel

Beef, Lamb, or Turkey Burgers
Topped with goat cheese, mushrooms, spinach & onions

1 lb. grass-fed beef, lamb, or turkey
1 slice sprouted spelt bread made into
     breadcrumbs (using a food processor)
1/4 cup raw goat milk, raw cow milk or water
1 egg
1 tsp. virgin olive oil or coconut oil
1/4–1/2 tsp. of each: sea salt, pepper, garlic powder,
     and fresh or dried parsley
Sliced raw goat cheddar cheese

Mix all ingredients except cheese in a bowl and divide meat into four burgers. Cook on a George-Foreman-type indoor grill, outside grill, or in a frying pan until medium well. Cook grass-fed meat slowly and not well done. Top with sliced cheese and cover to melt.

8 oz. sliced mushrooms or fresh spinach
1 large onion, thinly sliced
3 Tbsp. butter
     or 2 Tbsp. coconut oil
1 clove of garlic, minced
Sea salt to taste
Sprouted spelt buns

Sauté sliced mushrooms and/or spinach and onion slices in butter until onions are soft and translucent.

Top burger with mushrooms and onions, or spinach and onions. Serve with or without sprouted spelt bread or buns, toasted and buttered.

Lentil Burgers

2 lb. lentils
1 onion, finely chopped
2 fresh garlic cloves, minced
3 eggs
1/4 cup breadcrumbs, homemade
1/4 tsp. oregano
1/4 tsp. basil
1/4 tsp. parsley

Wash, clean, and soak lentils overnight. Cook until soft. Drain and mash. Sauté onion; adding garlic at the end. Mix with mashed lentils. Add eggs, breadcrumbs, and seasonings. Shape and fry in butter on medium heat until done. Turn once.

Homemade Pizza

1 pkg. yeast (or 1 Tbsp.)
1 cup warm water (105–115°)
1 tsp. Rapunzel whole cane sugar
1 tsp. sea salt
2 Tbsp. coconut oil
2 1/2 cups sprouted spelt flour

Muir Glen organic pizza sauce
Raw goat milk cheese

Preheat oven to 350°. Dissolve yeast in warm water. Stir in remaining ingredients one at a time until you have a nice ball of dough. Knead. Let stand 30 minutes. Meanwhile, grease and flour your pans. Roll out dough. Top with sauce and cheese. Bake 20 minutes. If baking two pizzas, rotate pans after 10 minutes. Serve with a large tossed salad. Enjoy!

Additional Toppings:
Sautéed mushrooms, bell peppers, spinach, onions and/or recommended meats.

Marinara Sauce

3 sprigs fresh parsley (or 1 1/2 tsp. dried)
6 basil leaves, chopped (or 1 1/2 tsp. dried)
1 1/2 tsp. oregano (optional)
8 cloves garlic, minced
1 small onion, diced
3–4 Tbsp. olive oil/butter combo
2 cans crushed tomatoes

Sauté veggies in oil for about 5 minutes. Add tomatoes. Let simmer for 1/2 hour or longer, while you prepare pasta.

Option: Add zucchini to first 4 ingredients and sauté for 10 minutes before adding tomato sauce. Add fresh spinach 5 minutes before serving over whole-grain pasta.

Bolognese Sauce

Use Marinara Sauce ingredients (above), plus:

1 lb. Italian sausage
1 lb. ground beef
1/4 to 1/2 cup red wine (optional)

Sauté garlic and onion in oil for 5 minutes. Add Italian sausage and ground beef. After 5 minutes of sautéing, peel off sausage casings and dice into bite-sized pieces. Sauté until beef is browned. Add spices, tomatoes, and wine. Cover and cook on low for at least one hour. Serve over whole grain spelt spaghetti, or other whole grain pasta.

Option: When on Stage 1 or 2, serve sauce over acorn or spaghetti squash.

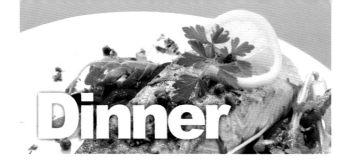

Dinner

Crock Pot or Oven Roast Beef

2–4 lbs. beef chuck, rump, sirloin, or Pike's Peak roast
Sea salt and pepper
3 large carrots, peeled and sliced
2 medium onions, sliced
2 stalks of celery, sliced
2–3 large potatoes, quartered or diced
1 lb. fresh mushrooms, sliced (optional)
1–1 1/2 cups of beef broth
1 cup red wine (optional)
2 cloves garlic, minced
3 sprigs fresh thyme, stemmed
    or 1 1/2 tsp. dried thyme
1 bay leaf

Place meat in crock pot or roasting pan and season with salt and pepper. Add remaining ingredients. *In crock pot:* Cover and cook on low for 10–12 hours, on high for 6–8 hours, or until meat is tender. *In the oven:* Set oven for 350°. Cover and cook for 2 1/2–3 hours or until meat is tender.

Crockpot Beef Stew

2–4 lbs. beef chuck stew meat, cut into 1" cubes
1/2 cup sprouted flour
Sea salt and pepper
3 cups beef broth
1 Tbsp. Worcestershire sauce
3 cloves garlic, minced
2 bay leaves
6 small potatoes, quartered
2–3 onions, chopped
3 celery stalks, chopped

Sprinkle flour, salt, and pepper over meat in crockpot. Add remaining ingredients and stir well. Cover and cook on low for 8–10 hours or on high for 5–6 hours, or until meat is tender. Stir thoroughly before serving.

Grilled Garlic Butter Shrimp

1 1/2 lb. large, wild-caught shrimp,
    peeled and deveined (1/2 lb. per person)
1/2 cup butter
2 Tbsp. extra virgin olive oil
1/8 cup orange juice, freshly squeezed
    (omit in Stage)
3–4 cloves garlic, minced
1 Tbsp. dry, white wine or fresh lemon juice
1 Tbsp. fresh, flat-leaf parsley, chopped
1 1/2 tsp. fresh basil, finely chopped
Sea salt and black pepper

Place shrimp in a large bowl. Combine remaining ingredients. Divide sauce in half. Pour 1/2 of the sauce onto shrimp. Toss to coat, cover, and place in refrigerator for 30–60 minutes. Heat grill to medium heat. Heat reserved sauce in pan on low until warm. Put shrimp onto skewers. Place onto grill and cook 2–3 minutes per side. When shrimp is no longer translucent, remove from heat, pour heated sauce over top, and serve.

Liver & Onions

Buy liver that is organic and fresh. The butcher should remove the surrounding filament; otherwise, the edges will curl when it is cooked. Liver should be sliced about 1/4-inch to 3/4-inch thick. The taste is greatly improved if the liver slices are first soaked in lemon juice for several hours before cooking. This draws out impurities and gives a nicer texture.

1 1/2 lbs. sliced liver
Juice of 2–3 lemons
1 cup sprouted spelt flour
1/2 tsp. sea salt
1/2 tsp. pepper
4 Tbsp. butter
4 cups onion, finely sliced
2 Tbsp. butter
2 Tbsp. extra virgin olive oil

Marinate liver slices in lemon juice for several hours. Pat slices dry and dredge in a mixture of flour, salt, and pepper. In a heavy skillet over high heat, sauté slices, two at a time, in butter. Transfer to a heated platter and keep warm in the oven. Meanwhile, in a separate pan, sauté the onions in butter and olive oil over medium heat for about 1/2 hour or until golden brown. Pour over liver and serve.

Variation: Liver and Mushrooms

Instead of onions, sauté 1 lb. of fresh mushrooms, washed, patted dry, and sliced.

Nourishing Traditions

Basic Beans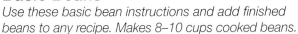

Use these basic bean instructions and add finished beans to any recipe. Makes 8–10 cups cooked beans.

2 cups beans (black, kidney, pinto, or white beans;
    or lentils or black-eyed peas)
Warm, filtered water
2 Tbsp. whey or lemon juice
4 cloves garlic, peeled and mashed (optional)
Sea salt and pepper

Cover beans with warm water. Stir in whey or lemon juice and leave in a warm place for 12–24 hours, depending on the size of the bean. Drain, rinse, and add water to cover beans. Bring to a boil and skim off foam. Reduce heat and add optional garlic. Simmer, covered, for 4–8 hours. Check occasionally and add more water as necessary. Season to taste.

Nourishing Traditions

Taco Salad or Tacos

2 Tbsp. butter
1 small onion, finely chopped
1 small green pepper, finely chopped
1 garlic clove or 1/2 tsp. garlic powder
1 lb. ground beef, lamb, or turkey
2 Tbsp. fresh cilantro leaves
2 Tbsp. organic tomato paste diluted in 1/2 cup water
    or 1/2 cup plain tomato sauce
Chili powder to taste
Sea salt and pepper to taste

Toppings:

    1 cup cooked sprouted brown rice
    Shredded romaine lettuce
        (or other green, leafy lettuce)
    Goat or cow cheddar cheese, grated
    Avocado slices or guacamole
    Tomatoes, diced or your favorite salsa

Tortilla or Wrap:

    Coconut wrap
    Sprouted corn, Einkorn, or spelt tortilla

Sauté onion, green pepper, and garlic in butter. Add meat and brown. Add tomato sauce and spices. Simmer for a few minutes. Layer on a plate—brown rice, meat, shredded cheese, lettuce, tomato, and avocado. Or serve in a coconut wrap or sprouted tortilla.

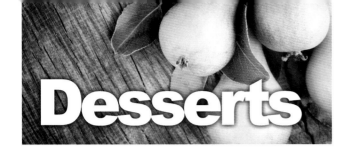

Desserts

All desserts should be consumed occasionally.
All desserts are recommended after the 48 days.

Baked Pears

1/2 cup lemon juice
1 cup red wine
1/2 cup honey or maple syrup
8 whole pears
1/2 cup sweet cream sauce, optional

Preheat oven to 350°. Combine lemon juice, wine and honey (or syrup) in a small pan and simmer. Peel pears and core from bottom end. Set on sides in buttered pyrex dish and pour wine mixture over them. Bake for 30 minutes, turning and basting frequently. Carefully remove pears to a bowl and chill well. Pour syrup into a small saucepan and boil down until it thickens. Let cool. Pour optional sweet cream sauce over chilled pears.

Nourishing Traditions

Sweet Cream Sauce

(Creme Anglaise)
2 cups heavy cream, preferably raw,
   not ultra-pasteurized
1/2 cup maple syrup or honey
1 Tbsp. grated ginger, optional
1 Tbsp. vanilla extract
5 large egg yolks

Combine cream, syrup or honey, optional ginger and vanilla in a bowl. Heat until quite warm to the touch, but not burning, by placing the bowl in a pan of simmering water. Meanwhile, place egg yolks in a double boiler and heat for several minutes until pale. Over a low flame, add the warm cream mixture to yolks very gradually, stirring constantly, until the mixture thickens slightly. Chill well. Serve with fresh berries or other fruit.

Nourishing Traditions

Oatmeal Raisin Cookies

1 1/4 cups sprouted spelt flour
1 tsp. baking soda
1/2 tsp. sea salt
1/2 tsp. cinnamon
1 cup butter, softened
1/3–3/4 cup honey
2 eggs
1 tsp. vanilla
3 cups oatmeal. soaked
1 cup raisins
1/2 cup crispy nuts, optional

Preheat oven to 350°. Mix dry ingredients and set aside. Beat butter, honey, eggs, and vanilla. Blend in dry ingredients, then add the oatmeal, raisins, and nuts. Drop by spoonfuls onto a baking sheet. Bake for 7–8 minutes. These freeze well.

Real Peanut Butter Cookies

Yummy!! These are my personal favorites!!!

1 cup organic peanut butter
2/3 cup honey
1/4 cup expeller-pressed coconut oil
1 egg
1/4 tsp. sea salt
1/2 tsp. vanilla
1 1/2 cup sprouted spelt flour or whole spelt flour
1 tsp. aluminum-free baking powder

Preheat oven to 375°. Beat together peanut butter, honey and oil until smooth. Beat in egg, salt, and vanilla. Mix together flour and baking powder and add to mixture. Using hands if necessary, form a thick, but not dry, dough. Add up to 1/4 cup extra flour if dough is too soft. Form into 1 1/2" balls and place on greased baking sheet. Flatten with a fork. Bake for 10–12 minutes or until slightly browned. Cool on a rack.

From the Heart Cookbook
Revised by Michele Menzel

Coconut, Carob & Peanut Butter Balls

A favorite with kids!

1/2 cup organic peanut butter
1/2 cup virgin coconut oil
1/2 cup shredded coconut (more if necessary)
1/4 cup raw cacao, carob, or cocoa powder
1 Tbsp. honey

In a bowl, combine the peanut butter and oil and mix thoroughly. Stir in the coconut, carob powder and honey. If necessary, use additional coconut to thicken. Form into balls. Cover and chill in refrigerator or freezer. Serve chilled.

Variations: Add 1/4 cup raisins or 1/4 cup walnuts

Chocolate Pudding

2 medium, ripe avocados,
    quartered, peeled, and pitted
3/4 cup unsweetened raw cacao, cocoa,
    or carob powder
1/2 cup raw milk, raw cream,
    or homemade almond milk, more as needed
6 Tbsp. or less raw honey
1/4 tsp. pure vanilla extract
Fine sea salt, to taste

Blend together avocados, cacao powder, milk, honey, and vanilla until smooth. Add more milk as needed to reach the desired consistency. Add salt to taste. Transfer the pudding to serving bowls and serve immediately or chill before serving.

Revised by Michele Menzel

Holly's Chocolates

1 cup crispy almonds (p. 172)
1 cup organic, unsweetened coconut flakes
4 oz. raw organic 100% cacao baking bar
1/2 cup organic virgin coconut oil
2 Tbsp. raw local honey (or to taste)

Grind nuts and coconut flakes in a food processor until it resembles chunky dirt. Melt cacao and coconut oil in saucepan over low heat. Add honey. Mix in the nut mixture and stir well.

Drop into mini cupcake papers in a mini muffin pan or drop into heart-shape molds. Freeze for 10 to 15 minutes. Transfer to a container with a lid. Keep refrigerated or frozen until ready to eat.

Holly Moulder

Chocolate Delight

1/2 cup coconut oil
1/2 tsp. vanilla
1/2 cup Rapunzel cocoa or raw cacao powder
Honey to taste

Melt oil and whisk in other ingredients until smooth, or use a blender. Pour into ice trays and freeze. Pop out of ice tray and keep frozen in a covered container.

Rebecca Pound

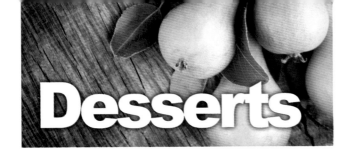

Desserts

Chocolate Cake

1 2/3 cups sprouted spelt flour
3/4 cup Rapunzel whole cane sugar
1/4 cup Rapunzel cocoa or raw cacao powder
1 tsp. baking soda
1/2 tsp. sea salt
1 cup water
1/3 cup virgin coconut oil, melted
1 tsp. apple cider vinegar
1 tsp. vanilla
1 cup Rapunzel organic chocolate chips or
    1 Rapunzel chocolate bar (or other acceptable bar),
    broken into very small pieces

Preheat oven to 350°. Mix dry ingredients, then add wet ingredients. Mix well. Use food processor, if desired. Grease (with coconut oil) and flour the pan. Bake for 30 minutes or until toothpick comes out clean. Let cool. Refrigerate leftovers. Serve this cake alone, with fresh strawberries or blueberries, or with hot fruit topping.
    Bake in an 8"x8" pan; a 9"x13" pan can hold a double batch.

Chatfield's
Revised by Michele Menzel

Pumpkin Pie

2 eggs
2 cups pumpkin, cooked and pureed
1/2 cup honey
1/4 cup butter, softened
1/2 cup raw milk
1/2 tsp. sea salt
1 tsp. vanilla
2 Tbsp. sprouted spelt flour or whole spelt flour
1 tsp. cinnamon
1/2 tsp. nutmeg
1/4 tsp. ginger
Dash cloves or allspice, if desired
9" unbaked pie shell (Company Pie Crust)

Preheat oven to 425°. Beat eggs. Add pumpkin and remaining ingredients, blending well after each addition. May be mixed in a blender. Pour into pie shell. Bake for 15 minutes. Turn oven down to 350° and bake for 45 minutes or until knife inserted in the middle comes out clean.

Company Pie Crust

1 3/4 cups sprouted spelt flour or whole spelt flour
1 tsp. sea salt
10 Tbsp. cold butter
3–5 Tbsp. cold water

Mix flour and salt. Cut in butter until dough resembles rolled oats. Sprinkle in just enough water to hold the dough together. Form into a ball, handling as little as possible. Roll out on floured waxed paper and turn into pie pan. For a flakier crust, refrigerate 2 hours before filling. This recipe will make a small 2-crust pie or a large 1-crust pie. Bake according to the pie recipe you are using.

From the Heart Cookbook,
Revised by Michele Menzel

Apple Cranberry Crisp 🍂

Filling:

4 cups chopped apples, with skins
2 cups cranberries, fresh or frozen
1 1/2 tsp. lemon juice
1/2 cup or less Rapunzel whole cane sugar
1 tsp. cinnamon

Topping:

1 1/3 cups rolled or steel cut oats
1 1/3 cups warm filtered water
1 Tbsp. yogurt or kefir
1 tsp. cinnamon
1 cup crispy walnuts, chopped
1/3 cup Rapunzel whole cane sugar
1/2 cup butter, melted

Soak oats overnight in water with yogurt or kefir in a warm place. If using sprouted oats, omit the overnight soaking.

Preheat oven to 325°. Strain excess liquid from the oat/water mixture. Add cinnamon, walnuts, whole cane sugar, and melted butter. Mix and set aside.

Lightly grease 9"x13" pan with coconut oil. Mix the filling ingredients and place in the pan. Pour the topping over the apple mixture. Bake for one hour.

For a special party, put the apple mixture and topping in individual mini muffin pans with mini holiday papers. Bake 20–30 minutes.

Susan Lampman
Revised by Michele Menzel

Banana Bread 🍂

2 cups sprouted spelt flour
1 tsp. aluminum-free baking powder
1 tsp. baking soda
1/2 tsp. sea salt
1/4 cup Rapunzel whole cane sugar
1 1/2 cups mashed ripe bananas, about 3–4
1/4 cup plain goat yogurt
1 tsp. vanilla
1/2 cup Rapunzel whole cane sugar
3 Tbsp. unsalted butter, softened
2 eggs
1/4 cup crispy walnuts or pecans (p.172),
    broken into pieces

Preheat oven to 350°. Combine dry ingredients. Set aside. Mash bananas and combine with yogurt and vanilla. Set aside. Beat together sugar and butter until light and fluffy (3–5 minutes). Add eggs, one at a time. Reduce mixer speed to low.

Beat in 1/2 flour mixture, 1/3 banana mixture, 1/4 flour, 1/3 banana, 1/4 flour mixture, and 1/3 banana. Do not over-mix. Batter should be thick and chunky. If it is too runny because the bananas were very ripe, add more flour. Pour into greased 5"x9" loaf pan. Sprinkle top with nuts. Bake for 55 minutes or until golden brown and toothpick comes out clean. Cool in pan for 10 minutes, then cool on a wire rack. Will keep at room temperature for 3 days, or longer in the fridge. Freezes well.

Tip: While measuring dry ingredients, make two extra batches and store in glass, quart-sized jars for next time!

Karen Munger

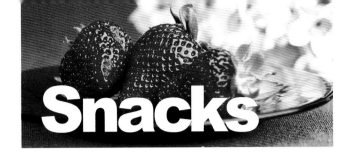

Snacks

Fruit & Milk or Cheese

1/2 cup strawberries or other sliced fruit
6 to 8 oz. glass of raw goat's milk
 or 2 oz. raw cheddar cheese

Raw Veggies & Almond Butter

Raw vegetables such as carrots, celery, tomatoes,
 zucchini, or summer squash
Raw almond butter

Anytime Energy Smoothie

6–8 oz. raw goat milk *or* yogurt *or* kefir
 or full-fat coconut milk (Thai brand)
 or raw cow milk
1–3 tsp. virgin coconut oil (optional)
1–2 raw eggs
1 Tbsp. flax seed oil (optional)
1 tsp.–1 Tbsp. raw honey
1–3 tsp. Essential Living Whey protein powder
1/2 cup fresh or frozen fruit (berries are best)
1–2 scoops digestive enzyme powder (Formula 30-P)
1 tsp. vanilla extract (optional)

Blend all in a high-speed blender (Vita-Mix).

Crispy Nuts

These are the best nuts you will ever have!
Kids, family, and friends will rave about them.
It is a really easy recipe and worth the wait!

4 cups of nuts (almonds, peanuts, hazelnuts, walnuts,
 cashews, pecans, etc.)
1 Tbsp. sea salt
Filtered water

Mix nuts with salt and filtered water and soak in a
warm place for at least 7 hours or overnight (except
for cashews, maximum soaking time is 6 hours). Drain
in a colander.

Oven Drying: Spread nuts on a stainless steel baking
pan and place in a warm oven (no higher than 150°)
for 12–24 hours, stirring occasionally, until completely
dry and crisp. Store in an airtight container.

Dehydrator: Spread nuts on trays and place in
dehydrator. Set temperature at lowest setting (usually
145–150°) for 12–24 hours, stirring occasionally, until
completely dry and crisp. Store in an airtight container.
 Nourishing Traditions. Revised by Michele Menzel

Zesty Popcorn

3 Tbsp. coconut oil   Sea salt
1 cup popcorn   Herbamare to taste
3 Tbsp. butter, softened

Use a Stir-Crazy Popcorn Popper. Put coconut oil in
the popper, and add popcorn. Cover and add softened butter on the top of dome lid. Plug in. Pops in
6 minutes. Salt and season to taste.

Peanut Butter Popcorn

1/4 cup peanut butter   2 Tbsp. butter
1/4 cup honey

Melt in saucepan over low heat until smooth. Pour
over popcorn and toss.

 Jessica Menzel Brown

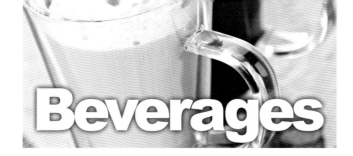

Beverages

Healthy Hot Chocolate

1 cup raw milk
1 heaping tsp. raw cacao or cocoa powder
2 tsp. honey
1 drop pure extract such as vanilla, peppermint,
    almond, hazelnut (optional)
Sprinkle cinnamon or nutmeg (optional)
Pinch of salt (optional)

Heat milk in small saucepan over medium heat
(3–4 minutes). Slowly whisk in cacao and honey. Do
not boil. Add a drop of flavoring if desired. Serve plain,
top with fresh whipped raw cream, or sprinkle with
cinnamon or nutmeg.

Jessica Menzel Brown

Lemonade

8 cups filtered water
4 whole lemons, squeezed
Honey or other approved natural sweetener to taste

Combine, add ice, and enjoy!

Amazing Almond Milk

*Almond milk is delicious and can be used in place of
milk in most recipes. Try it in coffee or tea, as well as
in desserts, including puddings.*

4 cups filtered water
1 cup raw almonds
Sweeteners and/or flavorings, such as pinch of salt,
    raw honey, vanilla, nutmeg

Soak almonds overnight in water. Place water and
soaked almonds in blender. Blend on high speed for
one minute. Pour contents from blender through nut
milk straining bag. Close bag and strain almond milk
by squeezing milk through bag. If desired, sweeten
with raw honey or vanilla.

Nut milk bags can be found online. You can also
use cheesecloth, any bag made of fine mesh, or a fine
stainless steel strainer.

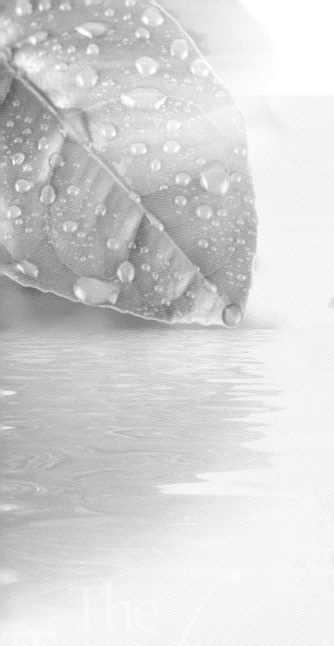

Organic & Locally Grown

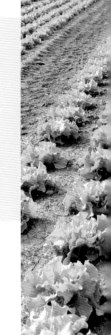

Always Buy Organic
Foods with the Highest Pesticide Load

Apples   Blueberries   Celery   Cherries   Cucumbers   Grapes   Lettuce
Nectarines   Pears   Peaches   Potatoes   Spinach   Strawberries   Sweet Bell Peppers

Organic produce has higher levels of beneficial minerals like iron and zinc.
Organic fruits and vegetables contain up to 40% more antioxidants!

I believe there is a misconception that there would not be enough meat in each state to be sustainable. After talking with many of our local farmers, this is not true. There is plenty of land and farmers who are willing to farm for the needs of the people. Buying your meat locally will not only support them in their efforts to supply healthy products, but be more economical for you as well. When you purchase a whole, half, or quarter of a cow, the price per pound is more affordable than when buying individual cuts. Purchasing an extra freezer for the garage is what we have done, and this works really well. You can also split a whole animal with friends or family members! And don't forget to always ask the processor for the bones to make stock and the extra fat to make tallow/lard.

Eating organic food grown in your region of the country is very beneficial to the body.

Seasonal food is the perfect match for the design, energy, and vitality of our biological system. Cultures from around the world and for thousands of years have eaten organic and local. They hunted and gathered and then learned how to grow their own food. They always ate in season because they had to gather, hunt, and grow what was available. Their food was in its original design, and chemicals and fertilizers did not exist. We have digressed in this area. Modern (big) agriculture, food preparation, and the refining processes have made hunting, gathering, and growing our own food a thing of the past. Progress is good (I love my washer and dryer), except when it affects the natural function of the human body.

We have come to realize the devastating effects of man-made chemicals to our environment, to us, and to our animals. The health consequences of factory farming techniques and the inhumane treatment of animals has caused great alarm. There is an increase of allergies, asthma, ADHD, gastrointestinal problems, and other chronic illnesses. People are finding healing from these as they change to an organic diet of whole foods.

It takes time and effort to change shopping habits, read labels, and search for local farmers. However, the benefits of selecting pure, whole food outweigh the adjustment it might take. The extra time is minimal compared to the devastating effects on your health from eating convenience food. The growing number of farmers who have become organic food pioneers,

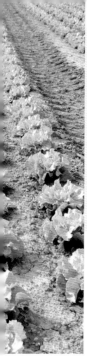

Use a Vegetable Wash to Clean Fruits with No Lowest Pesticide Load

Asparagus   Avocado   Banana   Broccoli   Cabbage   Cantaloupe
Eggplant   Grapefruit   Kiwi   Mango   Mushrooms   Pineapple   Onion
Sweet Peas   Sweet Potatoes   Watermelon

It is important to read the labels of all produce! You do not want to buy GMO produce. *Genetically modified will carry the 5-digit code: "84011." Conventionally grown produce carries a 4-digit code: "4011," and organic produce carries a 5-digit code beginning with a "9": "94011."*

reverting to natural cultivation have made pure, whole food more readily available.

If you are like me—a city girl without a green thumb—or do not have the time to devote to start your own garden, raise your own meat, or milk your own goat, then buying locally from farmers is the way to go. The majority of us are not able to produce all of the food we need. Buying local will help individual families and support the nationwide effort to become sustainable.

The freshest organic food is grown closest to you. By purchasing in-season local foods, you also eliminate the environmental damage caused by long-distance shipping. Your food dollar goes directly to the farmers supporting your area. You and your family will enjoy the health benefits of eating fresh, unprocessed fruits and vegetables. Buying seasonal produce also provides an exciting opportunity to try new foods and experiment with seasonal recipes.

This change does not have to be burdensome and boring. Everything is what we make of it. The Internet didn't exist when I started my search for pure, whole foods, so I asked a lot of questions when shopping at my local health-food store. Many health-food stores supply local produce, meat, and honey, and can be a great resource of farms and co-ops in the area. I also talked to people at the farmers' markets and with friends. Today, the search is so much easier, and the food is more available.

Here are a few ideas to help in your search for organic, local, pure, and whole foods:

1. Find a local Weston A. Price Foundation (WAPF) **chapter leader.**

Visit www.westonaprice.org, for more information. Local chapters help you find locally grown organic and biodynamic vegetables, fruits, and grains; and milk products, eggs, chicken, and meat from pasture-fed animals. They also represent the Weston A. Price Foundation at local fairs and conferences and may host cooking classes, potluck dinners, and other activities to help you learn how to integrate properly prepared whole foods into your lifestyle. Some local chapters are also able to put you in touch with health practitioners who share the foundation's philosophy and goals.

2. Find local, raw milk.

Visit the www.realmilk.com website. A Campaign for Real Milk is a project of the WAPF. Enter your city and state to find local sources of raw milk. This site is also a wonderful resource of information on the safety and benefits of raw milk.

3. Find local meat.

Visit the www.eatwild.com website. Eat Wild is a U.S., Canadian, and international site of farms and ranches dedicated to organic and natural methods. They also provide wonderful information regarding the health benefits of grass-fed farming.

4. Plant your own garden.

This can be an individual project or a project for the whole family. It is a wonderful way to incorporate many of the laws of wellness—sunshine, fresh air, grounding, and exercise. You can begin enriching your soil through composting and start out with a few herbs and vegetables. However, be sure to always purchase organic, heirloom seeds or plants. Some wellness centers and health-food stores provide gardening classes, and there are many good organic gardening books on the market.

5. Shop local farmers' markets.

This is one of my favorite things to do! It is probably the oldest form of marketing local produce, and is a great benefit to you and your family. Our farmers' market provides all types of handmade items and food, like eggs, breads, herbs, plants, honey, homemade dips and sauces, and personal care products. Make sure you read ingredients to avoid white sugar and harmful preservatives. Most markets mandate farmers to sell only what they have grown or created. If you are purchasing from a vendor for the first time, ask the origin of their product and their farming practices.

Establishing a good relationship with your local farmer is essential. Start by asking about his farming techniques. Is his farm organic? Some farms have not gone through the process of becoming certified, but follow organic farming principles. When buying eggs or meat, are they using genetically engineered feed for their animals or growing GE plants such as corn? Most local egg farmers have not switched to non-GMO feed. (If you are not able to find a local source, my favorite store-bought brand is Vital Farms eggs.)

If the farm is not organic, ask about the chemicals they spray on their plants. Beware of glyphosate, the active ingredient in Roundup—it is extremely dangerous to our system. Many farmers are using more organic methods, but we must do our homework before purchasing. Any man-made chemical sprayed on plants has the potential to enter our system and wreak havoc on our health.

6. Join a community-supported agriculture (CSA) program.

CSA members pay a weekly, biweekly, or monthly subscription. In return, they pick up a box of produce and/or other locally produced foods like cheese, eggs, and breads. To find a CSA in your area, visit www.localharvest.org.

7. Visit pick-your-own farms.

Pick-your-own farms allow customers to pick their own produce. It is usually weighed and sold by the pound. Similarly, gleaning programs have been established where volunteers harvest leftover produce and donate it to local food banks for distribution. In New Jersey, we enjoyed picking blueberries, strawberries, apples, and peaches

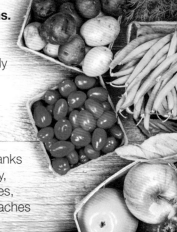

every year—the kids loved it, and it was an opportunity to teach them the value of growing/picking our food and knowing its origin.

8. Join a local food co-op.

Food cooperatives are customer- and worker-owned businesses where the customer pays a nominal annual fee and is provided with high-quality, local food products. There are many local cooperatives available. There are also food co-ops that make monthly bulk orders. This can be a good source to buy beans, nuts, and grains. Read the labels and ask questions to make sure the food items only contain natural sugars and correctly prepared whole grains. White flour, white sugar, and high-fructose corn syrup are highly processed and unnatural.

9. Shop local grocery and health-food stores when markets and farms are not an option.

Many grocery stores, private health-food stores, and nationwide health-food stores like Whole Foods, Sprouts, and Trader Joes offer local and organic produce, organic chicken, 100% grass-fed meat, raw cheeses, organic free-range eggs, coconut oil, bulk herbs and spices, organic beans, grains and nuts, etc. Always shop the perimeter of the store and remember to read labels. The center aisles (even at health-food stores) usually carry processed, denatured, and devitalized products.

10. Read food labels and know the origin.

Labeling regulations require retailers to list the place of origin for seafood, meat, produce, and nuts. On pages 176–177 is a list of produce with the highest and lowest pesticide load, as well as the identifiable codes for GMO, organic, and conventional produce. Buy food with "non-GMO" labels and stay away from harmful preservatives and chemical ingredients. These chemicals are not only in our food, but personal care products as well.

11. Buy fair trade.

Search for fair trade certified products if local is not an option. Fair Trade USA uses a market-based approach to empower farmers to receive a fair price for their work and harvest, and contribute to their local economies.

13. Buy in bulk.

I used this method for many years. Ordering a large amount is an initial investment, but more economical and convenient in the long run. An ideal situation is for families and friends to split bulk items. This is a great method to buy meat, beans, nuts, and grains. Always store dry goods in airtight containers, preferably glass jars. For bulk fruit and vegetables, you can freeze, or make salsa, sauce, or jam. Your fresh food can be enjoyed all year—nothing is wasted!

12. Research your restaurants.

Unless specified, 75% of the food served in restaurants is genetically modified. This makes eating out a challenge when you are trying to heal your body and are concerned for the health of your family. In recent years, farm-to-table cooking has become one of the hottest restaurant trends. Visit CleanPlates at www.cleanplates.com to find local restaurants that serve pure, whole foods. Your local chapter leader and your natural health care practitioner are other sources of information.

Have fun on this wonderful shopping journey!

Seasonal Produce

Spring Vegetables
Asparagus
Cabbage
Greens
Lettuce
Onions
Peas
Spinach

Spring Fruit
Apricots
Blueberries
Cantaloupes
Casaba melons
Cherries
Currants
Figs
Nectarines
Papayas
Pineapple
Raspberries
Rhubarb
Strawberries

Summer Vegetables

Beans
Bell peppers
Carrots
Corn
Eggplant
Okra
Onions
Potatoes
Tomatoes

Summer Fruit
Apples
Blueberries
Cherries
Figs
Grapes (red)

Kiwis
Mangos
Melons
Nectarines
Papayas
Peaches
Pears
Plums
Pineapples
Raspberries
Strawberries
Valencia oranges
Watermelons

Fall Vegetables
Avocados
Beans
Beets
Bok choy
Broccoli
Broccoli rabe
Brussel sprouts
Cabbage
Carrots
Cauliflower
Celery root (celeriac)
Chestnuts
Collards
Garlic
Jerusalem artichokes
Kale
Leeks
Lettuce
Parsnips
Pumpkins
Rutabaga

Salsify
Snow peas
Spinach
Squash (winter)
Sweet potatoes
Swiss chard
Turnips
Watercress

Fall Fruit
Apples
Bananas
Clementines
Cranberries
Grapefruit
Grapes
Kiwis
Kumquats
Oranges
Pears
Persimmons
Quinces
Satsuma Mandarin oranges
Tangerines

Winter Vegetables
Artichokes
Avocados
Bok choy
Broccoli
Broccoli rabe
Brussel sprouts
Cabbage
Cauliflower
Celery root

Chestnuts
Jerusalem artichokes
Kale
Lettuce
Parsnips
Radishes
Rhubarb
Rutabagas
Salsify
Snow peas
Squash
Sweet potatoes
Turnips (white)
Watercress

Winter Fruit
Bananas
Blood oranges
Clementines
Cranberries
Grapefruit
Grapes (red)
Kiwis
Kumquat
Oranges
Passion fruit
Pears
Persimmons
Pomegranates
Pummelos
Rhubarb
Satsuma oranges
Tangelos
Tangerines
Ugli fruit

For a list of seasonal produce in your state, visit www.eatwellguide.org.

182 ENERGETIC WELLNESS

Why No GMOs?

Studying food and its nutritional content has been a passion of mine for over 20 years. Food was created to be our medicine and medicine our food. In its natural and organic state, it is a perfect match for the human body. Food gives the body energy and the nutrients it needs to function as designed by our Creator.

Genetically modified (GMO) or engineered (GE) food is not a natural design. Genetically modified organisms have had specific changes introduced directly into their DNA. One technique, in particular, creates an herbicide-tolerant variety which is designed to survive high doses of toxic weed killers, like Roundup. We call this variety "Roundup Ready". Roundup, or the active ingredient glyphosate, wreaks havoc on human health. It is a very dangerous herbicide.

Why No GMOs?

Genetically modified foods or biotech foods are foods derived from genetically modified organisms (GMOs). Genetically modified organisms have had specific changes introduced into their DNA through genetic engineering techniques.

In agriculture, there are two types of GM crops. The herbicide-tolerant variety is designed to survive high doses of toxic weed killers. Such weed killers are themselves linked to a string of health disorders, such as birth defects, cancer, and hormone disruption. When used on highly resistant crops, some of these toxins end up in our food.

Other GM foods are designed to produce their own insecticide in every cell throughout the plant. For example, BT-toxin is an insecticide that breaks open the stomachs of insects in order to kill them. It has been reported that BT-toxin can also break the walls of human cells. According to one study, the BT-toxin from genetically modified corn was found in the blood of 93 percent of pregnant women and 80 percent of their unborn fetuses.

GMOs are leading to a massive increase in human exposure both to the Roundup herbicide, and to the BT-toxin that has been genetically engineered into corn and other plants.

Research gathered by a physicians' group called the American Academy of Environmental Medicine (AAEM) reports that lab animals fed GMOs suffered from these symptoms:

- Premature aging
- Reproductive disorders
- Gastrointestinal problems
- Organ damage
- Insulin & cholesterol disorders
- Immune imbalance & allergies

Shortly after GM soy was introduced in the UK, food allergies shot up by 50 percent. Now more than ever, medical organizations like the AAEM are telling us to stop eating GMOs.

- Genetically modified foods are new, and have not been in use long enough for the risks to be known.
- Genetically modified foods have not been subject to thorough research and testing.
- Foods that are genetically altered can involve risks of unknown toxins and allergens never before seen in humans.

In my opinion, GE food is ten times more harmful than food grown conventionally, which is harmful in and of itself because of the pesticide load. GE crops have not only been altered from their original design, but are resistant to Roundup. This means that they are typically far more contaminated with glyphosate than conventionally grown crops, because they are heavily sprayed to kill the surrounding weeds. Nearly 75% of all food in the grocery store and in restaurants is genetically engineered! Unfortunately, most people don't even know that GMOs exist, let alone how they are affecting our health and the health of our children.

A 2013 study confirmed why I believe GMOs and glyphosate are contributing to most, if not all, modern chronic conditions, and inhibiting the body's ability to heal itself. This peer-reviewed report authored by Anthony Samsel, a retired science consultant, and Dr. Stephanie Seneff, a research scientist at the Massachusetts Institute of Technology (MIT), reveals how glyphosate wrecks human health. Glyphosate causes systemic toxicity and nutritional deficiencies. Dr. Seneff states that GE foods consumed by most Americans such as GE sugar, corn, soy, and wheat, "enhance the damaging effects of other food-borne chemical residues and toxins in the environment to disrupt normal body functions and induce disease."

Glyphosate systematically disrupts the life and function of our gut bacteria. We have more microorganisms (microbes) in our body than we have cells. Trillions of them outnumber our cells by 10 to 1. Monsanto (the Roundup chemical company and owner of most GMO seeds) claims that Roundup is harmless to animals and humans because it is designed to kill weeds through the shikimate pathway

Nearly 75% of all food in the grocery store and in restaurants is genetically engineered!

which is absent in all animals. However, the shikimate pathway *is* present in bacteria (your microbes), which is the key to why it can lead to such widespread systemic harm in both humans and animals. The disruption of the gut bacteria can cause a host of gastrointestinal conditions such as bloating, gas, irritable bowel syndrome (IBS), inflammatory bowel disease, chronic diarrhea, colitis, leaky gut, and Crohn's disease. The consumption of glyphosate-contaminated GE foods causes other pathway disruptions to key components of the body. These include enzymes, amino acids, cholesterol, vitamin D, sulfur, calcium, manganese, cobalt, and zinc. These disruptions have been linked to allergies, autism, cancer, immune imbalances, multiple sclerosis (MS), Lou Gehrig's Disease (ALS), Alzheimer's disease, Parkinson's disease, depression, insulin and cholesterol disorders, obesity, infertility, and organ damage, just to name a few.

It is of vital importance that we are aware of GMOs in our food supply, and, to the best of our ability, stay away from them! This especially applies to our children. Their little systems are extra vulnerable. The rate of autism has risen quickly and it can be directly linked to environmental causes. The latest statistics released by the U.S. Center for Disease Control and Prevention (CDC) indicate that 1 in 50 children in the U.S. fall within the autism spectrum, with a 5:1 boy to girl ratio. In 2012, the reported rate was 1 in 88. If the numbers continue to grow at the same rate, in five years 1 in 2 children will be dealing with autism. This is a far cry from 30 years ago when the incidence of autism in the U.S. was only 1 in 100,000. We must turn the tide and stop consuming these foods.

In my opinion, genetically modified organisms are poisoning our food supply and are one of the most dangerous threats to our existence. For example, GMO corn contains more than 18 times the "safe" level of glyphosate set by the Environmental Protection Agency (EPA), compared to **zero** in non-GMO corn.

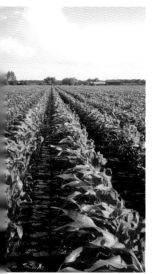

Many foods sold in the U.S. have been genetically modified. These include:

- 86% of corn (oil)
- 93% of soy (oil)
- 93% of canola (oil)
- 93% of cottonseed (oil)
- 95% of sugar beets
- Sugarcane
- 80% of Hawaiian papaya
- 13% of zucchini and yellow crookneck squash
- Sweet peppers (small quantities grown in China)
- Tomatoes (small quantities grown in China)
- Rice

Just Label It

It is time to label GMOs. Once thought to be an answer to poverty and hunger, they are turning out to be a consolidation of power by big agri-chemical companies—with profound and disturbing implications for our soil, our health, and our farmers.

A poll taken identified 93% of Americans want labeling of GMO foods and 53% of Americans say they wouldn't eat GMOs if they were labeled.

www.justlabelit.org

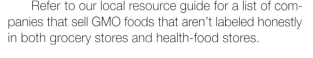

Refer to our local resource guide for a list of companies that sell GMO foods that aren't labeled honestly in both grocery stores and health-food stores.

How You Can Stay Away From GMOs

Very few vegetables sold in the produce section of your grocery store are genetically modified. Some papayas grown in Hawaii are genetically modified, and you should be aware of this when buying them. But produce is not a huge problem.

Most of the time, GMOs will be found in highly processed foods with long ingredient lists on the box. Many consumers purchase "natural" products and think they are organic. But *natural* means very little in the marketplace. Most "natural" foods are not only grown or produced using pesticides but also contain genetically engineered ingredients.

Since it is difficult to know which foods have GMOs, consider the following:

- Buy foods labeled 100% organic.

- Make your own homemade foods from non-GMO ingredients.

- Buy foods labeled non-GMO.

- Follow the recommended foods and supplements in this book.

- Buy local, and get to know your growers. You can ask them what they grow, or even visit their farm.

- Growing your own food definitely assures that it is GMO-free, as long as you are certain to purchase non-GMO seeds or plants.

- Know the main crops that are GM, and avoid buying foods if you

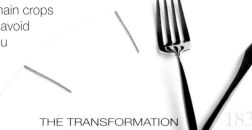

are uncertain as to whether or not they contain genetically modified ingredients.

Any other type of food can contain ingredients that you may not want in your diet. Download the True Food Shoppers Guide to Avoiding GMOs at www.truefoodnow.org.

When Eating Out

Good questions to ask are: "What oil do you cook with?" If they use soy, cottonseed, canola, or corn oils, they are likely GM unless they are organic. Ask what they have that is cooked without oil, or ask if they can use butter or olive oil. If they say it is "vegetable oil" or margarine, it will almost always be soy, cottonseed, canola, or corn oils. If they have olive oil, make sure it is not a blend. Many restaurants blend canola and olive oils.

Since most processed foods contain GM derivatives (corn and soy, for example), ask what foods the chef prepares fresh, and choose from those items. Check whether packaged sauces are used.

Avoid processed foods with the oils mentioned above, or with soy and corn derivatives, including soy flour, soy protein, soy lecithin, textured vegetable protein, corn meal, corn syrup, dextrose, maltodextrin, fructose, citric acid, and lactic acid.

Other potential sources of GM foods at restaurants include salad dressings, bread, mayonnaise, and sugar from GM sugar beets.

Genetically modified food additives, enzymes, flavorings, and processing agents, including rennet used to make hard cheeses are harder to avoid. It is also difficult to avoid meat, eggs, and dairy products from animals that have eaten GM feed, unless the restaurant uses organic, 100% grass-fed meat, and wild-caught fish.

In restaurants, you will likely have to avoid items with dairy, unless the restaurant uses organic dairy. Dairy products are usually from cows treated with recombinant bovine growth hormone (rBGH). This hormone is genetically engineered and marketed to dairy farmers to increase milk production in cows. Industrialized nations outside the U.S. have not approved rBGH.

Avoid all tabletop sweeteners but especially aspartame (NutraSweet® or Equal®, AminoSweet®).

If you plan ahead, you can call or email the restaurant you plan to visit and ask for a list of ingredients. Going through this process not only gives you a hopeful list of healthy eating options, but also informs the restaurant that you prefer healthier, non-GMO options when you dine out.

When shopping at the Grocery Store

Some foods that may contain GM Ingredients: Infant formula, salad dressing, bread, cereal, hamburgers and hotdogs, margarine, mayonnaise, cereals, crackers, cookies, chocolate, candy, fried food, chips, veggie burgers, meat substitutes, ice cream, frozen yogurt, tofu, tamari, soy sauce, soy cheese, tomato sauce, protein powder, baking powder, alcohol, vanilla, powdered sugar, peanut butter, enriched flour, and pasta. Honey and bee pollen may have GM sources of pollen.

The Grocery Manufacturers of America estimated that 75 percent of all processed foods in the U.S. contained a GM ingredient. Currently, the USDA does not require that GMOs be labeled.

BOTTOM LINE: The only way that you can eliminate your exposure to genetically modified organisms is to buy only 100% organic foods and those that are specifically labeled as non-GMO.

PLEASE SEE THE SOURCE ACKNOWLEDGMENTS ON PAGE 272 FOR A LIST OF RESEARCH, BOOKS, AND WEBSITES USED FOR THIS SECTION.

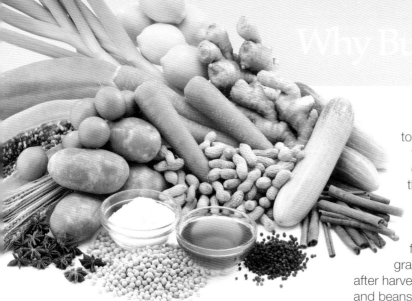

Why Buy Organic?

There are many reasons to buy organic.

It's better for the environment.

No pesticides means healthier soil, water, and wildlife. Buying organic supports small local farmers. Organic farmers can earn a fairer price for organic produce compared to factory farming. Organic farming is good for biodiversity. Organic farmers are growing a wide variety of non-GMO fruits and vegetables. Where factory farming has shrunk our choices in the supermarket to one or two produce varieties, organic farmers are resurrecting many heirloom varieties.

Organic foods are cleaner and healthier for you.

No pesticides and no GMOs means fewer toxins in the body. USDA tests show that most non-organic produce contains residual pesticides, even after washing. The long-term effects of consuming these pesticides has not been sufficiently studied, but common sense tells us organic food is better.

Eating organic provides more vitamins and minerals, especially vitamin C, magnesium, and iron. Soil Association writes, "A U.S. study found that organic crops had higher average levels of all 21 nutrients analyzed."

Unfortunately, we must go to great lengths to find organic pure whole foods to nourish the body. Read labels! Choose fresh, certified-organic foods and foods that have the non-GMO label. Purchase 100% grass-fed beef, organic pastured chicken, organic or non-GMO eggs and organic dairy products to assure the animals were not fed GMO corn or soy feed. All conventional grains and beans are sprayed with glyphosate after harvest. So seek out organically raised grains and beans as well.

An "All Natural" label does not mean it has organic standards. It is frequently misused by GE products and processed food companies. An organic product must be grown *without* synthetic pesticides, bioengineered genes, petroleum-base fertilizers, or sewage sludge-based fertilizers.

Organic foods in their natural state are the foods God intended for us to eat and use as our medicine! These foods are the perfect design for the body. They provide the body with nutrients that nourish and heal. Chemical-laden food causes disruption in the natural function of the body. We have the choice. ***Choose to go organic!***

BOTTOM LINE:

Here are some reasons why you might buy organic:
- Hormone-free - Antibiotic-free
- Pesticide & herbicide free - Non-GMO
- Higher nutrient levels - Prenatal benefits
- Better for the planet - Higher levels of antioxidants
- Support your local economy

Once you start eating organically, you will realize that organic food tastes better!

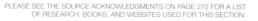

PLEASE SEE THE SOURCE ACKNOWLEDGMENTS ON PAGE 272 FOR A LIST OF RESEARCH, BOOKS, AND WEBSITES USED FOR THIS SECTION.

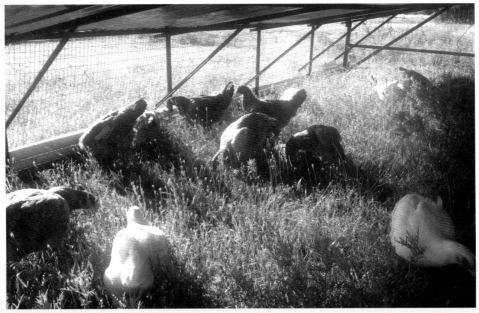

In the 1930s,
animal scientists were trying
to determine the best diet
for cows, pigs, and chickens
raised in confinement. It was
a time of trial and error.

In a 1933 experiment
conducted by the U.S.
Department of Agriculture,
breeding hens were taken off pasture and fed a wide variety of feed ingredients. When the birds were fed a diet
that was exclusively soy, corn, wheat, or cottonseed meal, the chickens didn't lay as many eggs and the chicks that
developed from the eggs had a high rate of mortality and disease.

But when birds were fed these same inadequate diets and put back on pasture, their eggs were perfectly normal.
The pasture grasses and the bugs made up for whatever was missing in each of the highly restrictive diets.

The Effect of Diet on Egg Composition. *Journal of Nutrition 6(3) 225-242. 1933.*

PLEASE SEE THE SOURCE ACKNOWLEDGMENTS
ON PAGE 272 FOR A LIST OF RESEARCH, BOOKS,
AND WEBSITES USED FOR THIS SECTION.

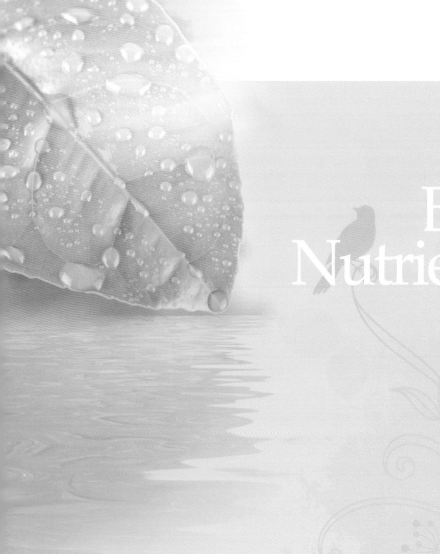

Benefits of Nutrient-Dense Food

Fats & Oils

Grass-Fed Beef

Pastured Poultry, Eggs & Pork

Raw Dairy

Fermented Foods

Wild-Caught Fish

Bone Broths

Whole Grains

Sugar

Salt

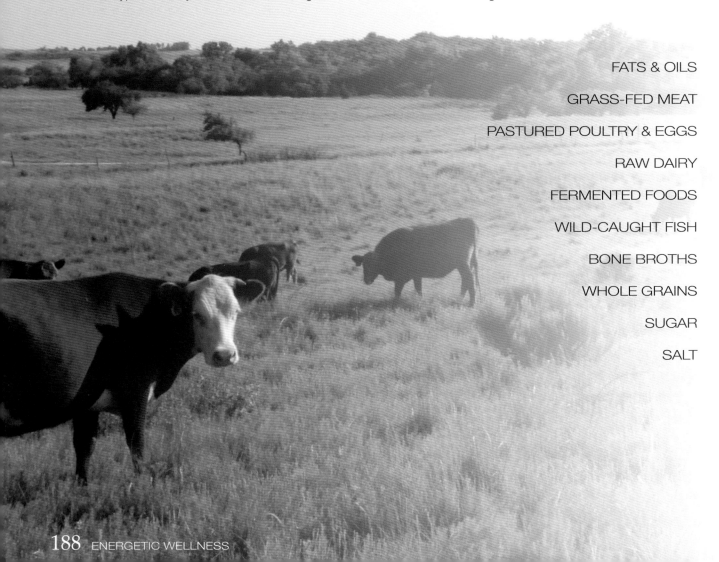

Benefits of Nutrient-Dense Foods

In this section, I share with you the benefits of nutrient-dense "real food" —
the type of food you have been learning about in this book. *So here we go!*

FATS & OILS

GRASS-FED MEAT

PASTURED POULTRY & EGGS

RAW DAIRY

FERMENTED FOODS

WILD-CAUGHT FISH

BONE BROTHS

WHOLE GRAINS

SUGAR

SALT

Fats & Oils

Recognize the counterfeits.

Most allopathic and naturopathic health care providers seem to have the same advice: *avoid saturated fat!* This would include whole foods like eggs (especially the yolks), real butter, whole milk, raw dairy products, and especially red meat. The replacements they offer are highly processed, industrial-made vegetable oils, egg beaters, low-fat or fat-free dairy, soy or rice products, and lean meats. These substitutes are fake, highly processed foods and lack the balance of essential fatty acids. Twenty years ago, I adopted this philosophy and fell prey to a vegan diet. However, it soon became apparent that the elimination of these vital fats left me completely overwhelmed, fatigued, extremely emotional, nutrient-deficient, and unable to heal.

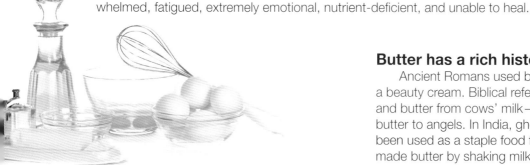

When students learn how to recognize counterfeit money, they do not study the counterfeit, they study the original. Let's study real food from history, learn what our ancestors ate, and understand how we have been deceived to eat the counterfeit.

Prior to the introduction of modern processing, our ancestors consumed fats from animals in the form of milk, butter, cheese, meat, and oils naturally extracted from fruits, nuts, and seeds. They ate what was created and available for food. (It certainly wasn't Crisco, margarine, or refined vegetable oils!)

Fats from animal and vegetable sources provide a concentrated source of energy, the building blocks for cell membranes, and a variety of hormones and hormone-like substances. Fats, as part of every meal, slow down nutrient absorption so that we are satisfied and can go longer without feeling hungry. They are also important carriers for the fat-soluble vitamins A, D, E, and K (which is the missing link to our current deficiency of vitamin D in the body), vital for the conversion of carotene to vitamin A, for mineral absorption, and for a host of other very important processes.

Butter has a rich history.

Ancient Romans used butter to treat burns and as a beauty cream. Biblical references include goats' milk and butter from cows' milk—Abraham even served butter to angels. In India, ghee (clarified butter) has been used as a staple food for 3,000 years. People made butter by shaking milk in bags of animal skins or in hollow logs. My daughter's favorite childhood book, *Little House on the Prairie*, describes a time of making butter in a wooden churn. You might even remember your grandmother making butter. It is real food, and has been enjoyed for thousands of years by many cultures. They benefited and thrived from butter and all animal products containing saturated fat—butter, raw milk, cheese, and meat.

Both butter and olive oil are made by a natural process. The fat is separated from the whole milk and churned until it forms into butter. Olive oil is made by pressing the olives to extract the oil. They are real food. There is no need to use chemicals to clean and deodorize them as in our modern oil process. Today butter is made in big machines, but the process still resembles that of our great-grandmothers—churning cream until it turns to butter.

Somewhere along the way, we switched from enjoying the rich taste of butter in our dishes to using margarine and refined vegetable oils. We have adopted the notion that a healthy diet is one with minimal fat. Fats that were once considered sacred in many cultures are now claimed to be harmful contributors to a host of health conditions.

How did this happen?

In 1837, William Procter and James Gamble (Procter & Gamble) joined as partners making and selling soap and candles. In 1870 they extended their manufacturing and marketing efforts to include lard.

In 1911, Crisco was conceived to provide an economical alternative to animal fats like butter and lard. It was made from leftover seeds from the cotton industry. Crisco was the first solidified shortening product made entirely of vegetable oil. It was also the first hydrogenated oil—a new process that produced solid shortening at room temperature.

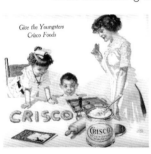
Give the Youngsters Crisco Foods

In 1912, advertising for Crisco took off in a very popular women's magazine. The ads focused on the benefits of Crisco over butter and lard. Crisco could be heated to much higher temperatures than lard and Crisco did not pick up the flavor of food and could be used again and again, saving the consumer money.

They created a cookbook to introduce cooking with Crisco to every American home. For two decades, P&G hired home economists to lead cooking schools around the country to teach homemakers how to use the vegetable shortening. They also found a growing market in bakeries, restaurants, and hotels. In 1969, the first liquid vegetable oil was introduced. It didn't require melting as the shortening did, and was introduced to be perfect for salads and salad dressings.

At the turn of the century, heart disease was rare. But by 1960, it was considered the number one cause of death. Butter consumption had decreased from eighteen pounds per person per year to four pounds per person per year. And yet they blamed butter and animal products for heart disease. This came as a result of researcher Ancel Keys' 1950 study called the lipid hypothesis theory. The theory is based on a relationship between the amount of saturated fat and cholesterol in the diet and the incidence of coronary heart disease. Many subsequent researchers have pointed out the flaws in his data and conclusions, but the vegetable oil and food processing industries worked behind the scenes to promote further research that would support the lipid hypothesis.

Modern technology and the underlying belief system of convenience foods for the modern lifestyle gave no thought to the harmful effects of industrial processing. In the name of progress, we failed to recognize the consequences of chemical substitutes that replace real food.

Although there has not been a move to reverse this advice, evidence shows that health risks are higher with refined, unsaturated, and polyunsaturated fats (vegetable oils).

Trans-fats are formed as a result of chemical hydrogenation—they are artificially created. Margarine may be made of up to 45 percent of these harmful fats. Only in recent years have trans-fats formed a significant part of our diet. They are found in fried and processed foods, and have detrimental effects on our health—including a risk for type 2 diabetes, elevated cholesterol, and reduced blood vessel function.

The majority of our population has been deceived in

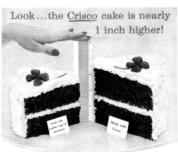
Look...the Crisco cake is nearly 1 inch higher!

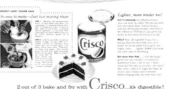
2 out of 3 bake and fry with Crisco...it's digestible!

thinking butter is bad for us. Can food containing such high levels of trans-fats be better for us than butter? Real food or chemically processed industrial food?

Canola oil is known today as the healthiest oil because it has the lowest saturated fat content, even though the process to create this oil uses chemical solvents, industrial steaming, de-waxing, bleaching and a deodorizing process. There is quite a difference between a real food (butter) and a chemical substitute.

"...canola oil hydrogenates beautifully, better than corn oil or soybean oil, because modern hydrogenation methods hydrogenate omega-3 fatty acids preferentially and canola oil is very high in omega-3s. Higher levels of trans mean longer shelf life for processed foods, a crisper texture in cookies and crackers—and more dangers of chronic disease for the consumer."
—Sally Fallon Morell and Mary G. Enig, PhD

Everyone is familiar with the USDA dietary recommendations and food pyramids. These have changed numerous times since the U.S. Department of Agriculture first published its dietary recommendations in 1894.

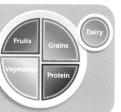

The most recent change is the creation of MyPlate. This new version of the ideal American diet is virtually void of fats! Except for a small portion of fat-free or low-fat dairy, fats are missing entirely. There is no mention of the importance of dietary fats, even the "politically correct" mono-unsaturated fats in olive oil and nuts. The only oil advised is canola oil (which, in my opinion, should be completely avoided).

Dr. Joseph Mercola recently constructed his version of the food pyramid. This is a pyramid we can follow. It is wonderfully balanced and will assist us in the purpose of *The Transformation* and the Foods for Life.

At the base of the pyramid are **Healthful Fats & Veggies.** The fats include coconut oil, olive oil, butter, and raw nuts. For vegetables, he recommends raw, organic vegetables. For the best absorption of nutrients, be sure to properly prepare the nuts. (See Crispy Nuts recipe on p. 172)

There are a number of vegetables that can be enjoyed raw, but there are many that are intended to be cooked. See the Stage 1 food list (p. 110). The minerals in these vegetables are better absorbed by the body when lightly cooked in butter.

The second level on Dr. Mercola's pyramid is **Protein**. He recommends grass-fed, organic meat and poultry, organic, pastured eggs, safe fish such as wild Alaskan salmon, and raw dairy products. I would also add fermented dairy in the form of raw milk yogurt, kefir, and buttermilk.

The third level is **Fruit**. He recommends organic fruit in moderation.

At the top of the pyramid, for minimal or no consumption, are **Grains & Sugar.** This includes complex carbohydrates—like bread, cereal, pasta, potatoes, corn, rice, and grain products. After helping many people through *The Transformation*, I agree with this recommendation. Many of us have very little tolerance for processed grains. As you work through *The Transformation*, you learn what whole grains in this category work best for you. White sugar should be avoided and natural sugars should be limited to an occasional treat.

Saturated fats play many vital roles in the body.
- They provide integrity to the cell wall.
- They promote the body's use of essential fatty acids.
- They enhance the immune system.
- They protect the liver and help to dump its fat content.
- They contribute to strong bones by helping incorporate calcium into bone.
- They are essential for hormonal balance.
- The airspaces of the lungs are coated with a thin layer of lung surfactant; the fat content of which is 100% saturated fatty acids.
- They assist kidney function.
- They provide nourishment for the brain— which is mainly fat and cholesterol.
- They play a role in proper nerve signaling.

Saturated fats do not cause heart disease. In fact, saturated fats are the preferred food for the heart. When there are not enough fats in your diet, your body makes them out of carbohydrates and excess protein.

Fats also contain essential fatty acids (Omega-3 and 6) which are only available from food sources. When depleted, your body is not able to produce them out of anything else. Recent scientific research is uncovering the host of health problems created by a lack of Omega-3 and -6.

Mental Wellbeing

Our brains are 60% fat! This fat needs to be maintained for proper brain function. Therefore, unrefined fats and oils are essential for such conditions as depression, emotional disorders, ADHD, and autism— to name just a few. A low-fat diet can lead to a host of neurological disorders.

For Weight Loss

Eating fat can actually keep you slim. By adding unrefined essential fatty acids to a healthy diet, normal weight can be restored. In order for this to work, all refined oils and margarine must be removed from the diet.

The right fats and oils are essential for your well-being—include them in your diet!

The Best Fats to Consume
- Organic raw butter*
- Ghee (clarified butter)
- Organic extra virgin olive oil (unfiltered)
- Virgin coconut oil
- Unrefined palm oil—red
- Organic, grass-fed lard
- Organic, grass-fed tallow
- Raw, whole milk dairy products
- Organic, free-range eggs
- Grass-fed meats, especially the fatty cuts
- Grass-fed pork bacon
- Avocados

Raw butter cannot legally be sold in U.S. stores. You can make your own by purchasing cream from your local farmer. If raw cream is not available, I would only recommend butter from grass-fed cows such as Kalona Supernatural butter, Kerrygold butter, and Organic Valley pastured butter.

Cold-Pressed Oils (for occasional use)

Sesame	Flax
Sunflower	High oleic safflower oil
Peanut	Expeller-pressed palm oil
Macadamia	Expeller-pressed coconut oil
Avocado	Filtered extra virgin olive oil

Avoid These Highly Processed Commercial Fats & Oils:
- Vegetable oils: cottonseed, soy, corn, canola, rice bran, hemp, grapeseed
- Margarine, Crisco, spreads
- Partially hydrogenated vegetable shortenings
- Egg beaters
- Conventional meat
- Pasteurized dairy products, especially low-fat and non-fat
- All processed food—especially fat-free food

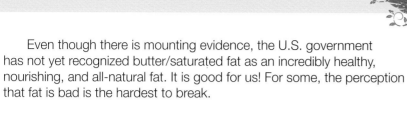

Even though there is mounting evidence, the U.S. government has not yet recognized butter/saturated fat as an incredibly healthy, nourishing, and all-natural fat. It is good for us! For some, the perception that fat is bad is the hardest to break.

Your great-grandmother knew better.

A word about fish oil supplements. *Omega-3* has become the latest buzzword in health, and many people are taking an abundance of fish oil. These oils become rancid very quickly and are hard for the liver and gallbladder to process. There are only two brands of fish oil I recommend: Blue Ice™ Royal Butter Oil / Fermented Cod Liver Oil and Vital Choice Salmon Oil (along with a nutrient-dense diet as outlined in this book). Please note that those without a gallbladder should only take fermented cod liver oil.

Butter & Your Health

Heart Disease: Butter contains many nutrients that protect against heart disease including vitamins A, D, K2, E, lecithin, iodine, and selenium. A medical research council survey showed that men eating butter ran half the risk of developing heart disease as those using margarine (*Nutrition Week* 3/22/91, 21:12).

Cancer: The short- and medium-chain fatty acids in butter have strong anti-tumor effects. Conjugated linoleic acid (CLA) in butter from grass-fed cows also gives excellent protection against cancer.

Arthritis: The Wulzen, or "anti-stiffness" factor in raw butter and the vitamin D2 in grass-fed butter protect against calcification of the joints and pineal gland as well as hardening of the arteries and cataracts. Calves fed pasteurized milk or skim milk develop joint stiffness and do not thrive.

Osteoporosis: Vitamins A, D, and K2 in butter are essential for the proper absorption of calcium and phosphorus, which are necessary for strong bones and teeth.

Thyroid Health: Butter is a good source of iodine in a highly absorbable form. Butter consumption prevents goiter in mountainous areas where seafood is not available. In addition, vitamin A in butter is essential for proper functioning of the thyroid gland.

Digestion: Glycosphingolipids in butterfat protect against gastrointestinal infection, especially in the very young and the elderly.

Growth & Development: Many factors in butter ensure optimal growth in children—especially iodine and vitamins A, D, and K2. Low-fat diets have been linked to a failure to thrive, yet they are often recommended for youngsters!

Asthma: Saturated fats in butter are critical to lung function and protect against asthma (Thorax, Jul 2003;58(7):567-72).

Overweight: CLA and short- and medium-chain fatty acids in butter help control weight gain.

Fertility: Many nutrients contained in butter are needed for fertility and normal reproduction.

Why Butter Is Better

Vitamins: Butter is a rich source of easily absorbed vitamin A, which is needed for a wide range of functions such as maintaining good vision and keeping the endocrine system in good order. Butter also contains all the other fat-soluble vitamins (D, E, and K2), which are often lacking in the modern, industrial diet.

Minerals: Butter is rich in important trace minerals, including manganese, chromium, zinc, copper, and selenium (a powerful antioxidant). Butter provides more selenium per gram than wheat germ or herring. Butter is also an excellent source of iodine.

Fatty Acids: Butter provides appreciable amounts of short- and medium-chain fatty acids, which support immune function, boost metabolism, and have anti-microbial properties by fighting against pathogenic microorganisms in the intestinal tract. Butter also provides the perfect balance of omega-3 and omega-6 essential fatty acids. Arachidonic acid in butter is important for brain function, skin health, and prostaglandin balance.

CLA: Cows that are allowed to feed on green grass produce butter that contains high levels of conjugated linoleic acid (CLA), a compound that gives excellent protection against cancer and helps the body build muscle rather than store fat.

Clycospingolipids: These are a special category of fatty acids that protect against gastrointestinal infections, especially in the very young and the elderly. Children who drink reduced fat milk have higher rates of diarrhea than those who drink whole milk.

Cholesterol: Despite all of the misinformation you may have heard, cholesterol is needed to maintain intestinal health. It is also vital for the development of the brain and nervous system in children.

Stigmasterol / Wulzen Factor: This hormone-like substance that prevents arthritis and joint stiffness is only found in raw butter and cream. It ensures that calcium in the body is utilized by the bones rather than by the joints and other tissues. The Wulzen factor is destroyed by pasteurization.

BOTTOM LINE:
Fat does not cause you to be fat!
Make good fats a part of your meals every day.
Purchase real butter from grass-fed cows,
use coconut oil, use olive oil as a base for
homemade salad dressings, and consume avocados!

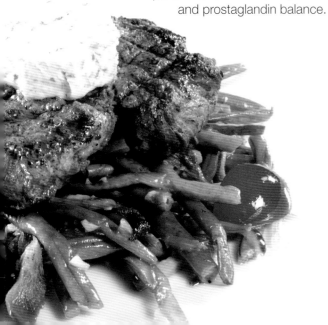

PLEASE SEE THE SOURCE ACKNOWLEDGMENTS
ON PAGE 272 FOR A LIST OF RESEARCH, BOOKS,
AND WEBSITES USED FOR THIS SECTION.

Grass-fed Meat

Animal Products

Raising animals on pasture is dramatically different from the status quo. Virtually all the meat, eggs, and dairy products you find in the supermarket come from animals raised in confinement in large facilities called "Confined Animal Feeding Operations." These highly mechanized operations provide a year-round supply of food at a reasonable price. Although the food is cheap and convenient, there is growing recognition that factory farming creates a host of problems, including:

- Animal stress and abuse
- Air, land, and water pollution
- Low-paid, stressful farm work
- The loss of small family farms
- Food with less nutritional value
- The extensive use of hormones, antibiotics, and other drugs

Grass-fed Beef & Lamb

Grass-fed meat is humane.

Just as for humans, good health for animals is assisted by what they eat, fresh air, sunshine, clean water, and freedom to move about. Animals that forage over a large landscape are eating the way nature intended. Because they graze over long distances in the great outdoors, they are lean, fit, and healthy. Fresh pasture and a mix of dried, wild grasses and herbs supply their bodies with what is needed for life.

The difference between grain-fed and grass-fed animal products is dramatic.

An animal's diet has a profound influence on the nutrient content of its products. First, grass-fed products tend to be much lower in total fat than grain-fed products. A sirloin steak from a grass-fed steer has about one half to one third the amount of fat as a similar cut from a grain-fed steer. In fact, grass-fed beef has about the same amount of fat as skinless chicken, wild deer, or elk.

In factory farms, animals are switched to an unnatural diet based on genetically modified corn and soy. But many large-scale dairy farmers and feedlot operators also save money by feeding "byproduct feedstuffs." This can mean waste products from the manufacture of human food—from floor sweepings from factories that manufacture animal food, bakery wastes, and potato wastes to sterilized city garbage,

candy, bubble gum, or a scientific blend of pasta and candy. (ByProduct Feedstuffs in Dairy Cattle Diets in the Upper Midwest, *College of Agricultural and Life Sciences at the University of Wisconsin at Madison, 2008.*)

Until 1997, U.S. cattle were also being fed meat that had been trimmed from other cattle, turning herbivores into carnivores. This unnatural practice is believed to be the underlying cause of bovine spongiform encephalopathy (BSE) or "mad cow disease."

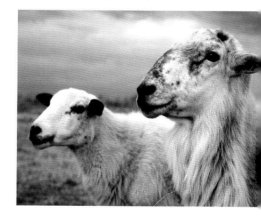

Grass-fed beef is more nutritious and healthy.

Most beef is pastured in grass fields for a short time and "finished" on grain in feeding areas that are confined and unclean. Since grain is unnatural to them, this can boost *E. coli* counts in their intestines. This is a direct result of the body's response to eating unnatural food. This has become a major problem in factory-farmed cattle and one that is beyond control. Much of the meat in the grocery store will contain high levels of *E. coli*.

Grass-fed Meat, *cont.*

True grass-fed cows are pastured for their entire lives. Not only are grains not an option, grass-fed cows do not have their life cycle accelerated with hormones, which allow them to mature naturally. This extended life and nutrient-rich diet ends up benefiting the meat consumer.

Some studies suggest grass-fed beef has more nutrients, as much as 10 times more beta-carotene, three times more vitamin E, and two to four times more omega-3 fatty acids.

Omega-3s are formed in the chloroplasts of green leaves and algae. Sixty percent of the fatty acids in grass are omega-3s. When cattle are taken off omega-3-rich grass and shipped to a feedlot to be fattened on omega-3-poor grain, they begin losing their store of this beneficial fat. Each day that an animal spends in the feedlot, its supply of omega-3s is diminished.

Omega-3s are much-needed fats lacking in the standard American diet. They play a vital role in every cell and system in the body. Of all the fats, they are the most heart-friendly. People who have ample amounts of omega-3s in their diet are less likely to have high blood pressure or an irregular heartbeat. Omega-3s are essential for your brain, since the brain consists of 60 percent fat. A lack of this good fat in the brain could contribute to depression, schizophrenia, hyperactivity in adults and children, multiple sclerosis, or Alzheimer's.

The body has a better chance to heal from any condition when consuming sufficient amounts of omega-3 foods. One of the best benefits of this fat is a reduction of inflammation and increased weight loss. A higher level of good fats in the diet will help the adipose tissue release stored fat, leading to weight loss.

Conjugated linoleic acid (CLA) is a newly discovered fat that has gained great attention as a potent cancer-healing agent. In animal studies, it is known to block the initiation and promotion of cancer. Most anti-cancer synthetic agents block only one of these stages. CLA has also slowed the growth of an unusually wide variety of tumors, including cancers of the skin, breast, prostate, and colon.

Since the study of CLA is fairly new, few human studies have been conducted. These studies show similar benefits in people. A recent survey determined that women with the most CLA in their diets have a 60 percent reduction in the risk of breast cancer.

Many people are taking synthetic versions of CLA promoted as a diet-aid and muscle-builder. This may have some potentially serious side effects, including promoting insulin resistance, raising glucose levels, and reducing HDL cholesterol. Anything taken in synthetic form is contrary to our design. Few people realize that CLA is found in nature, and this natural form does not have any known negative side effects!

The most abundant source of natural CLA is in the meat and dairy products of grass-fed animals. Research conducted since 1999 shows that grazing animals have from 3 to 5 times more CLA than animals fattened on grain in a feedlot. You will greatly increase your intake of CLA by switching from grain-fed to grass-fed products!

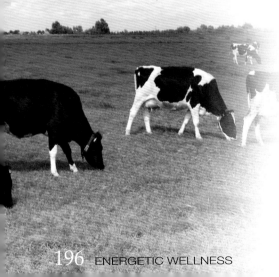

Grass-fed is tastier.

Any product resulting from the animal being raised on pasture will taste better. Their products take on a distinct flavor based on the terrain, grasses, weather, soil, and water.

In order for grass-fed beef to be succulent and tender, the cattle need to forage on high-quality grasses and legumes, especially in the months prior to slaughter. Providing this nutritious and natural diet requires healthy soil and careful pasture management so the plants are maintained at an optimal stage of growth. Because high-quality pasture is the key to high-quality animal products, many pasture-based ranchers refer to themselves as "grassfarmers" rather than "ranchers." They raise great grass; the animals do the rest.

Grass-fed means less waste.

Animal pastures take up a lot of land. Typically, there is a wide variety of vegetation growing through-out these fields. As the ranchers rotate their herds through the seasons, they preserve soil fertility by building organic matter in the soil, whereas grain farming destroys organic matter with the use of tillage, chemical fertilizer, and herbicides. By maintaining a diverse plant life, they ensure a healthy ecosystem and balanced nutrition for the animals, reduce erosion, and eliminate the waste-management problems associated with industrial feedlots. A major problem today is water pollution from runoff.

A 2009 joint study between the USDA and Clemson University in South Carolina compared grass-fed beef to grain-fed beef. Here are some of the differences they found:

- Lower in total fat
- Higher in beta-carotene
- Higher in vitamin E (alpha-tocopherol)
- Higher in the B-vitamins thiamin and riboflavin
- Higher in the minerals calcium, magnesium, and potassium
- Higher in total omega-3s
- A healthier ratio of omega-6 to omega-3 fatty acids (1.65 vs 4.84)
- Higher in CLA (cis-9 trans-11), a potential cancer-fighter
- Higher in vaccenic acid (which can be transformed into CLA)
- Lower in the saturated fats linked with heart disease

BOTTOM LINE: Find a local 100% grass-fed farmer. When you are shopping, ask for 100% grass-fed beef, bison, and lamb. Choosing products from grass-fed animals supports small farmers, safeguards the environment, and promotes animal welfare.

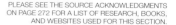

PLEASE SEE THE SOURCE ACKNOWLEDGMENTS ON PAGE 272 FOR A LIST OF RESEARCH, BOOKS, AND WEBSITES USED FOR THIS SECTION.

Pastured Poultry, Eggs & Pork

Pastured meat includes pigs and poultry. They are not strictly called *grass-fed* because these animals' natural diet includes grain. When living in their natural environment, they are allowed to field-graze on pesticide-free and herbicide-free pasture just like grass-fed animals. They are also usually fed pesticide-free, antibiotic-free, non-GMO (genetically modified organism) rations.

Chickens

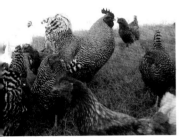

Chickens were first domesticated in Asia about 8000 years ago, and came to the U.S. by way of Europe in the 15th century. The average American eats about 80 pounds of chicken per year, which makes it by far the main source of animal protein in the American diet.

Pastured, organic chickens raised the old-fashioned way are still available throughout the U.S. from family farms who care about their animals and provide them with good, healthy diets. Their meat is much healthier and tastier than industrial chicken.

High demand has created massive factory farms where most of the nation's chickens, turkeys, and pigs are raised in close confinement. Typically, they suffer an even worse fate than the grazing animals. Tightly packed into cages, sheds, or pens, they cannot practice their normal behaviors, such as rooting, grazing, and roosting. Laying hens are crowded into cages that are so small there is not enough room for all of the birds to sit down at one time. An added insult is they cannot escape the stench of their own manure. They are kept alive pumped full of antibiotics and chemicals, and genetically engineered to grow quickly. Meat and eggs from these animals are lower in a number of key vitamins and omega-3 fatty acids.

Since the 1960s, large-scale poultry producers have added arsenic to their poultry feed. Although inorganic arsenic is toxic, small amounts speed the growth of the birds, make their breast meat pinker, and kill certain bacteria. Is this practice harmful for humans? Chronic exposure to high levels of arsenic has been linked with cancer, heart disease, diabetes, and a decline in brain function. The USDA has decreed that it is safe as long as poultry meat has fewer than 0.5 parts of arsenic per million.

That ruling, set in the 1950s, should be revised. Within the past few years, studies show that arsenic is a more potent cancer promoter than first believed. It has to do with its effect on blood vessels.

The reason that arsenic makes white meat pinker is that it increases the growth of blood vessels in the meat. The more blood, the pinker the color. That process, called "angiogenesis" also plays a key role in cancer promotion. Cancer cells speed up their growth with the creation of new blood vessels to fuel them.

The European Union banned the use of arsenic in poultry production in 1999. Several large U.S. producers have stopped the practice on their own. Some have not. Arsenic should be banned in all animal feed. Organic poultry should be free of arsenic and other potentially harmful chemicals.

A Bit About Eggs

Eggs are the perfect food! They are exceptionally nutritious which is not surprising since they contain everything needed to build a chick!

Eggs are a sacred food in China. A nursing or pregnant woman in China will eat up to ten eggs a

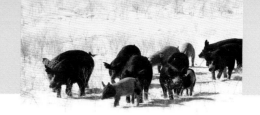

day, if she can afford them. The Chinese recognize that eggs are a brain food, ensuring the child will be very intelligent if he or she gets the nutrients through the mother's prenatal diet or through her milk.

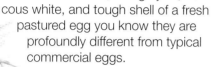

But not all eggs are created equal. If you have ever seen or tasted the tall, orange yolk, viscous white, and tough shell of a fresh pastured egg you know they are profoundly different from typical commercial eggs.

Pastured hens' diets are naturally complemented with bugs, earthworms, and other such critters that give their eggs a huge nutritious boost! They should also have freedom to spend their days scratching for bugs and taking plenty of dust baths.

Pastured hens, like all animals raised naturally, are much healthier and happier than their space-restricted and antibiotic-pumped industrial cousins. It is ecologically sustainable, humane, and produces the tastiest, most nutritious eggs.

Eggs from pastured hens contain up to 20 times more healthy omega-3 fatty acids than those from factory hens. Pastured eggs also have 10 percent less fat, 40 percent more vitamin A, and 34 percent less cholesterol than eggs obtained from factory farms.

Additional nutrients in pastured eggs compared to factory-farmed eggs include:

- 1/4 less saturated fat
- 2/3 more vitamin A
- 2 times more omega-3 fatty acids
- 3 times more vitamin E
- 7 times more beta carotene

Unless chickens are out in bright sunlight there will be no vitamin D in the egg yolks. In fact, most of the nutrients in the egg are in the yolk—the very thing we have been told to stay away from. All of the nutrients—including A, D, K2, beta-carotene, and omega-3 fatty acids—are in the yolk. So don't ever throw the yolks out!

Pork

Pork is a wonderful tasting meat and one of the most commonly consumed meats worldwide, with evidence of pig husbandry in China dating back to 5000 BC. Europeans began raising pigs by 1500 BC. The commonly hunted wild boar was probably the ancestor of today's modern species of pigs.

In the United States, the domestication of the pig can be traced to Hernando de Soto who arrived in Florida in 1539 with the original 13 pigs. Native Americans and succeeding generations have benefited from their arrival. The typical farmer at the end of the Seventeenth Century produced his own salt pork and bacon using the family pig.

I have fond memories of eating pork roast on Sundays at our home growing up—one of my mother's favorite dishes! When she visits, I like to serve a nice pastured pork roast or pork bacon.

My friend Kim Barker and his family at Walnut Creek Farms in Waynoka, Oklahoma, raise grass-fed beef and lamb, pastured pork and chickens. In confinement, he says that breeding pigs live their entire lives on concrete in crates. Meat hogs are raised with 20–30 in small pens which become very tight when they are full grown with "little to no room for them to move."

In contrast, local pasture farmers raise pigs that are not confined. Selecting their breed of choice, many farmers like Kim choose from old breeds that have never been confined like Duroc, Berkshire, or Mangalitsa—commenting that "the chefs really like them."

Look for your local farmers that are buying pure-breed animals and not using GMO feed.

BOTTOM LINE: You want to ask for pasture-raised, GMO-free, free-range and/or organic birds and pigs!

PLEASE SEE THE SOURCE ACKNOWLEDGMENTS ON PAGE 272 FOR A LIST OF RESEARCH, BOOKS, AND WEBSITES USED FOR THIS SECTION.

Raw Dairy

The History of Raw Milk

Milk and milk products have been part of man's diet for centuries. Scripture is full of passages about milk and its uses. In Genesis 18:8, we are told that Abraham took butter/curds and milk. Exodus 3:8 states God's assurance to deliver the nation of Israel to the promised land—a land flowing with milk and honey. In 1 Peter 2:2, there is an analogy that children require milk to grow strong.

In ancient times, milk was not heated to high temperatures—it was consumed straight from the animal. There was no fear of disease from raw milk. So where have we gone wrong?

From 1790 to 1840, New York grew from a small town of 33,000 to 400,000—a 1,200% increase in 50 years. Immigrants poured into the city to find a better life for their family. Most of them were accustomed to raw milk—especially for their children. Many kept family cows, but as the city grew, cows were kept in common pastures. Boston Commons is one of the most famous—cows grazed there as late as 1850.

As New York and other cities grew more crowded, the grazing land was lost. Those who wanted fresh milk had to send a messenger into the country to obtain it. There was a great demand for milk, but there were not enough farmers or proper transportation to meet the growing need. Raw milk became a commodity of the rich.

The War of 1812 led to swill milk dairies.

The war with England resulted in the permanent severance of America's supply of whiskey from the British West Indies. As a result, grain distilleries began to spring up throughout the country and in every major city.

The refining process extracted the starch and alcohol from the grains and left behind an acid waste of grain and water known as distillery slop. Owners built adjacent dairy barns and began feeding cows the hot slop as it poured off the stills. Thus was born the

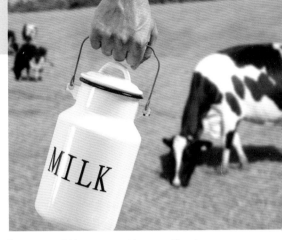

slop or swill milk system. What initially began as an experiment became a huge industry. This system proved to produce more milk at a lower cost than any other method.

The cows were kept in foul air with no other food. The grain slop had little nutrition, but it was plentifully supplied, and cows yielded an abundance of milk. They stood or rested in their own manure and grew sick until their tail rotted off and their skin broke out in gangrenous ulcers. The cows that died were removed and replaced by others to continue this inhumane cycle. The cows were left in these conditions and the milk was unfiltered and often unsafe to drink. It was also of very poor quality—it could not even be made into butter or cheese.

This was the milk that reached households. It was white or bluish and dirty. It was rarely strained before drinking and often mixed with the impure water available in the cities.

Certify or pasteurize?

By the last decade of the 19th Century, America had a major problem. The yearly death rate of infants who lived in the city was 50%. Children died from diarrhea, typhoid fever, cholera, diphtheria, and tuberculosis. Many doctors believed that unsanitary milk helped to spread the diseases.

In 1889, Dr. Henry Coit asked the Medical Society of New Jersey to formally investigate how to secure clean raw milk for his patients and the public. His own wife was experiencing difficulty nursing their infant son and he found the available milk an unacceptable substitute.

In April of 1893 Dr. Coit and 41 other physicians formed the Essex County Medical Milk Commission, which birthed the certified milk movement. Certified Raw Milk was endorsed by a significant number of medical professionals, legislators, and the public.

Crusader for Pasteurization

Nathan Straus was most responsible for popularizing pasteurization at the turn of the century. He made his fortune in business as a co-owner of Macy's department store. He dedicated thirty years of his life to championing the pasteurization of the milk supply in New York and other cities throughout America and Europe. He had a powerful ally in Dr. Abraham Jacobi, MD, who served for many years as president of the American Medical Association.

Conditions of the distilleries and nearby dairies had only marginally improved by 1893 when Straus established the first of his "milk depots" for the distribution of low-priced pasteurized milk. Changing the conditions of the dairies and the nutrition given to the cows seemed too difficult a task, so they focused their efforts on making the milk safe.

Dr. Straus did not consider that the poor quality milk failed to nourish and contributed to the problem.

In the absence of official action, Straus began his own crusade to pasteurize the milk supply of New York City. For Straus and the officials who backed him, pasteurization was a matter of economics and practicality. The enforcement of strict rules of hygiene on the forty thousand independent dairy farms that supplied milk to New York City seemed impossible. Pasteurization promised a quick, technological fix that would make New York's milk safe to drink.

Most recognized that certified raw milk was safe and healthy, but it was expensive to produce and sold for two to four times the cost of pasteurized milk.

Infant death rates dropped after pasteurization, but officials had also been working to clean up the water supply and the polluted city streets from horse excrement.

Straus saw milk as the problem because it was the only animal food taken in its raw state. They thought raw milk contained living germs. It seemed logical for health officials to embrace pasteurization as the solution to unsanitary dairy conditions, but proponents of pasteurization failed to understand fundamental nutritional principles. They did not realize that germs were not the problem, and that every traditional culture had emphasized the importance of raw animal foods in the maintenance of human health.

The pasteurization of this nutrient-devoid milk only created a deeper problem. The heat of pasteurization fundamentally alters the nutritional value of milk—all the live enzymes and nutrients are killed, leaving it indigestible to the human body. This not only fails to nourish, but causes our bodies to pull nutrients from our reserves to properly digest and assimilate.

This natural response causes additional mucus in the respiratory tract. The extra mucus is not an allergic reaction, but the body's attempt to rid itself of the counterfeit milk. Raw milk does not cause mucus or upper respiratory problems.

Contrary to popular belief, pasteurization of milk is not a step forward in nutrition and health. It is a step backward. Certain important nutritional elements such as vitamins, enzymes, and minerals are lost. Louis Pasteur developed pasteurization in 1864 to help French winemakers. It is reported that Pasteur sadly lamented when informed that pasteurization was being used for milk, "What are they doing to my wonderful food?"

Is Raw Milk Safe?

There have been no clinical studies of people drinking raw milk to prove or disprove the theory that the bacteria in raw milk can cause disease in humans. Even beneficial nutrients found in raw milk have been falsely blamed for ill effects.

"The powerful crusade against raw milk has been lethal to the empirical evidence that raw milk and raw milk products are probably the most nutritious food most people can consume." www.rawmilk.org

Factory-farmed cattle have 300 times more pathogenic bacteria in their digestive tracts than cattle that are allowed to openly graze in pastures.

Proven Farm History of Raw Milk Safety

Organic Pastures Dairy Farm: Since 1999, there have been over 40,000,000 servings of raw milk—without one confirmed illness. In over 1,300 tests, no pathogens were found in the milk, milking area, or in any of the dairy cows.

Claravale Dairy: During Claravale Farm's 80-year history, no consumers of their milk have ever gotten sick and no pathogens have ever been detected in the milk.

Pasteurized Outbreaks: Since 1999, there have been several recalls of pasteurized milk products and one publicized outbreak of illness due to pasteurized milk—an outbreak of Campylobacter that sickened 1,300 people.

Benefits of Raw Milk & Dangers of Pasteurized Milk

Pasteurization is a process that slows microbial growth in food. It is not intended to kill all pathogenic microorganisms in the food or liquid, but aims to reduce the number of viable pathogens so they are unlikely to cause disease.

Two Main Types of Pasteurization Used Today:
- High Temperature / Short Time (HTST): 161°F for 15–20 seconds
- Ultra-Heat Treated (UHT): 280°F for a fraction of a second

Rapid Heating: Both treatments involve rapid heating by forcing the milk between heated stainless steel plates.

Raw milk's *antimicrobial* properties have been detailed only recently, but its properties were recognized as early as 1938 in studies showing that raw milk did not support the growth of a wide range of pathogens.

Researchers noted that heating milk inactivates *inhibins*—factors that inhibit bacterial growth. Pasteurization destroys enzymes, diminishes vitamin content, denatures fragile milk proteins, alters vitamin B12 and vitamin B6, kills beneficial bacteria, promotes pathogens, and is associated with allergies, increased tooth decay, colic in infants, growth problems in children, osteoporosis, arthritis, heart disease, and cancer.

The pasteurization process was mainly created to increase the shelf life of milk for transport across the country. This process has not only caused a decline in our health, but has taken away the livelihood of many small farmers who could be safely supplying milk to nearby cities.

Pottenger's Cats

In the early 1930s, parallel to the studies of Dr. Weston A. Price, Dr. Francis Pottenger began a ten-year study of cats fed entirely different diets.

Dr. Pottenger classified the cats as the *normal cats, deficient cats,* and *regenerating cats*. The normal (healthy) cats were only fed raw food, including raw meat, raw milk, and cod liver oil. These cats continued to reproduce and were very healthy. In fact, some generations of Pottenger's healthy cats still exist today. These cats had well-operating lymph and circulatory systems and healthy fur and skin. They had a moderate heart size, good liver, firm intestines, and resting uterus.

The first generation of deficient cats were fed a diet of raw meat, *pasteurized* milk, and cod liver oil. These cats had thin hair, slight fatty atrophy of the liver, lack of intestinal tone, moderate distention of the uterus, and their skin had a purplish discoloration due to congestion. Also, the internal organs of the female cats were noted to have poor skin tone.

The diet of subsequent generations of deficient cats

consisted of cooked foods, raw or cooked meat, pasteurized milk, vitamin D milk, condensed milk, sweetened condensed milk, and cod liver oil. These cats showed serious health deficiencies in just one generation, and the severity increased with each generation. The cats had many issues—musculoskeletal, organs, quality of skin and fur, reproductive, and behavioral. Most of the deficient cats also had severe allergies and thyroid conditions.

The regenerating cats were first, second, or third generation deficient cats that were put back on the raw diet to see if they would return to better health. When the female cat of the first deficient generation was placed back on a raw diet after giving birth to a deficient litter, her next kittens benefited from her improved diet. However, it required four generations to regenerate the cats to a state of good health.

There were never more than three generations of deficient cats because the third generation was unable to produce healthy, viable offspring.

If we continue to eat fake, denatured, highly processed food, how many generations will it take before mankind ceases to exist? Could it be, as Dr. Katz stated in his studies, that the children born after the year 2000 will be the first to not outlive their parents? We have to stop the madness and return to pure, whole foods—future generations are at risk.

Clean, raw milk from pastured cows is a complete, balanced food. You could exclusively live on it if you had to. It supplies the body with enzymes, good bacteria, raw fat, raw protein, omega-3 fatty acid, CLA, fat-soluble vitamins, and needed minerals. Milk is not just a beverage—it is a food.

People all over the world have consumed raw milk directly from the cow, sheep, or goat for centuries—and still do. In America, many dairy farmers drink raw milk. We consumed raw milk for thousands of years before pasteurization—and they did not even have a complete understanding of sanitation. Why do we hesitate now? We should not think twice about drinking raw milk.

Dan Buettner, a research reporter, traveled the world searching for people who lived long lives. In his book, *The Blue Zones*, he describes an Italian man from Sardinia, Italy. I am of Italian descent, so this was of great interest to me. The man was 75 years old and still strong and healthy enough to climb the hills of Sardinia to tend his sheep. His main diet was raw cheese, vegetables, fava beans, and raw goat milk. The men of that region appeared to retain their vigor and vitality longer than men almost anywhere else.

Asthma & Raw Milk:

We have an asthma crisis in America. According to the Center for Disease Control (CDC), asthma is the second most prevalent chronic condition among children. It results in approximately 14 million days of missed school each year. Asthma in children increased from 3.6% in 1980 to 7.5% in 1995—approximately 5 million children.

A study done on asthma and raw milk revealed that long-term and early-life exposure to raw milk induced a strong protective effect against the development of asthma, hay fever, and rashes. The benefits are the greatest when we start our children on raw milk when they are young.

Researchers in London concluded that children who even infrequently drank raw milk had significantly less eczema and a greater reduction in allergic hypersensitivity. Raw milk is a strong factor in reducing the risk of asthma and allergies.

Since ancient times, an exclusive raw milk diet has been used to cure many diseases. In the early 1900s, the "Milk Cure" was used at the Mayo clinic to successfully treat cancer, weight loss, kidney disease, allergies, skin issues, urinary tract infections, prostate problems, chronic fatigue, and many other serious conditions.

Clean, raw milk from pastured cows is a complete, balanced food.

The Milk Cure only works with raw milk—pasteurized milk does not have the same curative powers.

Raw Milk: The Beverage That Is a Food!

My family started drinking raw milk after I learned about its many benefits. We all loved it immediately and now I don't like going a day without it. I feel stronger when I drink it; it helps me fall asleep at night, and it gives me an overall sense of wellbeing. One of my sons has benefited the most. As a child, he experienced frequent fevers and bronchitis, as well as some learning difficulties. When we started drinking raw milk, he became a different child and even he felt the difference.

Raw milk has the most comprehensive immune-supporting qualities to protect and assist the body in its natural function. It contains the perfect balance of raw fat, raw protein, vitamins, minerals, and enzymes. Raw milk is a wonderful composition of whole food nutrients in a form that is instantly digested—and is able to independently sustain life.

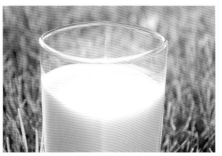

Raw milk—the perfect, complete storage food—contains calcium, phosphorus, CLA, minerals, and vitamins B12, A, D, E, K2, and C.

- **Raw Fat**—Grass-fed raw milk has a wonderful combination of essential fatty acids, saturated fat, and conjugated linoleic acid (CLA) very similar to that of grass-fed meat. Refer to Grass-Fed Meat (p. 195).
- **Raw Protein**—The protein in raw milk consists of amino acids, casein, and whey. It is one of the easiest proteins to digest and utilize in the body. The raw proteins in milk are very fragile and, when pasteurized, are unrecognized by the body—it requires an immune response to eliminate them. This puts an unwanted burden on the body and explains some of the digestive problems of most Americans.
- **Immunoglobulins**—Also known as antibodies, immunoglobulins are an extremely complex class of milk proteins. They protect and control immune responses in the body to keep us healthy. Lactoperoxidase is a natural bacterial defense—levels are 10 times higher in goat milk than in breast milk. Lactoferrin regulates microbes, balances the inflammatory process, and stimulates the immune system. The layers of the lungs are loaded with these wonderful workers to protect us when we inhale something unhealthy. Raw milk is the perfect remedy for upper respiratory conditions. Lactoferrin is believed to cut belly fat and is now being sold as an isolated nutrient supplement (not recommended). Nothing compares to the real thing—drink your milk. These powerful helpers are almost nonexistent in pasteurized milk.
- **Carbohydrates**—The main carbohydrate in milk is lactose. It is made of the simple sugars glucose and galactose. When people become lactose intolerant, their bodies fail to produce the enzyme lactase to digest milk sugar. This is only a problem with pasteurized milk. I have found that even those who are lactose intolerant do very well on raw milk. All the wonderful enzymes and bacteria are intact in raw milk—making it easily digestible.
- **Vitamins**—The most wonderful benefit of raw milk is the host of beneficial vitamins, including B12, A, D, E, K2, and C, which are all absent in pasteurized milk. Grass-fed raw milk contains the fat-soluble vitamins that work together with minerals to build strong bones. Dr. Weston A. Price discovered that the body requires high levels of minerals and vitamins beginning in utero for optimum health. America is on the 4th or 5th generation of processed food—food that has been altered from its original state.
- **Minerals, Minerals, Minerals**—Most of my patients are very deficient in minerals. Calcium is abundant

in raw milk. It works in synergy with other minerals required to build a strong bone structure in both children and adults. Children and pregnant and nursing mothers have the greatest need for milk. Many argue that the vitamin and mineral content is the same in pasteurized milk and raw milk. However, the heating process alters the structure of the food and the added synthetic nutrients are not assimilated by the body. Although the U.S. consumes the largest amount of dairy products in the world, we are vitamin D deficient and suffer from a host of musculoskeletal conditions. Drink the real thing to get the perfect balance of nutrients for the natural body.

• **Enzymes**—Raw milk is loaded with digestive enzymes. Drinking a little raw milk with each meal helps the utilization of nutrients and creates less work for our pancreas, which releases digestive enzymes. Enzymes and minerals are the catalysts to every function in the body. There are 60 active enzymes in raw milk. Some are inherent in the milk, some come from the bacteria growing in raw milk, and some protect the milk from unwanted bacteria, which makes it very safe for us to drink.

• **Bacteria**—Most food goes bad as it ages, but raw milk only gets better. The nutrients increase in raw milk, raw cheese, raw yogurt, and raw kefir. It has self-protective properties and a host of nutritional benefits. Raw dairy is the most easily digestible food. If you cannot obtain raw milk, it is essential you eat good quality raw cheese, yogurt, or kefir.

• **Immunity Powerhouse**—There are many immune system boosters in raw milk. The natural hormones and growth factors in raw milk stimulate the strength and maturity of the gut lining which can prevent "leaky" gut.

Old Paradigm: Healthy human body is sterile and microbes attack it, making us sick.

New Paradigm: Healthy human body lives in a symbiotic relationship with microorganisms.

Arguments for pasteurization are based on this discredited medical paradigm. For generations, medical authorities have enslaved and imprisoned the human mind with a fear of "diseases."

It is a challenge to convince some of my patients to switch to raw milk. The strong grip of the old paradigm still causes fear. History has made it difficult for people to understand the benefits of raw milk. We fear what we do not understand.

BOTTOM LINE: Raw milk is a support system powerhouse that benefits everyone. I would not advise anyone to drink or eat pasteurized dairy products.

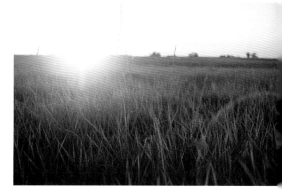

For more information on the benefits of raw milk, refer to www.realmilk.com, www.westonaprice.org, or read *The Untold Story of Milk* by Ron Schmid, ND.

PLEASE SEE THE SOURCE ACKNOWLEDGMENTS ON PAGE 272 FOR A LIST OF RESEARCH, BOOKS, AND WEBSITES USED FOR THIS SECTION.

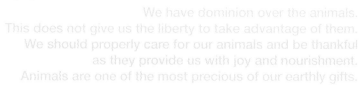

We have dominion over the animals.
This does not give us the liberty to take advantage of them.
We should properly care for our animals and be thankful
as they provide us with joy and nourishment.
Animals are one of the most precious of our earthly gifts.

Fermented Foods

Raw, Fermented Foods Are Rich in Enzymes

Only recently have fermented foods begun to disappear from our plate. Modern pickles and sauerkraut are made with vinegar instead of the **traditional method of lacto-fermentation using salt**. Bread and pasta are made with commercial yeast instead of being naturally leavened with wild yeast (sourdough). Wine, beer, and cheeses are being pasteurized, killing off all the good bacteria.

There are many advantages to the traditional ways of our ancestors, including fermented foods. Humans all over the world have been fermenting food since ancient times.

The earliest evidence of winemaking dates back 8000 years in the Caucasus area of Georgia between Asia and Europe. 7000-year-old jars, which once contained wine, were excavated in the Zagros Mountains in Iran. There is evidence that people were making fermented beverages in Babylon circa 5000 BC, in ancient Egypt circa 3150 BC, in Mesoamerica circa 2000 BC, and in Sudan circa 1500 BC. There is also evidence of leavened bread in ancient Egypt dating back to 1500 BC and of milk fermentation in Babylon circa 3000 BC.

Fermenting foods before we eat them is like partially digesting them before we consume them. People that have a hard time digesting milk can usually tolerate yogurt. The lactose in milk is broken down as the milk is fermented.

Your body needs enzymes to properly digest, absorb, and make full use of your food. Eating processed food cuts down on the body's supply of enzymes. This has caused many scientists to hypothesize that if you could guard against enzyme depletion, you could live a longer, healthier life.

Fermentation of milk breaks down casein, one of the most difficult proteins to digest. Culturing restores many of the enzymes destroyed during pasteurization, including *lactase*, which helps digest *lactose*. Lactase produced during the culturing process allows many people who are sensitive to fresh milk tolerate fermented milk products.

Both the vitamin B and vitamin C content of milk increases during fermentation. Regular consumption of cultured dairy products lowers cholesterol and protects against bone loss. And most importantly, cultured dairy products provide beneficial bacteria and lactic acid to the digestive tract. They aid in the fullest possible digestion of all food we consume!

Kefir is a delicious probiotic cultured milk drink. It is tangy and sour, like a more liquid version of yogurt. Drink it straight, or put it in a blender and add a little fruit and maple syrup to make a kefir smoothie.

Making kefir at home is so easy. And it is very good for you. In fact, kefir made from raw milk from grass-fed cows is a magical drink. As a probiotic, kefir is much more powerful than yogurt.

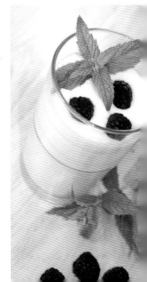

Most bowel conditions have been linked to a lack of "good bacteria" in the gut. The microorganisms in our gut are 80 percent of our support system. They are our little friends that come to the aid of our body every day and keep us healthy.

So the answer is to stop eating dead, devitalized food and replace it with nutrient-dense food rich in enzymes found in fermented foods. Nothing can compare to fermented foods. Many traditional societies value them for their health-promoting properties and insist on giving them to the sick, the aged, and nursing mothers.

Raw-milk cheese is made with milk that is unpasteurized. Since 1949, the U.S. government has forbidden the sale of cheeses made from unpasteurized milk unless the cheese is aged at least 60 days. So you will not see any raw cheese sold retail that does not follow this law.

Some cheesemakers believe that using raw milk creates more flavorful and more healthful cheeses. Many cheesemakers believe there is no reason to be fearful of raw milk and no reason to wait 60 days to eat cheese made from it.

Fermented Vegetables & Fruits

Traditional cultures knew how to preserve vegetables and fruits for long periods without freezers or canning machines. This process is called lacto-fermentation. Lactic acid is a natural preservative that inhibits putrefying bacteria.

Starches and sugars in veggies and fruits are converted into lactic acid by the species of lactic-acid producing bacteria. Lactobacilli are present on the surface of all living things and especially numerous on leaves and roots of plants growing in or near the ground. The proliferation of lactobacilli in fermented vegetables enhances their digestibility and increases vitamin levels. These beneficial organisms also produce numerous helpful enzymes.

Their byproduct, lactic acid, not only keeps vegetables and fruits in a state of perfect preservation but also promotes the growth of healthy flora throughout the intestine! Other byproducts of this process include hydrogen peroxide and small amounts of benzoic acid.

Traditional cultures use fermented vegetables on a daily basis.

Europe—Sauerkraut, cucumbers, beets, turnips, pickled herbs, sorrel leaves, and grape leaves.

Russia & Poland—Pickled green tomatoes, peppers, and lettuce.

Asian (Japan, China, & Korea)—Pickled cabbage, turnip, eggplant, cucumber, onion, squash, and carrot. Korean kimchi is cabbage with other vegetables and seasoning, eaten daily.

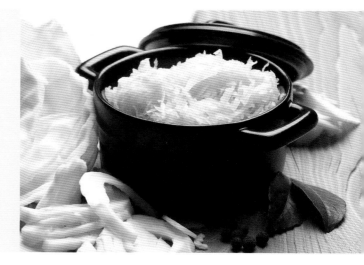

Fermenting food helps preserve food for longer periods of time. Raw milk lasts 7 days in the refrigerator but yogurt and kefir much longer. Sauerkraut, pickles, and salsa keep for months. And if you have a large batch of produce in your garden that you don't know how to use, ferment it! It will last for six months in the fridge!

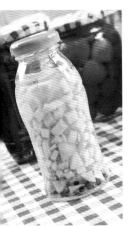

Fermenting food is inexpensive. There is nothing fancy required. You can use inexpensive cabbage to make sauerkraut, or purchase a kombucha scoby and with just pennies' worth of water, whole cane sugar, and tea, you've got a health elixir/soda pop.

Fermenting food increases the flavor. There's a reason we enjoy drinking wine and eating stinky cheese. There's a reason we like sauerkraut on our hot dogs and salsa on our tortilla chips. They taste good!

BOTTOM LINE: Delicious Fermented Foods

Dairy Products: cultured milk, cheese, cultured cream cheese, yogurt, kefir, whey, cultured cream, cultured sour cream (can be made into a Finnish culture called piima), and cultured buttermilk (into European-style sour cream, crème fraiche).

Vegetables & Fruits: cabbage, carrots, onions, garlic, cucumbers, beets, turnips, daikon radishes, red peppers, ginger, corn, tomatoes, cherries, mint, pineapples, papayas, raisins, lemons, oranges, apricots, and berries.

Eating fermented food helps us absorb the nutrients. You can ingest high amounts of nutrients, but unless your body actually absorbs them, they are useless.

Shopping Tips for Dairy Products

Since all of us live such busy lives, finding the time to prepare fresh homemade yogurt and kefir and other fermented foods can be a challenge. We can purchase certain brands of dairy products in health-food stores and grocery stores if we make wise choices.

I am very specific about the dairy products I recommend. Of course, **raw dairy products** are superior to any other dairy, and I highly recommend you avoid all pasteurized dairy. Search for raw milk from your local farmer (p. 178), some of them make fresh raw cheese, yogurt and kefir. Or learn how to make your own.

You can also purchase vat-pasteurized whole milk grass-fed dairy products from Kalona Supernatural. **Vat-pasteurization** is a low-heat method used so the dairy products can be sold in grocery stores. This is the only milk I recommend in health-food stores. Organic Valley now produces a Grass-Milk that is also acceptable.

Check local stores for **imported cheeses**—most imported cheeses are made from raw milk and are of high quality. Look on the label for the words "milk" or "fresh milk." Some are even labeling them "unpasteurized," which is great.

Buy plain, organic whole milk yogurt and kefir and dress them up yourself with fresh berries, nuts, and if needed, a minute amount of honey or other approved natural sweetener. Adding a small amount of digestive enzyme powder aids in the absorption of minerals. I recommend Redwood Hill Farms plain goat yogurt and kefir.

For a complete shopping guide, check with your local WAPF chapter leader or www.westonaprice.org (p. 260)

PLEASE SEE THE SOURCE ACKNOWLEDGMENTS ON PAGE 272 FOR A LIST OF RESEARCH, BOOKS, AND WEBSITES USED FOR THIS SECTION.

Wild-Caught Fish

Omega-3s are most abundant in seafood. One of the most significant benefits of eating fish is the high level of omega-3 fatty acids that it contains. We do not produce omega-3s on our own, so it is vital that we eat these foods.

People in various cultures have consumed seafood since the beginning of time. Many native cultures that Dr. Price visited survived mostly on seafood prior to the introduction of modernized food. In fact, inland tribes often traveled great distances to the nearest coast.

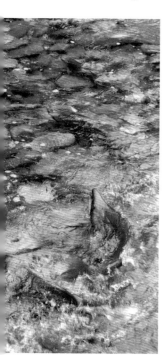

Other Beneficial Nutrients in Fish

Fish are also the richest food sources of three other valuable food factors:

- *Vitamin D* offers uniquely strong bone-building and anti-cancer benefits. Tuna and wild salmon are the richest food sources known.
- *Astaxanthin* is the powerful anti-inflammatory, carotenoid-class antioxidant that gives wild salmon its characteristic red-orange color.
- *Selenium* is an essential mineral needed to make enzymes that play key roles in the body's internal antioxidant network.

Fish farming presents many of the same problems as factory farms, including environmental pollution, unsanitary conditions, and an inferior final product. A typical fish farm may cram up to 90,000 fish in a single pen that's 100 feet long by 100 feet wide. Salmon, one of the most commonly farmed fish, must be fed a significant amount of smaller sea life such as sardines, anchovies, mackerel, and herring. Farmed salmon are typically fed pellets composed of these, along with wheat, soy, antibiotics, pesticides, and hormones. The salmon that are raised on this unnatural diet are a dull gray and are given the synthetic pigments canthaxanthin and astaxanthin to imitate their natural and vivid tone of pink.

Multiple studies have shown farm-raised fish to contain significantly higher amounts of pollutants, including mercury and PCBs. The unnatural conditions in which farmed fish are raised also promote the spread of disease and parasites, and even alter the content of omega-3 fatty acids, which negates the primary benefit of eating fish. Farmed fish also contain lower levels of vitamins A and D.

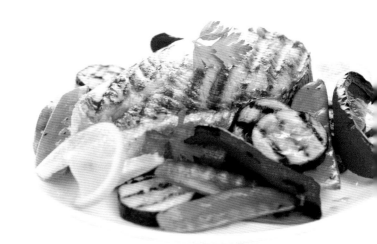

Fish Oil Supplements

Due to factory farming techniques, the American diet is very deficient in essential fatty acids—especially omega-3. The animals we eat no longer have access to pasture. When animals are confined and not allowed to live according to their design, the fatty acid ratio is out of balance. Animal products from grass-fed, pasture-raised animals and wild-caught fish, have the balanced amount of all essential fatty acids needed by the body.

Fish oils have become very popular and there are many to choose from. However, not all supplements are created equal. Virtually, all fish oils are rancid by the time they are purchased, and when not taken with a diet that is rich in saturated fat, the body is not able to properly absorb and utilize them.

Cod Liver Oil—A Super Food

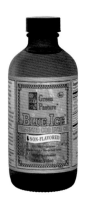

Fish liver oils (as opposed to fish oil) were once a standard supplement in traditional cultures. Fish liver oils were used medicinally to treat a host of conditions dating back to the recorded use by Hippocrates. Cod liver oil has an abundant natural form of the fat-soluble vitamins A and D. In the 1930s, Dr. Weston A. Price found that the diet of primitive people contained 10 times the amount of fat soluble vitamins than that of the typical American diet.

Cod liver oil is also rich in eicosapentaenoic acid (EPA) and docasahexaenoic acid (DHA). The body makes these fatty acids from omega-3 linolenic acid as an important link in the chain of fatty acids. This results in beneficial levels of prostaglandins, (localized tissue hormones) responsible for the proper function of the brain, nervous system, and for good eyesight. DHA is especially important for neurological function. Diabetics and people who consume large amounts of harmful oils have a difficult time producing EPA and DHA.

Cod liver oil is most beneficial when accompanied by a diet rich in what Dr. Price called "Activator X"—now thought to be vitamin K2. Vitamin K2 works synergistically with the vitamins A and D found in cod liver oil. Together, these fat-soluble vitamins ensure the efficient assimilation of minerals and water-soluble vitamins in our diet. Foods high in vitamin K2 are grass-fed butter, fish eggs, shellfish, and other grass-fed dairy products. Insects and organ meats are also considered good sources.

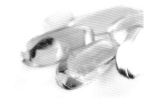

The combination of cod liver oil and grass-fed butter and other grass-fed dairy products assist in the natural function of the brain and nervous system.

The combination of cod liver oil and grass-fed butter assist in the natural function of the brain and nervous system. A diet rich in saturated fats such as lard, tallow, butter, and tropical oils ensures proper utilization of the omega-3 fatty acids in cod liver oil. The natural calcium in bone broth and grass-fed, raw dairy products works with vitamins A, D, and K2 to build strong bones and teeth. And foods rich in magnesium like green vegetables, nuts, whole grains, legumes, and organ meats work in synergy for the metabolism of vitamin D to strengthen our immune system. A combination of cod liver oil and these foods supports the natural function and design of the body.

Cod Liver Oil: A Key Source of Vital Nutrients

Vitamin A: Necessary for mineral metabolism, strong bones, immune system, normal growth, successful reproduction, healthy skin, and good eyesight

Vitamin D: Necessary for mineral absorption, nervous system function, insulin production, immune system health, and protection against depression

Vitamin K2 (found in fermented cod liver oil): Necessary for normal facial development, strong bones, healthy arteries, and optimal function of the brain and nervous system

Vitamin E: Necessary for normal reproduction and protection against free radical damage

DHA: Necessary for optimal visual and brain function, immune system health, and helps resolve inflammation

The best way to take cod liver oil is not by the spoon! Mix it with a small amount of warm water or organic, freshly squeezed orange juice. Stir and swallow quickly. Take immediately before a meal. Capsules are available but are expensive in comparison to the liquid.

I recommend Blue Ice Fermented Cod Liver Oil when choosing a Cod Liver Oil supplement, especially for those without a gallbladder. Salmon Oil is the only other fish oil recommendation but only from Vital Farms Seafood. Find both products at the EW online store.

BOTTOM LINE:
Always choose wild-caught seafood.
Even shrimp is farm raised now, so look for wild-caught shrimp!

When supplementing with fish oil, always choose
a fermented fish liver oil and don't bother with the rest.

PLEASE SEE THE SOURCE ACKNOWLEDGMENTS
ON PAGE 272 FOR A LIST OF RESEARCH, BOOKS,
AND WEBSITES USED FOR THIS SECTION.

Bone Broths

Bone broth is a medicinal food!
"Good broth will resurrect the dead."
—South American proverb

I'll never forget visiting my great Aunt Ethel years ago when an African woman was living with her. She was a beautiful woman with amazing skin, bright white teeth, and wide cheek bones. She was in the kitchen cooking soup and all I remember is seeing the feet in the pot! She was making this soup for herself because she didn't eat the standard American diet.

Today, broth is uncommon in American cuisine. Most traditional diets made use of bones, either ground up and made into a paste or cooked with water and made into a bone broth. Bone broths have been used throughout the world in Asian, African, European, French, Italian, South American, Middle Eastern, and Russian foods.

Nearly every traditional society boiled bones of meat animals to make a nutritive broth. It is deeply flavorful and versatile. It can provide the base for soups, sauces, gravies and a cooking medium for grains and vegetables.

Years ago, when butchers sold meat on the bone rather than as individual filets, and whole chickens rather than boneless breasts, our thrifty ancestors made use of every part of the animal by preparing stock, broth, or bouillon from the bony portions. Unfortunately, the use of homemade meat broths to produce nourishing and flavorful soups and sauces has almost completely disappeared from American food.

In 1908, the Japanese invented **monosodium glutamate (MSG)** to enhance food flavors, particularly meat-like flavors. Did you know we actually have glutamate receptors on our tongues? It is the protein in food that the human body recognizes as meat. With the ability to hydrolyze just about any protein to create free glutamic acid, manufacturers could now create intense, meat-like flavors without any meat present. Now industry had created a way to make food that tasted "just as good" at a fraction of the cost.

In a General Foods Company report issued in 1947, chemists predicted that almost all-natural flavors would soon be chemically synthesized. When the industry learned how to make the flavor of meat using inexpensive proteins isolated from grains and legumes, the door opened to a flood of new products, including bouillon cubes, dehydrated soup mixes, sauce mixes, TV dinners, and condiments with a meaty taste.

Even in finer restaurants, "homemade" soup often begins with a powdered soup base that comes in a package or can, and almost all canned soups and stews contain MSG, often in ingredients called hydrolyzed proteins. The fast food industry could not exist without MSG and artificial meat flavors to make "secret sauces and spice mixes" that trick consumers into eating bland and tasteless food.

But at what cost to our health?

The dangers of MSG have been well documented, but the industry has worked very hard to conceal it from the public. In 1957, scientists found that mice became blind and obese when MSG was administered by feeding tube. Monosodium glutamate is a neurotoxic substance that causes a wide range of reactions, from temporary headaches to permanent brain damage. In 1969, MSG-induced lesions were found in the hypothalamus region of the brain.

When homemade stocks were pushed out by cheap substitutes, an important source of minerals disappeared from the American diet. The thickening effect of gelatin could be mimicked with emulsifiers, but the health benefits were lost.

Benefits of Bone Broth

Grandmothers, midwives, and healers were right! Soup is the cure for when you are down. It is warm, easy to digest, and it can contain lots of immune-boosting herbs and spices. It is definitely healthier than the chemical-laden, canned stuff you buy in the supermarket.

Making soup with bone marrow stock is more than a mood cure; it enhances your **support system** and provides you with easy-to-assimilate minerals. The marrow inside the bones contains nutrients that feed your bone marrow. When your bone marrow is nourished, it creates more robust immune cells that can better support your body and rebuild health.

As the bones cook in water—especially if that water has been made slightly acidic by the inclusion of apple cider vinegar—minerals and other nutrients leach from the bones into the broth in a form the body can easily absorb.

Homemade broth is rich in calcium, magnesium, phosphorus, silicon, sulfur, and other trace minerals. Bone broth contains broken down material from cartilage and tendons containing **glucosamine** and **chondroitin**—which are thought to help mitigate arthritis and joint pain. Cartilage is formed from collagen and elastin proteins. Chondroitin sulfate is a structural component of cartilage and is essential in maintaining the integrity of the extracellular matrix. It lines the blood vessels, may play a role in lowering cholesterol, and is very good for the heart! Using cartilage-rich beef knuckles, chicken feet, trachea, and ribs in your stock will assure you get these great

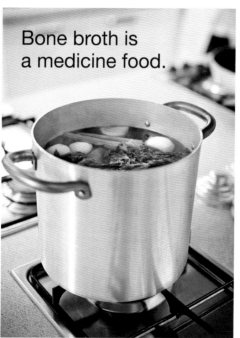

Bone broth is a medicine food.

benefits in your broth!

Fish stock, according to traditional lore, helps boys grow up into strong men, makes childbirth easy, and cures fatigue. Broth and soup made with fish heads and carcasses provide iodine and thyroid-strengthening substances.

Homemade bone broths are often rich in **gelatin**. So when the broth is cooled, it congeals. The use of gelatin as a therapeutic agent dates back to the ancient Chinese. Gelatin is not a complete protein, and contains only the amino acids arginine and glycine in large amounts. It acts as a protein sparer by helping to stretch less meat into a complete meal.

Gelatin aids the body in repairing degenerative joints. It also helps to support the connective tissue in your body and helps the fingernails and hair grow well and strong. Gelatin in nutrient-dense broth also helps the body assimilate protein so that you can stretch meat further.

Bone broth also contains **proline**. Proline is essential to the structure of collagen and is therefore necessary for healthy bones, skin, ligaments, tendons, and cartilage. Small amounts can be manufactured by the body, but evidence shows that adequate dietary protein is necessary to maintain an optimal level of proline in the body.

Collagen is basically the same as gelatin! We say "collagen" when referring to the body, and "gelatin" when referring to the extracted collagen used as food!

Most commercial gelatins are made from animal skin and often contain MSG!

Poor wound healing, bleeding gums, and bruising are often associated with a vitamin C deficiency; however, the problem is actually a collagen deficiency because vitamin C is needed to metabolize proline and synthesize collagen. Gelatin also helps heal the mucus membranes of the gastrointestinal tract in cases of inflammation.

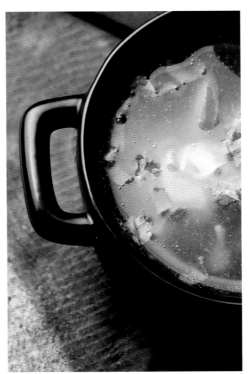

Glycine is a simple amino acid necessary in the manufacture of other amino acids. Glycine is a vital component in the production of hemoglobin, the part of the blood that carries oxygen. It is also involved in the manufacture of glucose, supports digestion by enhancing gastric acid secretion, and is essential for wound healing! It is a precursor amino acid for glutathione and large amounts are needed for the liver to detoxify after chemical exposure.

Both Glycine & Proline Are Needed For:
- Manufacture of glucose
- Enhancing gastric acid secretion
- Soft tissue and wound healing
- Healthy connective tissue
- Effective detoxification of the liver
- Production of plasma
- Maintaining a good memory

Collagen & Gelatin Are Needed For:
- Soft tissue and wound healing
- Formation and repair of cartilage and bone

- Healing and coating the mucus membranes of the gastrointestinal tract
- Facilitating digestion and assimilation of proteins

Minerals Found in Bone Broth

Minerals are essential for life! Minerals provide the basis for many important functions in the body. They are necessary for connective tissue and bone, create electrical potential that facilitates nerve conduction, and are catalysts for enzymatic reactions. Most Americans are very mineral deficient!

Calcium is necessary for strong bones, muscle contraction and relaxation, proper clotting and tissue repair, normal nerve conduction, and endocrine balance.

Mineral deficiency can lead to osteoporosis, brittle nails, periodontal conditions, muscle cramps and spasms, palpitations, depression, insomnia, and hyperactivity.

Phosphorus is necessary for the general production of energy in the body. It is a critical component of cell membranes and helps regulate intracellular pressure. A phosphorus deficiency can lead to fatigue, weakness, muscle weakness, celiac disease, and seizures.

Magnesium is the most common dietary deficiency in the U.S. It is involved in over 300 enzyme reactions, is a cofactor for vitamins B1 and B6, and is involved in the synthesis of proteins, fatty acids, nucleic acids, and prostaglandins. Proper nerve transmission, parathyroid gland function, and muscle contraction and relaxation are also dependent on magnesium.

So here's what's in your soup!

Calcium	Chondroitin sulfate
Phosphorus	Hyaluronic acid
Magnesium	Glycine
Potassium sulfate	Protein
Collagen	

Wonder why we sell so many synthetic supplements for arthritis and joints? I think it's because we've taken these rich mineral broths out of our diet. We eliminated one of our primary sources of calcium, as well as many vital nutrients for joint health. Then when we suffer from osteoporosis and arthritis, we assume it is just because we are "getting old." We spend a fortune on medicines and artificial supplements trying to undo the damage. So instead of buying glucosamine and chondroitin supplements, make bone broth a part of your regular diet and feel the difference!

The amounts and types of substances in your bone broth soup depend partly on the types of bones you use. Try to use organic, and try to use mixed bones. Bone marrow and cartilage provide the most beneficial ingredients.

Just one pint of soup can give you as much as 1,000 milligrams of calcium. Wow! Bone marrow soup stock is not only a great winter food, but also one of the best traditional foods for recuperation and rejuvenation. It is very beneficial for recovery from illness, surgery, and fatigue. If you are in any stage of healing, drink two cups of bone marrow broth a day.

Fasting & Cleansing

During fasting, because little or no food is consumed, protein tissues, such as muscle, often break down. If broth is consumed, the glycine in the broth limits or prevents degeneration during the fast and is also beneficial in the detoxification process.

Frugal Benefits

Bone broths are remarkably inexpensive to make. Many times you can prepare a decent broth for the cost of the energy used to heat your pot alone. By using the bones from leftover roast chicken and vegetable scraps you have saved, you can make a gallon of stock for pennies. Get to know your butcher or local rancher, and you can often acquire beef or lamb bones for free.

Boxed, canned broths and stocks are commercially available, and you can even purchase organic and free-range meat broths; however, these watery stocks pale in comparison to both the nutrient density and flavor of homemade bone broths. These commercially prepared broths are often aseptically packaged (70 percent paper, 24 percent polyethylene or plastic, and 6 percent aluminum) and highly processed, as well as expensive!

BOTTOM LINE: Save yourself money and maximize the flavor and nutrient density of your foods by incorporating broth into your diet!

PLEASE SEE THE SOURCE ACKNOWLEDGMENTS ON PAGE 272 FOR A LIST OF RESEARCH, BOOKS, AND WEBSITES USED FOR THIS SECTION.

Whole Grains

Whole Grains

Agriculture, as some estimate, first developed in the Middle Eastern and Mediterranean countries about 8000 B.C., starting with simple grass seeds. Eventually, wheat, barley, rye, oats, millet, rice, and sorghum were all cultivated. By about 4500 BC, grain had become a staple food.

The first method of *preparing* grains was to parch them and then boil them whole. The first *milling* was achieved by crushing wild grain with rocks. Then, people began to grind the grain with a mortar and pestle to make porridge or gruel.

Eventually, the first round, flat *loaves* of bread were made from heavy porridge-like pastes of flour and water that were baked in front of the fire. The nearest modern equivalents are the chapattis of India and Mexican tortillas.

The next development was *fermentation* to make the bread lighter and more digestible. This was probably an accidental discovery from leaving porridge in a warm place for a few days.

Phosphorus in the bran of whole grains is tied up in a substance called phytic acid. Phytic acid combines with iron, calcium, magnesium, copper, and zinc in the intestinal tract, blocking their absorption. Whole grains also contain enzyme inhibitors that can interfere with digestion.

Traditional societies usually soak or ferment their grains before eating them. This process neutralizes phytates and enzyme inhibitors and, in effect, pre-digests grains so all their nutrients are more available.

Three Ways to Prepare Grains for Maximum Absorption
- overnight soaking
- sprouting
- old-fashioned sour leavening

Sprouting, soaking, and genuine sourdough leavening "pre-digests" grains, allowing the nutrients to be more easily assimilated and metabolized. Soaking neutral-izes phytic acid, a component of plant fiber found in the bran and hulls of grains, legumes, nuts, and seeds that reduces mineral absorption.

Sprouting begins germination, which increases the enzymatic activity in foods and deactivates enzyme inhibitors. All of these benefits explain why sprouted foods are less likely to produce allergic reactions in those who are sensitive.

The Benefits of Sprouted Flour
- Easier to digest—Sprouting breaks down the starches in grains into simple sugars so your body can digest them like a vegetable (like a tomato, not a potato).
  - Increased Vitamin C
  - Increased Vitamin B—B2, B5, and B6
  - Increased Carotene—up to eight times
  - Increased Enzymes—The embryonic plant actually produces enzymes during sprouting.

Until the 20th Century, grain naturally sprouted in the field before it was milled into flour. The invention of the combine harvester during the Industrial Revolution changed everything. Grain could be harvested in the field and then moved to storage bins. The time-honored practice of sprouting was skipped by modern processing.

When whole grains are not allowed to ferment or sprout, they don't contain the same nutrients, and they retain the naturally occurring antinutrients, even when milled into flour.

Refined grains were virtually unknown in the human diet before 1600 and never used in great quantities before the 20th Century. Since grinding stones are not fast enough for mass-production, the industry uses high-speed, steel roller mills that eject the germ and the bran. Much of this "waste product"—the most nutritious part of the grain—is sold as "by-product" for animal consumption.

The resulting white flour contains only a fraction of the nutrients of the original grain. Even whole wheat flour is compromised during the modern milling process. High-speed mills reach 400°F, which destroys vital nutrients and creates rancidity in the bran and the germ. Vitamin E in the germ is also destroyed—a real tragedy because whole wheat used to be our most readily available source of vitamin E.

Nutrients Lost in the Refining Process

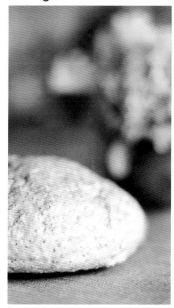

Thiamine (B1) 77%
Riboflavin (B2) 80%
Niacin 81%
Pyridoxine (B6) 72%
Pantothenic acid 50%
Vitamin E 86%
Calcium 60%
Phosphorus 71%
Magnesium 84%
Potassium 77%
Sodium 78%
Chromium 40%
Manganese 86%
Iron 76%
Cobalt 89%
Zinc 78%
Copper 68%
Selenium 16%
Molybdenum 48%

In nature, carbohydrates (the energy providers) are linked with vitamins, minerals, enzymes, protein, fat, and fiber—the body-building and digestion-regulating components of the diet. In whole form, starches support life. But refined carbohydrates have an adverse effect because they are devoid of body-building elements.

Dozens of dough conditioners and preservatives are added to modern bread, along with toxic ingredients like partially hydrogenated vegetable oils and soy flour. Soy flour—loaded with antinutrients—is added to virtually all brand-name breads today to improve rise and prevent sticking. The extrusion process, used to make cold breakfast cereals and puffed grains, adds high temperatures and high pressures that further destroy nutrients. Chemical preservatives allow bread to be shipped long distances and to remain on the shelf for many days without spoiling and without refrigeration.

People have become accustomed to mass-produced, gooey, devitalized, and nutritionally deficient breads, and have little recollection of how real bread should taste.

Ideally, you should buy organic or biodynamic whole grain berries and grind them fresh to make homemade breads and other baked goods. Since these farming methods do not allow synthetic chemicals and fertilizers, purchasing organic or biodynamic grain ensures you get the cleanest, most nutritious food possible. It also eliminates the possibility of irradiation and genetically engineered seed.

The second best option is to buy organic 100% stone-ground whole-grain flours at a natural food store. Slow-speed, steel hammer-mills are often used instead of stones, and flours made in this way can list "stone-ground" on the label. This method is equivalent to the stone-ground process and produces a product that is equally nutritious. Any process that renders the entire grain into usable flour without exposing it to high heat is acceptable.

If you do not make your own bread, there are ready-made alternatives available. Look for freshly baked or frozen organic naturally fermented sourdough or sprouted breads. If bread is made with 100% stone-ground whole grains, it will say so on the label.

When bread is stone ground and then baked, the internal temperature does not usually exceed 170 degrees, so most of the nutrients are preserved. Since they contain no preservatives, both whole grain flour and its products should be kept in the refrigerator or freezer. Stone-ground flour will keep for several months when frozen.

You have several options for preparing your grain. You can use a sour leavening method by mixing whey, buttermilk, or yogurt with freshly ground flour or quality pre-ground flour from the store. Or you can soak the grain whole for 8 to 22 hours, then drain and rinse. Some recipes use the whole berries while they are wet, ground right in the food processor. Another option is to dry sprouted berries in a low-temperature oven or dehydrator and then grind them in your grain mill.

Spelt Flour

I recommend spelt over wheat because many of my patients are very sensitive to wheat when they first come to see me. Naturally fermented spelt, sprouted, and sourdough breads are available—and delicious! You can also make your own baked goods at home using sprouted spelt flour.

Spelt in Comparison to Wheat

- Approximately 30% higher in thiamin (vitamin B1)
- Approximately 25% higher in B6
- Approximately 45% higher in vitamin E
- Higher in unsaturated fatty acids (mainly linol acid and linoleen acid), which are important for regeneration of nerve cells
- Supports good blood circulation
- Higher in water solubility, making it easier to digest and absorb
- Approximately 10–25% higher in protein, promoting fitness strength, muscle expansion, and endurance. Many endurance athletes find spelt to be invaluable during training.
- Higher percentage of amino acids
- Higher level of L-tryptophan, which in turn promotes and aids in the production of serotonin.

Einkorn

Einkorn is a newly discovered ancient grain. This original wheat was the first species grown by man more than 12,000 years ago. Einkorn has never been hybridized and is the most genetically pure wheat. It is a very good source of fiber and protein.

In 1991, two hikers came across a body protruding from a melting glacier in the Italian Alps. The body was that of Otzi the Iceman, named after the region where he was found. He was preserved in ice for over 5,000 years, and upon examination, they found his last meal consisted of ibex meat, roots, berries, and einkorn wheat.

Einkorn was the first species of wheat to be domesticated by humans during the Neolithic Revolution. This was a transitional time from hunter-gatherer to agriculture. Wild seeds were collected and farmed. Einkorn cultivation expanded from the Fertile Crescent (in the Middle East) to Central Europe. Einkorn grows best in cold climates. It entered the Bronze Age and then diminished over time as new, higher-yielding wheat varieties evolved.

Einkorn wheat has a protective layer (hull) that remains intact after harvesting. This requires an extra step to remove before milling. Einkorn can still be found in the wild in Turkey and in some parts of Europe.

The natural genetics of wheat has changed over the last 10,000 years through hybridization. Hybridization happens naturally in the wild, in the field, and through seed selection by farmers. The gluten content in wheat helps dough to rise. Plant breeders have produced wheat with a very high gluten value which

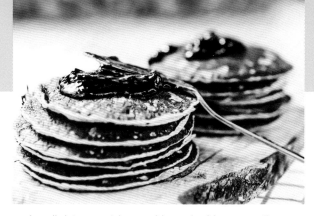

makes lighter pastries and breads. However, the higher gluten content, nutritional stripping, and added chemical "vitamins" that happens during processing has ushered in a host of gluten sensitivities. The gut is forced to pull from the body's resources to properly digest the nutritionally deficient baked goods. Once the body's reserves are used up, it begins to react to white flour products.

The website JovialFoods.com states, "Einkorn has always remained the purest form of wheat. Like einkorn, most plants are diploids, which mean they have one set of chromosomes from a male parent and one from the female parent. When other species of wheat were created, additional sets of chromosomes were added. Emmer wheat was created roughly 2000 years after einkorn by the hybridization of two wild grasses adding two sets of chromosomes. Kamut® and Durum wheat are descendants of Emmer. Spelt was the first wheat hybridization that occurred with the help of man between cultivated emmer and a wild grass, creating a species with six sets of chromosomes. Common bread wheat descended from spelt."

Although spelt is a hybrid of the original wheat, einkorn, in my opinion it is still a very good choice, especially for baking. This and other modern wheat is considered modified through cross hybridization, but that does not mean that it has been genetically modified. Genetic modification (GMO) integrates genes from other organisms in plants. GMO wheat is currently not grown anywhere in the world.

Nutritional Benefits of Einkorn:
- High in thiamin and essential minerals
- Good source of protein, iron, dietary fiber, and a number of B vitamins
- Contains a significant amount of the powerful antioxidant lutein
- Higher oxygen radical absorbance capacity (ORAC) than durum and bread wheat
- Higher content of proteins, tocols, and carotenoids than other species of wheat
- Lower percentage of nutrient loss during processing

Einkorn is considered to be the healthiest grain now being offered. Patients are testing very well for it—even those who are sensitive to wheat. However, this does not mean that those with celiac should consume it.

A small number of health-food stores are now carrying einkorn grain and pasta. You can purchase it from Energetic Wellness, through www.jovialfoods.com, or www.einkorn.com. Jovial 100% Organic Einkorn pasta is the best I've ever tasted.

Whole Grains
Considered gluten-free
- Amaranth*
- Barley*
- Buckwheat (kasha)
- Bulgur (cracked wheat)
- Corn (whole-grain corn or cornmeal)
- Einkorn (original wheat)
- Kamut® (Khorasan wheat)
- Millet*
- Oats (oatmeal, whole, rolled, or steel-cut oats)*
- Popcorn*
- Quinoa*
- Rice: black, brown, red*
- Rye
- Teff
- Spelt
- Sorghum
- Triticale (barley/wheat hybrid)
- Whole wheat
- Wild rice*

Gluten-Free Craze

In March 2013, I attended the largest Natural Foods Product Expo, held in California. There were 2,400 vendors ranging from large-scale retail stores to small stores like EW. Almost every company at the Expo had products with gluten-free labels—even the obvious gluten-free ones. Many companies are using "gluten-free" as a new marketing label to promote their products.

So, what is all the fuss about gluten?

Gluten-free is the latest buzzword in health. The term "gluten-free" means to eliminate grains and foods containing gluten. The gluten grains include wheat, barley, rye, and spelt. Unfortunately, many people who decide to eat "gluten-free" make very poor alternative choices.

Personally, I would not recommend any gluten-free baked goods on the market today. There was not one company at the largest Natural Products Expo that passed my whole food ingredients test!

Many people who are negatively affected by gluten don't fully understand why. Some choose to eliminate it because it is the latest health "discovery," but others experience digestive problems, allergies, fibromyalgia, chronic fatigue, ADD, or autism. And some don't really know what gluten is, but just feel better not eating it.

What is Gluten?

- Gluten (from Latin *gluten*, meaning *glue*) is a protein composite found in foods processed from wheat and related grain species, including barley and rye.
- Gluten gives elasticity to dough, helps it rise and keep its shape, and often gives the final product a chewy texture.
- Gluten may also be found in some cosmetic, hair, and other dermatological products.
- Gluten is usually defined as "a protein in wheat, barley and rye," but really, gluten is a mixture of two types of proteins: prolamins and glutelins.
- Gluten is found in all grains, but while the gluten's prolamins in rice and corn are safe for celiac patients, the prolamins in wheat (called gliadin), barley (called hordein), and rye (called secalin) have been found to cause a negative response in the body.

What is Celiac Disease?

Contrast this definition with the body's true response.

Standard Medical Definition:

Celiac disease is a disease of the digestive system that damages the small intestine and interferes with the absorption of nutrients from food.

Celiac disease occurs when the body reacts abnormally to gluten, a protein found in wheat, rye, barley, and possibly oats. When someone with celiac disease eats foods containing gluten, that person's immune system causes an inflammatory response in the small intestine, which damages the tissues and results in an impaired ability to absorb nutrients from foods.

The inflammation and malabsorption create wide-ranging problems in many systems of the body. Since the body's own immune system causes the damage, celiac disease is classified as an autoimmune disorder.

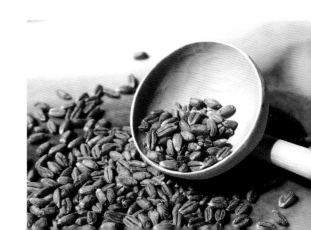

Body reacts abnormally to gluten—
The body responds exactly the way it was
designed to react. This is not "abnormal."
There is always a significant biological response.

Disease of the digestive system—
I do not believe in "diseases." The body was
created to assist us in times of distress—whether
from something we eat or an emotional crisis.
When we ingest something disagreeable or when
we face a difficult situation, our digestive system
and body immediately respond.

**Immune system causes an inflammatory
response**—This is not a negative response from
the immune system. An inflammation response
is always a sign of the body healing from the
indigestible-morsel situation.

**Body's own immune system causes
the damage**—The body was not designed to
cause damage, but to repair and renew itself
using its own natural healing abilities. The root of
the problem needs to be resolved—elimination
of the food (processed wheat) or the situation in
your life that is causing the indigestion.

Autoimmune Disease—In medical terms,
the autoimmune disease classification is used
when there is no other explanation for the body's
reaction. They blame it on the immune system
attacking itself. The body was ***not*** designed to
attack itself. It was designed to thrive and heal
itself.

Celiac and gluten sensitivity are new conditions.

"…whatever has happened with celiac disease has
happened since 1950," says Dr. Joseph A. Murray
of the Mayo Clinic. "This increase has affected young
and old people. It suggests something has happened
in a pervasive fashion from the environmental perspective."

In my practice, I conduct a food sensitivity test.
- 98% of my initial patients are gluten sensitive
- Of the 98% sensitive, 100% of them are only sensitive to wheat gluten (not barley, spelt, and rye)

Why are we sensitive to wheat gluten?
- Are we sensitive because the Standard American
Diet mainly consists of refined wheat products?—*Yes*.
- If we ate grains prepared correctly, would we still
be so sensitive?—*No*.
- Is it really the gluten *(no)* or is it the fact that we
have modified our wheat grain, sprayed it to death
with toxic chemicals, and refined and processed it to
create high-gluten flour without the nutrient base to
help us digest the gluten?—*Yes*.
- Could your digestive problems be related to a
situation in your life that needs to be resolved?—*Yes*.

Wheat contains the highest gluten content available
today. The Standard American Diet consists mainly of
refined wheat products like bread, pizza, rolls, pitas,
cookies, cakes, pies, muffins, bagels, pretzels, and
crackers—all snack foods.

I believe we have a generational effect. Those of
us who were raised on refined grain products seem to
be more sensitive. In my experience as a naturopath,
even those who do *not* think they are having a problem
with wheat test sensitive to it. They may not yet feel its
effects, but the body is reacting. Any denatured food
causes a response from the body to help us recover.
This reaction is not a disease—it is a natural response.

All food that has had minerals, vitamins, and enzymes removed is very difficult to digest—especially when chemical nutrients are added.

Whole food was created to be our medicine and medicine our food.

Gluten is an important source of nutritional protein when eaten in its natural state.

Are these whole food products?

Most "gluten-free" products are made with flours that are not prepared correctly. Rice, corn, tapioca, and soy often include other refined or synthetic ingredients like tapioca starch, potato starch, sugar (evaporated cane juice or white sugar), maltodextrin, calcium propanoate, xanthan gum, and GMO canola oil. The product itself might be gluten-free, but it is a far cry from being a whole, pure food.

Read Natural-Food Labels

Look for:
- Hidden salt
- Type of sugar
- Bad oils
- GMO ingredients
- Organic, but white flour and white sugar?
- Gluten-free—types of flours, additives, fillers
- Are these whole foods?

Many "all-natural whole-grain" products fool us into believing they are healthy. A processed food, whether organic or not, causes the body to respond the same way (e.g., an organic white flour cookie made with organic white sugar).

BOTTOM LINE: Choose organic whole grains to sprout, naturally ferment, or use a sourdough starter.

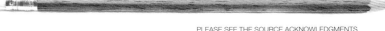

PLEASE SEE THE SOURCE ACKNOWLEDGMENTS ON PAGE 272 FOR A LIST OF RESEARCH, BOOKS, AND WEBSITES USED FOR THIS SECTION.

Sugar

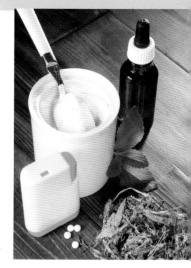

Most of us grew up with the occasional treat and soda pop. However, sugar was usually limited to desserts, and desserts were limited to special treats. Today, many Americans are addicted to sugar. Almost all prepared foods in the grocery store contain some form of refined sugar, high fructose corn syrup, or artificial sweetener—even some "salty" foods are sweetened. So what is the natural-minded consumer to do?

If we are conscious about eating pure, whole foods, what is considered a pure, whole sugar?

A pure, whole sugar comes from a natural food without being stripped of its original nutrient-dense state or individual nutrients through processing. Natural sweeteners are those used in their natural state.

Cultures throughout the world have used natural sweeteners for centuries. It is wonderful that we can satisfy our sweet tooth by consuming in-season, fully ripened fruit or a limited amount of wonderful, natural sugars that are high in vitamins and minerals: raw honey, maple syrup, maple sugar, date sugar, whole cane sugar (Rapunzel), whole stevia herb, and coconut sugar.

Natural, raw honey, without high-heat processing, is a pure, whole sugar. Organic maple syrup is tapped directly from a variety of maple trees. When this syrup is dried, it produces maple sugar. Date sugar is made from very finely chopped dry dates. The stevia plant is a beneficial herb sweetener, when used in its original or dried state. Coconut sugar, similar to maple sugar, is evaporated flower sap from the coconut trees.

Many of these natural sugars can be obtained from your local farmers' market, health-food store, or grocery store. You can use many of these natural sugars cup for cup in your favorite recipes. However, when using natural sugars, a good rule of thumb is to use less.

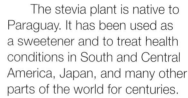

A pure, whole sugar comes from a natural food without being stripped from its original nutrient-dense state or individual nutrients isolated through processing.

Misconceptions About
Stevia & Agave

The stevia plant is native to Paraguay. It has been used as a sweetener and to treat health conditions in South and Central America, Japan, and many other parts of the world for centuries. It is a miraculous herb if used in its natural state. Stevia contains phytonutrients, trace elements, minerals, vitamins, and volatile oils, which give stevia its nutritional and medicinal properties. It is also high in chromium—a good choice for diabetics. As a poultice, it can be used for treating cuts, sun burns, rashes, and other skin conditions such as acne or eczema. Stevia will penetrate the cut, heal it quickly, and won't leave a scar. I've even heard of it vanishing wrinkles!

A number of studies show that stevia can be beneficial in the treatment of many health conditions because of its antibacterial, antiseptic, antimicrobial, antioxidant, antiglycemic, and anti-hypertensive properties. Consuming the whole stevia plant helps improve energy levels, strengthen the immune system, stimulate mental activity, and may also help ease withdrawal symptoms from tobacco and alcohol addiction.

Dried leaves and green stevia powder are the original whole food. They contain all of the nutrients from the plant and are developed through a natural drying process—no chemist needed! Teas that use the whole herb are fabulous and extremely nourishing. Wisdom of the Ancients brand teas have a selection of tea blends made with the whole stevia herb and are sold in the EW store and most health-food stores.

Initially, stevia leaves were consumed fresh or dried, but chemists eventually isolated the glycosides called stevioside and rebaudioside that give stevia its sweet taste. These isolated forms of stevia, which are white or liquid, are not in their natural form. Unfortunately, health companies market the white powder and liquid stevia as having the same health benefits. The process to create a white powder or liquid is similar to the process of making sugar alcohol. Therefore, I do not recommend either the liquid or white powder stevia options.

Manufacturers of agave nectar claim it is made from the sap of the agave plant and is a healthy, natural sweetener. However, it is actually made from the starch of the agave's giant root bulb. The root is mainly starch (similar to the starch in corn or rice) and a complex carbohydrate called *inulin* (which is composed of fructose molecule chains). About half of the carbohydrate content of agave is the highly indigestible inulin fiber. The agave glucose and inulin are subject to an enzymatic and chemical process that converts the starch into a fructose-rich syrup in the same manner that HFCS is manufactured. In fact, agave nectar is higher in fructose (70%) than high fructose corn syrup (55%). The process uses caustic acids, clarifiers, and filtration chemicals. Agave doesn't fit the picture of what constitutes a pure, whole food. Any process that isolates the sweetest part (fructose) or uses chemicals or high heat, changes the structure of the food and depletes the nutrients from its complex form. These processes make any food harmful to the body.

Refined Sugar

For generations, cultures have consumed natural fruits and sugars in moderation. Today, the average American consumes his weight in refined sugar each year—far more than the body can tolerate.

Refined white sugar is not a food, but a chemical—a drug! Studies have shown that sugar is more addictive than cocaine. The refining process leaves it void of any nutritional substance. It is void of vitamins, minerals, proteins, fats, and enzymes. It is very harmful to our body—especially in the quantities consumed by most Americans.

Dr. David Reuben, author of *Everything You Always Wanted to Know About Nutrition* says, "… white refined sugar is not a food. It is a pure chemical extracted from plant sources, purer in fact than cocaine, which it resembles in many ways. Its true name is sucrose and its chemical formula is $C_{12}H_{22}O_{11}$. It has 12 carbon atoms, 22 hydrogen atoms, 11 oxygen atoms, and absolutely nothing else to offer."

Why would we want to give such an addictive substance to our children? Why do we feel as though we are depriving them of a treat when it is the most harmful substance we can consume? And what is it doing to our body?

Refining means to make "pure" by a process of extraction or separation. Natural, whole foods, like sugarcane and sugar beets (often genetically modified) are first harvested and then chopped into small pieces. The juice is then squeezed out and mixed with water. This liquid is heated and lime is added. During the refining process, 64 vital food elements are removed or destroyed—some of which are potassium, magnesium, calcium, iron, manganese, phosphate, sulfate, A, D, and B vitamins, amino acids, enzymes, unsaturated fats, and fiber. Molasses, the chemical byproduct of sugar, is bottled and sold as a separate (and often "natural") sweetener. In this form, molasses is not in its natural state. *Read further comments under Whole Cane Sugar regarding natural molasses (p. 230).*

Today, we have a nation that is addicted to sugar. In 1915, the average sugar consumption (per year) was 15 to 20 pounds per person. Today, the average person consumes his/her weight in sugar *and* 20–60 pounds of corn syrup. The human body cannot tolerate this large amount of refined carbohydrates. The vital organs in the body are damaged by this gross intake of sugar.

• Because refined sugar is an incomplete food, your body must borrow vital nutrients from healthy cells to metabolize it. Calcium, sodium, potassium, and magnesium are depleted from various parts of the body to make use of the sugar. Often, so much calcium is used to neutralize the effects of sugar, that the bones become osteoporotic.

• The teeth are also affected as they are drained of calcium until decay occurs and hastens their loss. If sugar consumption is continued, an over-acid condition results, and more minerals are depleted from deep in the body to correct the imbalance.

• If the body does not have the nutrients needed to metabolize sugar, it cannot properly rid itself of the poisonous residues.

• Americans consume over 24 pounds of candy each year, and much of it is consumed by children on and around Halloween.

• One 12-oz. cola contains 11 teaspoons of sugar (and that's aside from the caffeine).

Sugar causes a rise in the blood sugar level and gives you quick energy— but only for a brief time. The body releases a rush of insulin to lower the blood sugar, causing a significant drop in energy and endurance. It is easy to see why America's health is in serious trouble.

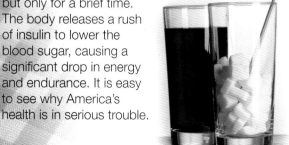

The Effects of Refined Sugar on the Emotions

Amino acids are the super-nutrients that your brain uses to make its most powerful pleasure chemicals. These regulate our appetites and moods:

Glucose—adequate levels stabilize our blood supply (fewer cravings and less moodiness)
Serotonin—our natural antidepressant and sleep promoter (like Prozac)
Catecholamine—our natural energizer and promoter of mental focus (like cocaine)
Endorphins—our natural comfort chemicals (stronger than heroin)
GABA (gamma-aminobutyric acid)—our natural tranquilizer (more relaxing than Xanax)

A brain that is fully stocked with these natural mood enhancers has no need for sugar highs. If we have enough of all five, our emotions are stable. When they are depleted or out of balance, "pseudo-emotions" can result. These false moods can be every bit as distressing as those triggered by abuse, loss, or trauma. They can drive us to relentless eating.

For some, sweet and starchy foods have a drug-like effect, altering the brain's mood chemistry and fooling us into a false calm or temporary energy surge. We become dependent on these drug-like foods for continued mood lifts. The more we use them, the more depleted our natural mood-enhancing chemicals become.

Prolonged stress uses up your natural sedatives, stimulants, and pain relievers. The emergency stores of precious brain chemicals can get used up if you continually need to use them to calm yourself.

Eventually, your brain can't keep up with the demand. We automatically try to "help" our brain by eating foods that have similar, drug-like effects. The cravings are legitimate, but using fake food and chemicals only makes the problem worse.

These natural brain chemicals can be thousands of times stronger than the hardest street drugs. As the supply drops, greater amounts of alcohol, drugs, or drug-like foods are needed to fill newly emptied brain slots.

Regular use of drug-like foods such as refined sugars and flours or regular use of alcohol or drugs (including some medicines) can inhibit the production of your brain's natural pleasure chemicals.

All of these artificial substances plug into your brain's empty receptors in place of your natural brain drugs—the neurotransmitters. Your brain senses that the receptors are already full, so it further reduces the amounts of neurotransmitters that it produces.

This vicious cycle ends when these chemical substances are no longer able to fill the empty receptors. Your brain's natural mood resources are now more depleted than ever, and you still crave the mood-enhancing drugs—whether it's sugar, alcohol, or cocaine. Unfortunately, our rehabilitation centers often facilitate the replacement of one addiction (like alcohol) with another (refined sugar).

If you have an addiction, you are most likely not eating enough protein. Your brain relies on protein—the only food source of amino acids—to produce each of its mood-enhancing chemicals. Protein is the building block for manufacturing those crucial chemicals. Eating the equivalent of three eggs, a chicken breast, a piece of fish, or small steak at every meal should provide enough protein to keep your brain in good repair.

Nancy Appleton, PhD, clinical nutritionist, has compiled a list of 146 reasons of how sugar is ruining your health in her book *Lick the Sugar Habit*. Here are some of them:

- Sugar can decrease growth hormone
- Sugar feeds cancer
- Sugar increases cholesterol
- Sugar can weaken eyesight

- Sugar can cause drowsiness and decreased activity in children
- Sugar can interfere with the absorption of protein
- Sugar causes food allergies
- Sugar contributes to diabetes
- Sugar can contribute to eczema in children
- Sugar can cause cardiovascular disease
- Sugar can impair the structure of DNA
- Sugar can cause hyperactivity, anxiety, difficulty concentrating, and crankiness in children
- Sugar breaks down the defense against bacterial infection
- Sugar greatly assists the growth of Candida Albicans (yeast infections)
- Sugar contributes to osteoporosis

Sugar and refined carbohydrates cause a spike in blood sugar, which makes the body produce insulin. Your body then craves food to balance the excess insulin, causing weight gain and a variety of other health conditions, including diabetes. Cutting out refined carbohydrates and sugar is the first step to bringing your weight and overall health into balance. You will be amazed how happy and healthy you can be without refined sugar!

Fructose

Fructose, the natural sugar found in fruit, is healthy when you get it from whole foods, like apples (about 7% fructose). When eaten in its natural state, fructose comes with a host of vitamins, antioxidants, and fiber. The body is able to process and use the nutrients without depleting vital stores. But when fructose is commercially extracted from fruit, concentrated, and made into a juice or sweetener, it has dangerous effects on the body.

Fructose causes insulin resistance and significantly raises triglycerides. It has been linked to non-alcoholic fatty-liver disease. Rats given high-fructose diets develop a number of undesirable metabolic abnormalities, including elevated triglycerides, weight gain, and extra abdominal fat.

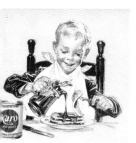

High Fructose Corn Syrup (HFCS)

The process of creating HFCS is similar to the destructive process of refined sugar. The problem with this highly processed, unnatural product is that it is often included under "all-natural" labels. And though it is calorie rich, it has no nutritional value. HFCS is a significant cause of the obesity epidemic! The Corn Refiners Association disagrees because it is inexpensive to make (due to America's massive corn subsidies). Food manufacturers, not growers, are bound to the product.

HFCS acts as a preservative, extending food's shelf life, yet it is cheaper than sugar or other natural sweeteners. While the Corn Refiners Association claims that high fructose corn syrup is made from corn, has no artificial ingredients, has the same calories as sugar, and is fine to eat in moderation, there is nothing "natural" about it. Does it originate in corn? Absolutely. But HFCS cannot be found in corn or anywhere else in nature.

Manufacturing HFCS requires a long series of mechanical processes and chemical reactions, including the introduction of three different enzymes to induce molecular rearrangements. Genetically modified corn is often used—corn that has been molecularly altered by genetically engineered enzymes. How can that be considered natural?

HFCS was introduced in 1970. By 1990, consumption of it had increased 1,000 percent. HFCS is now found in almost all caloric sweeteners added to foods and beverages in the U.S. It can be found in soft drinks and fruit drinks, candied and canned fruit, dairy products like ice cream and yogurt, bread and baked goods, cereals, jellies, ketchup, BBQ sauce, salad dressing, vitamins and supplements, and overwhelmingly in foods marketed to children.

HFCS is found in most processed foods and is difficult to avoid. Americans consume an average of 20–60 pounds of HFCS a year. Our bodies strongly react to it, leading to obesity, diabetes, and heart disease. Unlike glucose, fructose does not stimulate insulin secretion or enhance leptin production, which are both key processes in appetite regulation and fat storage.

Fructose causes us to overeat because we don't feel full. This leads our bodies to store more calories as fat. Part of what makes HFCS such a dangerous sweetener is that it is metabolized to fat in your body faster than any other sugar. Most fats enter our liver and are either stored, burned, or turned into fat. HFCS bypasses this process and our bodies turn it directly into fat.

Caustic soda and hydrochloric acid, two of the many chemicals used to make HFCS, often contain traces of mercury. These two chemicals are made in the same way as chlorine, and are produced in two ways. One involves pumping saltwater through a vat of mercury. As Dr. David Wallinga of the Institute for Agriculture & Trade Policy stated, "Mercury is toxic in all its forms. Given how much high-fructose corn syrup is consumed by children, it could be a significant additional source of mercury never before considered. We are calling for immediate changes by industry and the [U.S. Food and Drug Administration] to help stop this avoidable mercury contamination of the food supply." The good news is that the industry is heeding the call and moving away from the mercury-grade process.

Why No Artificial Sweeteners?

Aspartame

Aspartame is the technical name for the brands NutraSweet®, Equal®, AminoSweet®, Canderel®, Spoonful®, and Equal-Measure®. Aspartame was accidentally discovered in 1965 by James M. Schlatter, a chemist at G.D. Searle & Company. He was working on new drugs to treat ulcers, when he licked his fingers to pick up a piece of paper and accidentally tasted the intense sweetness of the compound he had created.

It was originally approved for dry goods in 1974. However, objections were soon filed by neuroscience researcher Dr. John W. Olney and consumer attorney James Turner. There was also an investigation of G.D. Searle's research practices. The FDA put their approval on hold until 1981. It was later approved for carbonated beverages in 1983.

In 1985, Monsanto purchased G.D. Searle and divided the company into Searle Pharmaceuticals and The NutraSweet Company.

Aspartame accounts for over 75% of the adverse reactions to food additives reported to the FDA. Many of these reactions are very serious—including seizures and death. A few of the 90 different documented symptoms caused by aspartame include: headaches/migraines, dizziness, seizures, nausea, numbness, muscle spasms, weight gain, rashes, depression, fatigue, irritability, tachycardia, insomnia, vision problems, hearing loss, heart palpitations, breathing difficulties, anxiety attacks, slurred speech, loss of taste, tinnitus, vertigo, memory loss, and joint pain.

According to researchers and physicians studying the adverse effects of aspartame, the following chronic illnesses can be triggered or worsened by aspartame: brain tumors, multiple sclerosis, epilepsy, chronic fatigue syndrome, Parkinson's disease, Alzheimer's, mental retardation, lymphoma, birth defects, fibromyalgia, and diabetes.

Aspartame is made up of three chemicals: aspartic acid, phenylalanine, and methanol.

In the book *Prescription for Nutritional Healing*, James and Phyllis Balch list aspartame under the category of "chemical poison."

Saccharin

Saccharin, the first artificial sweetener to be discovered, is chemically classified as an O-toluene sulfonamide derivative. It was originally synthesized from toluene, a colorless liquid hydrocarbon distilled from coal tar, which may account for saccharin's bitter, metallic aftertaste. Toluene is also used to manufacture certain dyes, pharmaceutical drugs, and trinitrotoluene (the blasting agent more commonly known as TNT).

Saccharin is currently manufactured by a more cost-effective method, beginning with synthetically produced methyl anthranilate, a compound that also occurs naturally in grape and other fruit juices. It is combined with nitrous acid, sulfur dioxide, chlorine, and ammonia. That combination doesn't sound like a natural sweetener, but a chemical cleaner! And yet millions of people consume saccharin every year.

Saccharin is the main ingredient in Sweet'N Low, which is 200–400 times sweeter than sugarcane. A 1/4 packet contains the sweetness of 2 teaspoons of sugar. It is added to some diet soft drinks, gum, toothpaste, and foods like canned fruits and salad dressings. Saccharin may be found in ingredient lists under three forms—acid saccharin, sodium saccharin, and calcium saccharin. Saccharin comes with a warning on the package: Use of this product may be hazardous to your health. Determined to cause cancer in laboratory animals.

Sucralose (Splenda®)

The fourth FDA-approved, non-nutritive sweetener is sucralose, chemically known as 1,6-dichloro-1,6-dideoxy-beta-D-fructofuranosyl-4-chloro-4-deoxy-alpha-D-galactopyranoside. Sucralose may have the strangest "accidental discovery" story of all.

In 1976, a British sugar company by the name of Tate & Lyle was conducting experiments in collaboration with Queen Elizabeth College at the University of London. They were searching for ways to use sucrose as a chemical intermediate. Shashikant Phadnis, a foreign graduate student working on the project, misunderstood a request for "testing" of a chlorinated sugar as a request for "tasting." This led to the discovery that many chlorinated sugars are hundreds or thousands of times sweeter than sucrose.

Following this discovery, Tate & Lyle arranged with Johnson & Johnson to develop and test a new sweetener from chlorinated sugars. In 1980, Johnson & Johnson formed a subsidiary company by the name of McNeil Specialty Products for this purpose. The product they created, at an impressive 600 times sweeter than sucrose, would be known as sucralose and marketed as Splenda®.

Consider the Research

- Diet sodas may double your risk of obesity
- Artificial sweeteners can stimulate your appetite, increase carbohydrate cravings, and stimulate fat storage and weight gain

Gaining weight is only one of the side effects of consuming these man-made chemical sweeteners. There is enough evidence showing the dangers of consuming artificial sweeteners to fill an entire book— which is exactly why Dr. Joseph Mercola wrote *Sweet Deception*. This book explains how we have been deceived about the truth of artificial sweeteners in diet beverages and diet foods—for greed, for profits…, and at the expense of our own health.

The Wonderful Benefits of Natural Sugars

Whole Sugarcane

Sugarcane originated in Papua New Guinea. After peeling the outer bark, natives chewed on the fibrous stalks. A press was later developed to extract the juice. This process preserves all of the nutrients, making the juice low-glycemic and beneficial to the body. Unlike table sugar, raw sugarcane juice is a complex carbohydrate.

Consuming sugarcane juice is vastly different than drinkng fruit juice. Fruit was created to be eaten as a whole, whereas the sugarcane is too fibrous to ingest. Fruit, in its complex form, comes complete with the needed ingredients for assimilation in the body.

Extracting the juice from fruit forces our body to find other ways to balance the fructose—usually pulling from our reserves. Also, fruit juice is usually pasteurized, which kills any remaining nutrients and creates an even sweeter product that is much higher in fructose.

Raw sugarcane juice contains only fifteen percent total sugar. The remaining content is water and an abundance of vitamins and minerals. Sugarcane is rich in calcium, chromium, cobalt, copper, magnesium, manganese, phosphorus, potassium, and zinc. It also contains iron and vitamins A, C, B1, B2, B3, B5, B6, a high concentration of phytonutrients (including chlorophyll), antioxidants, proteins, soluble fiber, and numerous other health supportive compounds. The synergy of this "whole food" juice is remarkably healthy.

Whole sugarcane juice has a beneficial healing role, including treating cancer, stabilizing blood sugar levels, assisting in weight loss, reducing fevers, clearing the kidneys, and preventing tooth decay. *Nutrition and Physical Degeneration*, by Dr. Weston A. Price, presents his research of men who spent their days cutting down the sugarcane and who chewed it on a regular basis. There was no evidence of diabetes or tooth decay in these men.

Rapunzel whole cane sugar is made by extracting the juice from the sugarcane (using a press) and stirring the juice with paddles under low heat to evaporate out the water. It is not boiled at high heat (like all other sugars), it is not spun to form crystals, and the molasses is not separated from the sugar. The polyphenols and the balance of vitamins and minerals are retained—no other sugar can make these claims.

Raw, whole cane sugar contains the perfect balance of sucrose, glucose, and fructose. In refined sugars, the fructose and glucose have been washed out. This leaves behind pure sucrose, which causes a rise in blood sugar. Rapunzel brand whole cane sugar is also organic and does not contain any chemicals or anti-caking agents.

To make refined sugar, the raw sugarcane juice is boiled to evaporate off the water. This leaves behind a dark, thick liquid, which is then separated from the sugar crystals. Most of the nutrients, including the polyphenols, end up in the thick, dark liquid, called molasses. Blackstrap molasses, made from the third boiling of sugarcane juice, is the most nutritious and concentrated form of molasses. It contains significant amounts of minerals, including iron, calcium, copper, potassium, magnesium, and manganese. Many sugarcane plants have been genetically engineered and heavily sprayed with pesticides. Unless the blackstrap molasses is organic, this concentrated form of nutrients also contains a host of chemicals.

Evaporating off the water from sugarcane juice does not produce the evaporated cane juice sold in grocery stores. Dee McCaffrey, CDC, spoke directly with those who sell raw sugar to the U.S. He states that, *"The term—evaporated cane juice—is wrongly used in the food industry. In reality, it is a very processed form of sugar, unequivocally the same as refined white sugar. The only difference is that is goes through one less processing step than white sugar, and has nearly zero nutrients in it."*

—www.processedfreeamerica.org

Evaporated cane juice is just a "healthy" term used by processed food companies to promote more natural product ingredients. Organic, whole cane sugar (Rapunzel) is the only raw, unrefined sugar that does not separate the molasses from the sugar crystals and retains the most nutrients, including the polyphenols found in the raw sugarcane juice. Whole cane sugar is "evaporated cane sugar," but not in the same way as it is being used in the natural product market.

Traditional cultures consumed the natural juice from pressed sugarcane. Benefits include:
- Sugarcane juice is a great natural remedy for a sore throat, cold, or flu.
- Sugarcane provides natural glucose to the body, which is stored as glycogen and burned by the muscles to provide energy.
- Sugarcane rehydrates the body after exposure to heat and strenuous physical activity. It also boosts athletic performance.
- It has no simple sugars and is considered a low-glycemic beverage. It will not elevate blood sugar levels, but diabetics should limit their consumption.
- It is an excellent substitute for cola.
- Fevers cause protein loss in the body. A liberal intake of sugarcane juice brings down high body temperatures and assists in febrile disorders.
- Helps replenish glucose levels after jaundice.
- The high potassium content helps digestion and constipation.
- Sugarcane juice is a vital drink for those with kidney problems. Regular intake strengthens the stomach, kidneys, heart, eyes, brain, and sex organs.
- Naturally lowers body cholesterol—both LDL and triglycerides.
- The juice has been found to be an effective remedy for prostate and breast cancer.
- To make your own juice, you can purchase a sugarcane press online.

Whole Cane Sugar Uses:
- Baking—cup for cup (I use a little less)
- Sprinkled on anything
- Drinks

Raw Honey

Raw honey is an ancient, natural sweetener. Honey is mentioned in many ancient documents. It is the most valuable food! Honey is an antiseptic, a natural antibiotic, antifungal, and antibacterial—it never spoils. Do not consume pasteurized honey. It has the same unhealthy benefits on the body as refined sugar.

The Benefits of Honey
There is not enough room to share the many benefits of honey, but here are a few.
- Oldest natural remedy mentioned in the Bible
- Promotes digestive health
- Its fatty acid content stimulates peristalsis laxative, lubricating qualities
- Contains the most usable carbohydrate compound in the body
- Strengthens the immune system
- Used in the treatment of ulcers
- Can be used for coughs as an expectorant
- Effectively treats respiratory conditions such as bronchitis and asthma

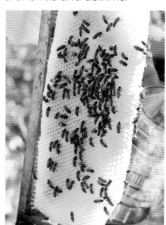

- Assists in healing seasonal allergies
- Calms the nerves
- Excellent remedy for skin wounds, rashes, and burns
- High in antioxidants
- Balances blood sugar
- Stabilizes blood pressure

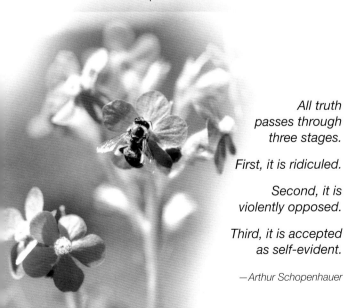

- Contains special anti-inflammatory properties useful for treating sore throats and reducing inflammation of the stomach, intestines, and other areas in our body
- There is no food or drug equal to the effects of honey for malnutrition

Honey Uses:
- Sugar replacement in recipes
- Tea and coffee
- Cough syrup (Olbas Cough or make your own)
- Moisturizer
- Bathing and antibacterial soap
- Hair and scalp treatment
- Natural preservative

All truth passes through three stages.

First, it is ridiculed.

Second, it is violently opposed.

Third, it is accepted as self-evident.

—*Arthur Schopenhauer*

Date Sugar

Dates are loaded with fiber, vitamins, and minerals. Date sugar is ground, dried dates. It has not been processed or refined.

Health Benefits:
- Good source of minerals essential for enzymatic reactions and proper metabolic processes (calcium, iron, magnesium, phosphorus, zinc, copper, manganese, and selenium)
- Rich source of potassium
- Moderate amount of B vitamins

Date Sugar Uses:
- Sprinkle on toast, oatmeal, etc.—does not melt
- Baking—replace 1 cup table sugar with 2/3 cup date sugar.

Coconut Sugar

Harvesting coconut sugar is similar to the process of tapping maple trees. The coconut palm flowers are cut by hand and the liquid sap is collected into containers. The sap is then placed under moderate heat until most of the water has evaporated. Coconut sugar retains many of the nutrients found in the coconut palm.

Health Benefits
- Whole food, unrefined sweetener
- Mineral rich—high in potassium, calcium, magnesium, zinc, and iron
- Full of short-chain fatty acids, polyphenols, and antioxidants
- Source of vitamins B1, B2, B3, B6, and C
- Unprocessed, unfiltered, and unbleached
- Zero additives and preservatives

Date Sugar Uses:
- Sweeten tea, coffee, oatmeal, baked goods, and desserts.

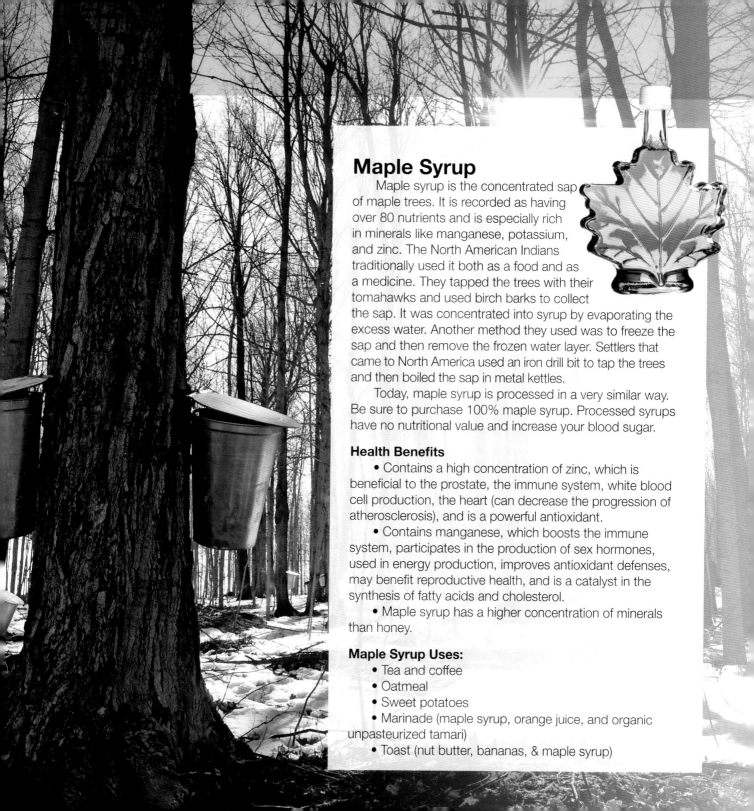

Maple Syrup

Maple syrup is the concentrated sap of maple trees. It is recorded as having over 80 nutrients and is especially rich in minerals like manganese, potassium, and zinc. The North American Indians traditionally used it both as a food and as a medicine. They tapped the trees with their tomahawks and used birch barks to collect the sap. It was concentrated into syrup by evaporating the excess water. Another method they used was to freeze the sap and then remove the frozen water layer. Settlers that came to North America used an iron drill bit to tap the trees and then boiled the sap in metal kettles.

Today, maple syrup is processed in a very similar way. Be sure to purchase 100% maple syrup. Processed syrups have no nutritional value and increase your blood sugar.

Health Benefits

• Contains a high concentration of zinc, which is beneficial to the prostate, the immune system, white blood cell production, the heart (can decrease the progression of atherosclerosis), and is a powerful antioxidant.

• Contains manganese, which boosts the immune system, participates in the production of sex hormones, used in energy production, improves antioxidant defenses, may benefit reproductive health, and is a catalyst in the synthesis of fatty acids and cholesterol.

• Maple syrup has a higher concentration of minerals than honey.

Maple Syrup Uses:

• Tea and coffee
• Oatmeal
• Sweet potatoes
• Marinade (maple syrup, orange juice, and organic unpasteurized tamari)
• Toast (nut butter, bananas, & maple syrup)

So-Called "Natural" Sugars to Avoid:

- Agave nectar
- Evaporated cane juice
  (Muscovado & Demerara)
- Florida Crystals
- Fructose
- Molasses
- Organic cane sugar
- Organic raw sugar
- Sugar in the raw
- Stevia—liquid or white powder
- Turbinado

Note: Evaporated cane sugars are boiled, dehydrated into crystals, and then spun in a centrifuge so the crystals are separated from the molasses. The clarifying process is usually done with chemicals, although sometimes through pressure filtration. The crystals are then reunited with some of the molasses in artificial proportions to produce sugars of varying colors of brown.

Chemical Sugars to Avoid:

- Acid saccharin
- AminoSweet®
- Aspartame
- Calcium saccharin
- Canderel
- Equal®
- High-fructose corn syrup
- NutraSweet®
- Saccharin
- Sodium saccharin
- Splenda®
- Sucralose
- Sweet'N Low®

BOTTOM LINE: Moderation is advised when heating any natural sweetener, as in baking. It should be a treat, not an everyday occurrence. The good news is that you and your family can enjoy your favorite recipes using pure, whole, natural sweeteners—with great health benefits to your body!

Dr. Menzel's Definition of a Pure Whole Sugar

Pure, whole sugar should come directly from a natural food. No form of processing should strip it of its original nutrient-dense state or isolate a certain nutrient. Pure, whole sugar is used in its natural state.

PLEASE SEE THE SOURCE ACKNOWLEDGMENTS ON PAGE 272 FOR A LIST OF RESEARCH, BOOKS, AND WEBSITES USED FOR THIS SECTION.

Salt

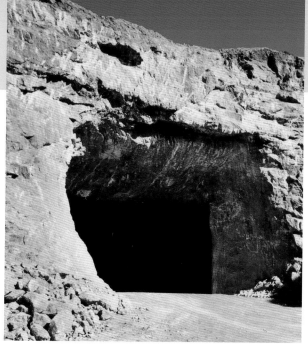

All salt originates from the sea.

Even the white table salt used by most Americans finds its origins in the ocean. It can come from a modern ocean, the Dead Sea, or an ancient sea. Researchers have debated the salt issue for many years—is it good for us?

People have consumed salt in its natural form for thousands of years. Civilizations were built around it and people prized, traded, and were paid with it. Salt was used to preserve food before refrigeration and it has been a wonderful part of many traditional cultures for flavoring food. Throughout the years, salt has made its claim to fame. We can't seem to live without it.

Scientists have long known that there is a secret to life in the sea. The salt content of the oceans is similar to the salt content of our own blood, tissues, and cells. The sac surrounding the embryo—where every human begins—is filled with this same saline solution called amniotic fluid.

Saltwater contains 84 mineral elements. The same 84 mineral elements are found in our bodies in perfect composition. Many of these trace minerals are in minute amounts, but they serve a very unique purpose in the function of the human body. The synergy of these elements is more than we will ever know or understand in our lifetime. The body is truly miraculous!

A loss or deficiency of any of these trace minerals can cause significant problems. *"Modern science has determined that 24 of the 84 elements are essential for life, although many believe that a proper balance of all 84 elements in our bodies is necessary for good health. Whenever a dietary deficiency of any of these elements occurs, the cells in our bodies lose ions. A loss of ions in our cells causes imbalances, a breakdown of the cell regeneration and growth process, and loss of the cells themselves, which leads to brain damage, muscle damage, or illness. Therefore, it is vital to your health to have the proper mineral balance in the saline and ion composition of your blood, and these compositions must be maintained within very precise limits. Many illnesses and poor health conditions have been traced to a deficiency of minerals, ironically the minerals that are found in sea salt." www.saltoftheearth.com.au*

The History of Salt

Circa 6000 BC—The earliest humans obtained their salt from meat and natural salt concentrations called licks. There are more than 30 references to salt in the Bible. Many relate to the cultural significance of salt in ancient Jewish culture.

Circa 3000 BC—Egyptians exported salted fish in return for other goods. Salt and salted animals are found buried in their ancient tombs.

Circa 2700 BC—A Chinese pharmacology treatise devoted a major portion to discussing more than 40 kinds of salt, including description of two methods of salt extraction. These methods are very similar to those used today.

Circa 2000 BC—The first salt tax was established in China by Emperor Hsia Yu. Profits were used to build the Great Wall. An early record describes salt production and trade during the Xia dynasty. It describes a technique of putting ocean water in clay

Salt, cont.

vessels and boiling it until it was reduced to salt crystals. This method was later spread through southern Europe by the Romans.

Circa 1450 BC—Egyptian art depicts salt-making. Ancient Greeks and Hebrews used salt during religious sacrifices.

20 BC–1400—The Romans built saltworks. Salt was an international currency and often was traded ounce-per-ounce with gold. Special salt rations given to early Roman soldiers were known as "salarium argentum," the forerunner of the English word "salary." During the time of the Roman Empire, shallow lead pans were used to boil salt water over open fires.

Circa 600—The Japanese developed a two-step process of the concentration and crystallization of salt using sea weed and clay pots. In areas where the climate did not allow solar evaporation, salt water was poured on burning wood or heated rocks. The salt left behind was then scraped off.

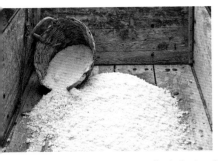

1770—Solar salt-making began in California using saltwater from the Pacific Ocean. Colonial Americans made salt by boiling brine in iron kettles.

Circa 1800—Salt also had military significance. For instance, it is recorded that thousands of Napoleon's troops died during his retreat from Moscow because their wounds would not heal as a result of a lack of salt. The U.S. began a large-scale salt production from drilling brine springs.

1830—Mechanical evaporation and purification began on Cape Cod. Open "grainer" pans were used, in which salt water was heated by steam running through pipes immersed in the water. This process is still used to produce certain types of salt.

Circa 1880—Open pans were replaced by a series of closed pans, in a device known as a multiple-effect vacuum evaporator, which had been used in the sugar industry for about 50 years. This process removed the minerals and added chemicals to produce a uniform product.

Circa 1900—Anti-caking agents, known as magnesium carbonate, were added to salt.

1924—Iodine was added to the mass-produced, refined salt to combat the iodine deficiency.

2013—The United States is now the world's largest producer of salt, followed by China, Russia, Germany, the United Kingdom, India, and France.

Civilization led to technological advances in salt-making. Modern salt production is vastly different from the sun drying process of old.

Refined Salt

Today, salt is made by several large, industrial companies. The largest, Cargill, currently sells 40 different types of processed salt. The process begins with salt from large, underground salt deposits or seawater. The salt "impurities" are removed to make it more attractive and uniform in appearance. Your salt may flow out of your saltshaker, but the refining process extracts 82 of the 84 mineral elements.

Industrial salt processors use the sodium chloride in salt and sell the extracted minerals for other uses. Boron is sold to make anti-knock petrol additives and chemical fertilizers; and magnesium is sold to manufacturers of light metal alloys and explosives. Some of the chemicals and minerals removed from salt are also used to make plastics.

This highly refined salt is the product of a high-temperature chemical process that removes all the valuable magnesium salts and naturally occurring trace minerals. Several harmful chemical additives are added (such as aluminum hydroxide and aluminum silicate) to bleach the salt and prevent water absorption while it is being packaged. These chemical additives also prevent the refined salt from being properly absorbed in your body.

To replace the natural iodine to salt, synthetic iodine in the form of potassium iodine is added in amounts that can be toxic. To stabilize the volatile iodide compound, processors add dextrose (sugar) which turns the iodized salt a purplish color. A bleaching agent is then necessary to restore whiteness to the salt. Table salt is not a natural, whole food—it is a dangerous chemical.

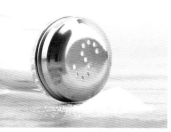

Synthetic iodine can become very toxic. The amount of iodine in refined salt is much higher than found in natural, unrefined sea salt. Iodine has been added to table salt since the 1920s to prevent the iodine deficiency. This has not been a successful attempt. Many people now suffer from thyroid problems as the body tries to metabolize the synthetic iodine. Most of my patients are on thyroid medication when they first come to see me. Those who choose to eat pure, whole foods and take additional whole food supplements are able to discontinue their medication or natural thyroid supplements within a relatively short amount of time.

I have also noticed similar results with my high blood pressure patients. Many of them have reduced or no longer need their blood pressure medication. Early research revealed salt as a culprit for increased blood pressure in some people. Studies of high blood pressure have been based on intake of commercially refined table salt.

Some sodium in the diet is beneficial as salt deficiency can lead to a loss of taste sensation, cramps, weakness, and respiratory distress from exertion. However, an overabundance of refined sodium can cause problems. Refined salt has a negative effect on the body. Therefore, I would recommend that anyone with blood pressure, thyroid, and/or hormonal issues switch to pure, whole salt.

A salt-restricted diet is not the answer!

* A salt restricted diet can raise or even lower your blood pressure. Many young adults suffer from low blood pressure.
* A lack of salt can cause aging, cellular degeneration, and starvation.
* A lack of pure, whole salt can impede proper organ function and chronic conditions such as weakened kidneys, stressed liver, and massive adrenal exhaustion.
* A salt-free diet leads to tiring heart valves due to a lack of essential minerals and trace elements found in natural salt.
* To pump properly, the heart needs magnesium.
* The healing powers of good salt equal those of vitamin C, vitamin E, and many other nutrients.

In 100% natural salt, there are over 80 trace elements that act as a buffer to protect us from sodium chloride retention. Natural sea salt lowers blood pressure by removing excess sodium from the tissues once it has completed its role within the cell matrix.

Americans receive most of their salt intake from processed foods. In his book, *Salt Sugar Fat*, Michael Moss states, "Americans are eating so much salt they are getting 10 times—even 20 times—the amount of sodium the body needs." This much salt is far more than the human body can handle. Although the food industry has been informed that sodium consumption should be lowered, processed food companies have not successfully lowered the amount in their products. The dead, fake, devitalized food would have no taste. Some processed food companies lowered the amount of sodium chloride and replaced it with other sodium-based compounds—which are just as bad or worse.

Chemical salt substitutes to avoid:

* Potassium chloride
* Sodium ascorbate
* Sodium diacetate
* Sodium lactate
* Sodium nitrate
* Sodium phosphates

In 2005, the Center for Science in the Public Interest came out with a report entitled *Salt: The Forgotten Killer... and FDA's Failure to Protect the Public's Health*. This consumer group was skeptical when the FDA asked manufacturers to go easy on the salt in 1983. The group began tracking the progress of 100 brand name products. In some years, the salt levels dipped, but from 1993 to 2005, the products became saltier. Their research conclusion stated that "Americans are consuming more—not less—salt. Thousands of packaged foods provide one-fourth or more of a day's maximum recommended intake."

Michael Moss, author of *Salt Sugar Fat, says,* "Without (refined) salt, processed food companies cease to exist."

Consumption of refined salt is not compatible with the human body—it is deadly. If you take into consideration the food industry's use of the wrong fats and sugars in their products, you have a triple whammy! Table salt lacks the valuable minerals to work in synergy with the natural body. It is a toxic substitute. The difference is its nutritional value, its taste, and the vast difference in the way your body responds.

The amount of sodium chloride in refined salt is 97.9%.

Fish from the ocean die quickly when placed in a solution of refined salt and water. Table salt—sodium chloride—is poisonous to them.

Unrefined Salt

Sea salt has the perfect balance of nutrients in its natural form. The body is able to utilize and absorb them and eliminate what it doesn't need. Unrefined sea salt contains 84 minerals. Some of them are in minute form, but they serve a specific purpose to meet the needs of the body.

Through my research, I have come to appreciate the purity of Celtic Sea Salt and Redmond Real Salt.

Celtic Sea Salt is harvested by hand. The salt is naturally dried by the sun and wind, then collected by farmers using long wooden tools. This is the only way to ensure all of the natural trace elements found in sea water are retained. Their salt is not altered by additives and nothing is removed. The sea salt supplies the body with over 80 vital trace minerals and elements, along with a proper balance of sodium chloride, the scientific name for salt. Sea salt contains twenty-four essential minerals for life. These minerals work in joint action to replenish the body and flush out any excess sodium chloride. Sea salt naturally enhances the flavor of foods and aids in digestion.

The brine and minerals found in Celtic Sea Salt are natural electrolytes that give your body a beneficial electrical charge. Our health depends on the abundance of these vital minerals to assimilate vitamins and nutrients to our cells. Celtic Sea Salt has a naturally occurring trace amount of iodine. This amount is not considered to be a significant source of iodine. However, it is a natural, pure source of iodine that is quickly absorbed and stored in your body.

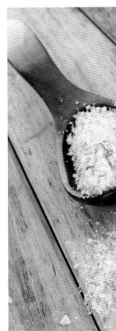

Redmond Real Salt comes from central Utah. The salt is extracted from an ancient sea bed deep within the earth, crushed, screened, and packaged without bleaching or refining. Real Salt has a unique "pinkish" appearance and flecks of color come from more than 60 natural trace minerals, including iodine. There is nothing added or taken away from this salt, and it is never chemically treated, bleached, or kiln dried—and it tastes great!

Caution: The sea salt in most grocery stores is not a pure, whole food. It is usually a refined salt with nutrients added back.

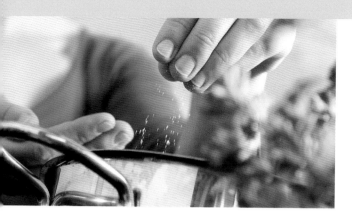

The accompanying minerals in unrefined sea salt provides the body with the whole picture. Table salt is an isolated nutrient in a synthetic form. As with any refined food, the body pulls from stored resources in an attempt to metabolize or rid itself of the chemicals. This becomes a constant adjustment.

Uses for Unrefined Sea Salt:

- Moderately salt food
- As a scrub to exfoliate and revitalize your skin
- Mixed with essential oils to create a therapeutic bath—relax after a long day
- Added to a neti pot for clearing out nasal cavity and sinuses
- Soak apples to freshen and preserve
- Mix with warm water and use as a mouthwash or throat gargle
- Use dry to preserve salad greens

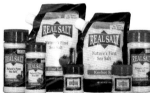

All salt originates from the sea but not all salt is created equal! Buy Celtic Sea Salt or Redmond Real Salt. Enjoy your seasoned food!

PLEASE SEE THE SOURCE ACKNOWLEDGMENTS ON PAGE 272 FOR A LIST OF RESEARCH, BOOKS, AND WEBSITES USED FOR THIS SECTION.

Naturopathic vs Allopathic Medicine Opinion

Both sides of the table have conflicting advice. We have been told to lower our salt intake to lower our risk of high blood pressure. Processes in the body are disrupted and problems occur when we introduce fake, devitalized food. However, we can find balance by removing processed foods from our diet and by living a natural lifestyle—the result is homeostasis.

We should eat pure, whole food in the way it was created, before man got a handle on it! A pure, whole food has not been through a chemical process and has not been stripped of its nutrients.

The American Heart Association believes there is no real health advantage of consuming unrefined salt. They believe the minute amounts of trace minerals found in sea salt are easily obtained from other healthy foods. They claim that the amount of sodium chloride is the same in both refined and unrefined salts.

The major difference lies within the body's response to the sodium chloride in refined salt and the unrefined sodium chloride in sea salt. I am not a chemist, but common sense tells me that any chemical process changes chemical composition. In terms of sodium chloride in sea salt and sodium chloride in table salt, one is in its natural form and one has been altered.

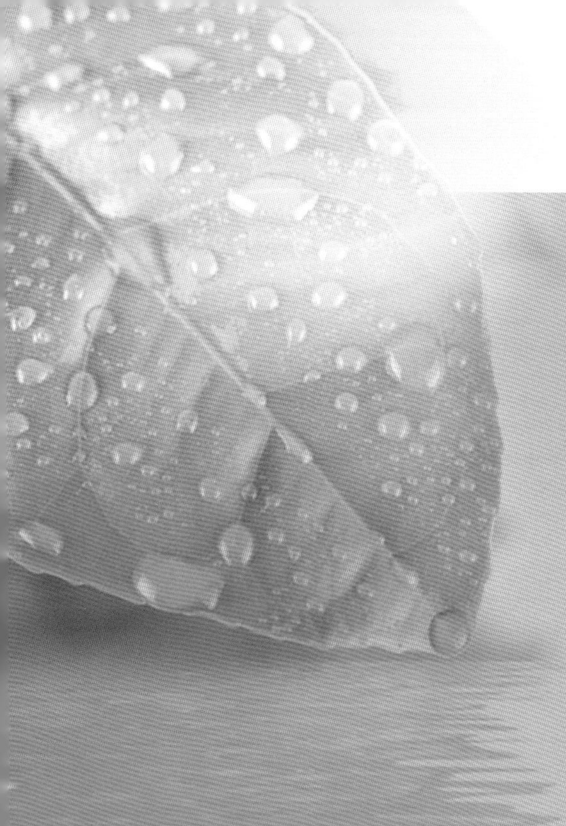

Therapies at Energetic Wellness

Wellness Appointments

German New Medicine

Body Balance Foot Bath

Far Infrared Sauna

Vitamin D Therapy

Esthetician & Spa Services

The Transformation

Wellness Appointments

My initial appointment with you is three hours long. I take the time to get to know you and understand what you hope to accomplish. Included in your appointment:

- Complete Health History Evaluation
- Introduction to German New Medicine®
- Wellness Counseling—The 7 Laws of Wellness
- SpectraVision™ Bio-Energy Balancing Scan
- Food Sensitivity Testing
- Biocompatible Supplementation Testing
- Individualized Homeopathic
  & Bach Flower Remedies
- Cold Laser Therapy
- Initial Appointment Wellness Folder
- Body Balance Foot Bath

SpectraVision™ Bionetic Stress Assessments

The SpectraVision™ technology is designed to eavesdrop on the body's responses using a specialized type of biofeedback known as "Non-Cognitive Bionetic Feedback." Because everything in life has a vibration, a Digital Pattern Array (DPA) can be created to see how your body reacts to various DPA signals for substances such as vitamins, minerals, flower essences, herbs etc. By measuring very small changes in the body's responses to the DPA matrix, the software can "read" how your body reacts and "see" your actual stress picture. This non-invasive process is comprehensive, painless, and easy. You will get an accurate picture of the things the body wants but doesn't have and what it has and doesn't want. It can also isolate what you might not be aware of regarding metabolism, elimination of toxins, nutrition,

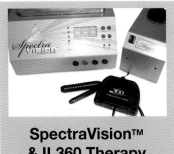

SpectraVision™ & IL360 Therapy

and levels of emotional stress. Determining how the body is working, and identifying where it can be optimized, is extremely valuable in creating a wellness plan for your overall health.

Stress & Its Impact

There are two types of stress: *background stress* (what a person isn't aware of) and *actual* or *perceived stress* (conflicts, jobs, money, children, etc.). Both types create a strain and place different demands on the body. Background stress uses up vital resources within the body (nutrition, vitamins, minerals, etc.). Actual stress causes fight-or-flight responses, activating the nervous system and releasing chemicals that, if not alleviated, become toxins in the body. Without understanding the stress demand from your overall stress picture, it is impossible to fully promote wellness. Stress affects all aspects of the person—the body, mind, and spirit. Due to the complexity of stress, it is difficult to completely support the body.

The Bionetic Stress Assessment (BSA) covers both aspects of stress and offers you a complete preventative approach to wellness.

When the stress load gets too high, it becomes a weight on the body's immune system, cardiovascular system, emotional and coping strategies, and impairs true healing due to lack of adequate sleep. This can compound itself, increase worry, and create a worse situation. In periods of high stress, we often make bad decisions such as poor food choices, neglecting exercise, and focusing on worry. By discovering why your body is reacting, the practitioner can help determine the best multi-dimensional solution (body-mind-spirit) to getting your body back into balance.

IL360 Low-Level Light Therapy

What is the history of laser therapy?

The use of light as a healing modality has been recorded as early as 2000 BC in ancient Egypt. Albert Einstein was the first person to theorize about lasers in 1917. Lasers were first invented in 1960 and have since been used for countless scientific and commercial purposes; including supermarket scanners, compact discs, vision repair, steel cutting, transmission of telephone messages, and the production of three dimensional images. Laser light is unique because it is monochromatic (one color), coherent (all waves are in phase with each other), and can be collimated (held to a small spot size at a great distance). Dr. Endre Mester was the first to observe its positive effects. He found that hair grew more quickly on shaved mice after their exposure to low levels of laser light.

How long have lasers been used by health care providers?

Therapeutic lasers have been used in Europe since Dr. Mester's discovery in 1967. The FDA approved the use of therapeutic lasers in 2002. Progressive physicians have since been offering laser therapy to their patients in ever-increasing numbers.

How do lasers work?

The photons of laser light penetrate through the skin and are absorbed by special components of the body's cells called chromophores. Just as photosynthesis creates energy for plants, the absorption of photons in the cells increases cellular energy. In areas of injury or damage, increased production of cellular energy improves the rate and quality of healing. This is referred to as bio-stimulation.

Because of its bio-stimulatory nature, laser therapy has the potential to help any situation wherein the body's cells are not working properly. Studies on tissue cultures reveal a wide range of beneficial effects, including increased levels of endorphins, prostaglandins, and other beneficial chemicals; reduced levels of harmful compounds, such as C-reactive protein and interleukin-1; pain modulation through a variety of mechanisms; and increased rate and quality of tissue healing. We are beings of light, and without it we lack the optimal promotion of healing and communication within the cells of our bodies.

IL360 addresses allergy-related illnesses such as:

- Eczema
- Psoriasis
- Asthma
- Seasonal allergies
- Environmental allergies
  (pollen, mold, dust, grass, trees, fungus)
- Pet dander allergies
- Food allergies
- Rashes & hives
- Locational allergies

"Many of the truths we adopt
we may not have verified for ourselves.
We come to believe what others have said,
or what we might have been taught.

We live adopted truths without conviction.
In some cases, this position is based on faith,
yet often, it is not based on faith
but is based merely on habit or laziness."

—*Lee G. Woolley,* CBP, BPA, BMD
Inventor of the SpectraVision™

The Value of MultiDimensional Products, Homeopathics & Natural Therapy

MultiDimensional products have been created to transform your being and address mental, emotional, physical, and refined energetic restrictions, which lie at the root of all illnesses. The value of a product comes from its ability to make changes that the body desires to make. Allopathic medicine fights to control symptoms, but symptoms are a sign of healing.

The principles of homeopathy include the recognition that symptoms must be encouraged so that their expression is enhanced and the duration is shortened. Add micro-dosing, flower essences for emotional support, and gemstone and vibrational therapy for mental support. High frequencies for spiritual and energetic pattern balancing bring homeostasis to the patient. Energetic imbalances exist before surfacing on the physical plane. All aspects must be addressed for complete healing to occur. Health and Harmony has created MutiDimensional products to help balance the entire being.

Health and Harmony begins with the highest quality nutrients, biodynamically grown, harvested at their greatest vitality, and free of toxins. These superior nutrients form the base of their products. They are then micronized into particles. This allows the micronutrients to become highly bioavailable, absorb sublingually directly through the lymphatic system, and eventually reach each of your cells. Sublingual absorption bypasses what is known as the *liver first pass effect*, which decreases the usable dosage by up to 90%. Micronized products deliver vital nutrients to every cell within twenty minutes!

Flower Essence Therapy

Much like homeopathy, flower essence therapy works on an energetic level to restore the equilibrium of the body, mind, and spirit. The particular specialty of flower essences is the realm of emotions and attitudes, which exert a powerful influence on health. Edward Bach, an English physician, homeopath, and the father of flower essence therapy, stated, "Behind all disease lie our fears, our anxieties, our greed, our likes and dislikes." By addressing underlying emotional issues and promoting energetic shifts in the mind and emotions, flower essences promote a return to health on all levels. In short, flower essences are the key to mind-body wellness.

Things to know:

- Extremely effective—results can be rapid, complete, and permanent
- Completely safe for children and women who are pregnant
- Can be taken alongside other medications.
- Uses all-natural ingredients
- Works in harmony with your immune system
- Non-addictive
- Treats the cause, not the symptoms

"The doctor of the future will give no medicine, but will interest her or his patients in the care of the human frame, in a proper diet, and in the cause and prevention of disease." —*Thomas A. Edison*

Emotox

A Closer Look at Emotox

The SpectraVision™ energetic balancing and assessment tool utilizes state-of-the-art technology with low-level light therapy. To date this is the best support for sensitivities. It works by balancing and supporting many systems of the body. The system provides an effective support system for addressing your specific sensitivities.

The therapy takes on average 10 visits and is completely painless. Once the sensitivities are identified, the SpectraVision™

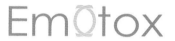

balances the patient by providing the correct frequencies of the sensitivity while simultaneously restoring "energetic blockages" in the body's nervous system and tissues. This is often times referred to as immune support.

Immune support is performed through low-level light therapy to stimulate specific areas of our nervous system in order to reprogram the body's immune response not to react when exposed to the original sensitivity.

For example, if we are working with a sensitivity to wheat, the unique software introduces the frequency for that particular wheat sensitivity into the body. If a stress response is detected, the system records it. From here, the practitioner utilizes low-level light therapy to stimulate specific acupuncture and auricular points, which releases endorphins and other chemicals, which in turn creates a new positive response.

So instead of the initial sensitivity causing your body to go into a reaction, the nervous system is now reprogrammed to respond normally when you eat wheat. Through this unique process, a reprogrammed nervous system response is developed that replaces the old pathway thus ridding you of that specific allergen.

Is it safe for children?

It is completely safe for children of all ages. Children, even infants, often benefit as much or more than adults as they respond very well at a time when their sensitivites seem to be the worst.

How many visits will I need?

Systemic conditions have generalized symptoms throughout the body, usually with inflammation, and are supported with a 10-series protocol. The Spectra-Vision™ Emotox protocol scans over 10,000 different items and substances. This protocol finds the underlying causes to most inflammatory conditions that ultimately compromise your immune system and increase our sensitivities to foods and other allergens.

Primary sensitivities are a simple error in the body associated with one major substance such as dog hair, nuts or pollen. These sensitivities are usually balanced and cleared within one to three visits, depending on the sensitivity.

Secondary sensitivities are symptoms of a bigger underlying issue that stimulates inflammation in the body, like infection, toxins, emotional traumas or other triggers. These allergies are generally resolved within the 10-series protocol.

Please keep in mind that natural healing can take time. You may not experience wellness overnight, but might notice slight changes in your health after just one visit, or manifest dramatic results within a very short period of time. Often, longstanding issues that have been present in the body for years can take several months to clear; however in our experience, they can be balanced!

Emotional CPR

Developed and taught by Lee G. Woolley, CBP, BPA, BMD – SpectraVision™ inventor and developer.

Emotional CPR is an adaptation and advancement of the work of Dr. Diana Mossop (England) and her Heart Lock technique.

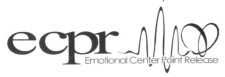

ecpr
Emotional Center Point Release

We all know that we bury away difficult feelings or don't process them fully. But have you considered how these buried emotions are affecting you on a subconscious level? They affect the way we view life; they create the filters we use to interpret and react to the experiences of life. For example, there is probably someone in your life that you always have problems with but you can't figure out why. This happens between family members all the time.

When people seek help for these feelings, they often turn to modalities like counseling, and psychological therapy. However, it can be difficult to discover deeply buried emotions and consciously talk through issues when they are hidden in the subconscious.

Emotional CPR gives us a way to identify and heal these buried, subconscious emotions. Years of research has found that these issues are actually stored within the muscle layers of the physical heart. The heart is a holographic holding point for our wounds. Using kinesiology or SpectraVision™ biofeedback as a guide, Emotional CPR finds where the emotional trauma is being stored, what it is about and gives us the tools to nudge the body to begin releasing and healing on a subconscious level. Emotional CPR does not involve hours of talking, excessive tears or emotional distress!

Here's a simple example how emotional hurt affects someone subconsciously:

A long time ago, when Johnny was 5 years old he had an awful stomach virus that he was just getting over. His younger brother just had his tonsils removed. Mom kept giving the younger brother ice cream to soothe is painful throat. Johnny really wanted the ice cream, but Mom said "No. It will upset your stomach." Johnny's five-year-old mind interpreted this event as "It's not fair! My baby brother gets all he wants!" Now, moving into adulthood, there is always this underlying bickering between Johnny and his younger brother. A seemingly benign childhood event created an emotional wound and programmed into Johnny's mind that "my brother always gets what he wants and I don't." Without anyone realizing it, that childhood event created long-lasting animosity between the brothers. This is the type of scenario that can be identified with the Emotional CPR, then the heart and mind are nudged to heal this event so that the brothers can have an easier and healthier relationship.

What happens during the office visit?

Muscle testing and SpectraVision™ biofeedback are the tools that can be used to find out where the emotional wound is stored within the heart. The heart is divided into 7 layers and we find the deepest layer that is ready for healing. This heart layer correlates with the basic conflict or emotion to be addressed. The heart is divided into 64 quadrants and the goal is to find the quadrant that is storing the emotional wound. By pinpointing the quadrant where the wound is stored, we can find:

1. How the mind interpreted the wound or event, and

2. The belief created in the mind from this trauma (usually a falsehood—like Johnny's belief that his brother always got everything. This false belief perpetuates a lack of healing or limits our growth.

3. We determine the specific lessons to be gained from the experience or trauma. What insights are possible from the experience as we post-process it with new information?

The Treatment

Once we obtain the specific area of the heart affected and the information about the wound or event, we then facilitate its release from the mind and body. The release is triggered by an energetic treatment that includes the therapies below. This treatment can be considered a form of psychological acupuncture.

Cold laser treatment of the heart and certain acupuncture points:

• Sound Therapy (tuning forks);
• Color Therapy (glasses);
• Essential healing oils may also be placed on certain acupuncture points; and
• An Emotional Profusion remedy is prescribed to be taken over the next 3–4 weeks.

Emotional Profusion Remedies
Continue the Healing

The healing begins during the office visit, but each patient is provided with a Profusion remedy so that processing and healing continues over the next three weeks. The formulas prompt the body to heal by using light, color, and vibration. Each remedy has an amino acid frequency that forms the key to unlock the physical process of getting the light frequencies all the way into the DNA of the cell nucleus. This lock-and-key process offers each formula their own unique pathway to work within the protein structure of the cells and tissues. Certain proteins regulate the cellular activities and cause growth and healing to occur. Each of the formulas can interact with thousands of regulating proteins to effect a change. The body uses light to carry information to the proteins acting as the carrier of information (healing) to stimulate the proteins to activate the cell membranes.

• Profusions are energetic delivery systems to access the body at the deepest molecular level. They utilize the latest technology in healing with light and laser.

• There are many different Profusion remedies. Each person's "lesson" from the treatment determines the Profusion remedy for them. Patients may take 1–3 Profusion remedies.

• The Profusion remedies last for 3–4 weeks. Patients should stay on the remedies until they are gone.

Profusions Will:

• Promote a general feeling of calmness.
• Stir up old memories or thoughts in a gentle third-party sense.
• Will stir up dreams. Dreams may be more frequent and more lucid.

Most of the healing occurs subconsciously in the "background" without any actual pain recollection and without any specific memories having to be relived. Journaling and stress reduction methods are encouraged while taking these remedies and healing.

Care Plan Options

Emotional CPR can be done every two weeks for a patient who desires to quickly resolve emotional stress issues and/or resolve health challenges. An aggressive care plan would be to alternate every two weeks between a SpectraVision™ balancing and an ECPR treatment. A moderate wellness plan would be to do ECPR a couple times in between quarterly SpectraVision™ sessions. Emotional CPR can certainly be done as a stand-alone treatment.

To make an appointment with Dr. Menzel, call 405-359-1245 Monday thru Friday, 9 a.m.–5 p.m.

If you live too far from Energetic Wellness, Oklahoma, and want to find a SpectraVision™ Practitioner in your area, contact Wellcare Health Services at 855-813-0884 or visit wellcaretechnology.com.

WellCare
Health Services

German New Medicine®

German New Medicine® encompasses the medical findings of Dr. Ryke Geerd Hamer.

Ten years ago, I came across the German New Medicine® website while doing studies on cancer. When I read the materials on the site, I knew I had found the answer to understanding the natural design of the body.

Dr. Hamer's work resonated so well with my belief that the body was created to self-heal that I was compelled to learn more. I studied and read the website frequently. But it wasn't until I went to study in Canada, under Caroline Markolin, that I grasped the truth of Dr. Hamer's remarkable discoveries.

On August 18, 1978, Dr. Ryke Geerd Hamer, MD—head internist in the oncology clinic at the University of Munich, Germany, at the time—received the shocking news that his son Dirk had been shot. Dirk died in December 1978. A few months later, Dr. Hamer was diagnosed with testicular cancer. Since he had never been seriously ill, he immediately surmised that his cancer development might be directly related to the tragic loss of his son.

Dirk's death and his own experience with cancer prompted Dr. Hamer to investigate the personal history of his cancer patients. He quickly learned that, like him, they all had gone through some exceptionally stressful episode prior to developing cancer. The observation of a **mind-body connection** was not really surprising. Numerous studies had already shown that cancer and other diseases are often preceded by a traumatic event. But Dr. Hamer took his research a momentous step further. Pursuing the hypothesis that all bodily events are controlled from the brain, he analyzed his patients' brain scans and compared them with their medical records. Dr. Hamer discovered that every disease—not only cancer—is controlled from its own specific area in the brain and linked to a very particular, identifiable, "conflict shock." The result of his

research is a scientific chart that illustrates the biological relationship between the psyche and the brain in correlation with the organs and tissues of the entire human body. (The English "Scientific Chart of GNM" is available through the GNM bookstore on the website.)

Dr. Hamer came to call his findings "The Five Biological Laws of the New Medicine®," because these biological laws, which are applicable to any patient's case, offer an entirely new understanding of the cause, the development, and the natural healing process of diseases. *(In response to the growing number of misrepresentations of his discoveries and to preserve the integrity and authenticity of his scientific work, Dr. Hamer has now legally protected his research material under the name German New Medicine® (GNM). The term "New Medicine" could not be copyrighted internationally.)*

German New Medicine® is a **true natural science**. This means that the Five Biological Laws are verifiable in each and every patient case. Since 1981, Dr. Hamer's findings have been tested more than 30 times by several physicians and professional associations through signed documents (you can view these verifications online). All documents attest to the 100% accuracy of Dr. Hamer's discoveries.

> German New Medicine®
> is a true natural science.
> The Five Biological Laws
> are verifiable in each and
> every patient case.

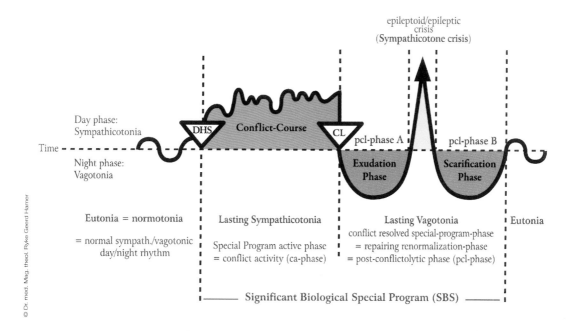

epileptoid/epileptic crisis
(**Sympathicotone crisis**)

Day phase:
Sympathicotonia

Time

Night phase:
Vagotonia

DHS **Conflict-Course** **CL**

pcl-phase A

pcl-phase B

Exudation Phase

Scarification Phase

© Dr. med. Mag. theol. Ryke Geerd Hamer

Eutonia = normotonia

= normal sympath./vagotonic
day/night rhythm

Lasting Sympathicotonia

Special Program active phase
= conflict activity (ca-phase)

Lasting Vagotonia
conflict resolved special-program-phase
= repairing renormalization-phase
= post-conflictolytic phase (pcl-phase)

Eutonia

— Significant Biological Special Program (SBS) —

The Biological Laws of the New Medicine are in perfect harmony with spiritual laws. Because of this truth, the Spanish call GNM "La Medicina Sagrada," the Sacred Medicine.

Standard Medical Theories

Modern medicine is largely based on theories, statistics, and countless "new studies" that are often contradicted by the "latest research." Even though medical doctrines, such as the concept of an "immune system" or of "malignant" and "metastasizing" cancers, have never been scientifically verified, the guardians of the existing medical paradigm have found effective ways to turn pure assumptions into "truths," leading the public to believe that the unproven results are "good science."

German New Medicine® is founded on natural laws rather than on theories, on inductive reasoning rather than on postulation. Dr. Hamer's discoveries offer a complete scientific system that serves as a basis for an entirely new understanding of "dis-eases."

This is real preventive medicine, an aspect of German New Medicine® that can hardly be emphasized enough. True prevention requires an understanding of the real cause of a disease, and that is what Dr. Hamer's research supplies in splendid detail. By understanding the Five Biological Laws of the cause and healing process of disease we can free ourselves from the fear and panic that often come with the onset of symptoms. This knowledge is more than power; it can save lives.

The 5 Biological Laws

1st **Every SBS (significant biological special program) originates from a DHS** (Dirk Hamer Syndrome), which is an unexpected, highly acute, and isolating conflict shock that occurs simultaneously in the psyche, the brain, and on the corresponding organ.

2nd **Every SBS runs in two phases**, provided there is a resolution for the conflict.

3rd **This law explains the correlation between the psyche (the brain) and the organ** within the context of the embryoic (ontogenetic) and evolutionary (phylogenetic) development of the human organism. It shows that neither the location of the ring configuration (Hamer Focus or HH) in the brain nor the cell proliferation (tumor) or tissue loss following a DHS are accidental, but embedded in a meaningful biological system inherent in every species.

4th **Law #4 explains the beneficial role of microbes** as they correlate to the three embryonic germ layers during the healing phase of any given Significant Biological Special Program (SBS).

5th **Every disease is part of a Significant Biological Special Program** created to assist an organism (humans and animals alike) in resolving a biological conflict. This law indicates that nothing in nature is meaningless or "malignant," as we have been taught. Each conflict (DHS) that catches an individual "on the wrong foot" triggers an SBS which assists the organism in resolving the actual conflict situation.

The Importance of a Healthy Diet

Dr. Hamer writes:

"An individual who eats properly is less susceptible to suffer biological conflicts. That is self-evident. It is a lot like why rich people don't get as many cancers as the poor, because the rich are able to resolve many conflicts simply by pulling out their cheque book and writing a cheque. But to prevent cancer (or any other disease) through diet is impossible, because even a healthy diet cannot stop conflicts from occurring. In Nature, the strong and healthy animal will naturally suffer fewer cancers than the one that is weak or aged. But this does not mean that being old is therefore carcinogenic."

It goes without saying that a healthy diet is essential for our wellbeing. **Eating healthy food** is particularly important when we are in a "biological program."

At the beginning of the healing phase, the appetite returns. Food now becomes true medicine. When an organ or tissue is in the stage of being repaired, the organism needs lots of nutrients that support the healing process. The **energy** we gain through a healthy diet makes healing so much easier. Conversely, foods containing toxins (pesticides, herbicides, preservatives, food additives, and the like) deplete the body of energy. This can prolong and even complicate the healing process.

When we fully recognize that it is the **psyche** where diseases begin and where they end, and that the brain functions as the biological control center of all bodily processes, including "pathogenic" changes, then we also learn to understand that our diet or nutritional supplements cannot per se prevent, let alone cure a disease. However, a healthy diet, ideally from organic sources, certainly accelerates the healing process.

If we live naturally to the best of our ability, as outlined in this guide, we will suffer fewer conflicts, and, therefore, fewer "diseases." When we take care of the natural function of our bodies:

We are more likely to experience life more abundantly

Our reactions to situations are much more controlled because we have a feeling of wellbeing

We respond better to challenges

We are not influenced by foods that create addictions

I have experienced this firsthand in my own life. The knowledge of GNM has given me confidence in the body's design. I can honestly say that I do not fear any condition.

I believe the true heart of GNM is that these biological programs are created in response to who we are and how we respond to circumstances, or the "conflict shock." When we have this knowledge, it helps us respond to situations that catch us off guard. If we can resolve it in the day it happens, or downgrade the situation, we help ourselves through the healing process.

I will be forever grateful to Dr. Hamer and my teacher, Caroline Markolin, for this wonderful knowledge. And I thank God for the design. We no longer have to fear symptoms, we can welcome them. Having peace in our design is what God intended.

I wholeheartedly believe in the truth of the discoveries of Dr. Hamer and the Five Biological Laws. There is no way in this short document to explain the intricate details of the biological processes. Please join me when I teach GNM in my Health Awareness classes, set a GNM consultation, or visit www.learninggnm.com.

Body Balance Footbath

Positive and negative ions are emitted that re-energize the body, including red blood cells. The detoxification process balances the body by extracting excess toxins that are stored in the kidneys, liver, bowels, and skin, not only during, but also after treatment.

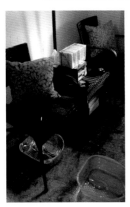

The footbath triggers the body, and continues to detoxify for the next 24 to 48 hours. The entire process takes 30–40 minutes for adults and is completely safe. It is, however, not recommended for pregnant women, anyone with a heart pacemaker, an organ transplant, or epilepsy.

The Sea-Onic footbath is one of the safest detoxification processes, as there is no electrical current injected into the body. The water in the footbath and the detailed configuration of the array plates ensure that the actual electrical current only flows between the narrowly spaced plates. This process produces tiny bubbles that safely penetrate through the feet and into the lymphatic system.

Through this process, there is a significant increase of negative ions. Ions are atoms or molecules that have lost or gained electrons. Free radicals are atoms with unpaired electrons.

The ionic technique of cleansing through the feet provides a full body purge to all vital organs, resulting in a reduction of menopause symptoms, menstrual cramps, sexual health problems, skin problems, acne, sleep problems, restlessness, stress, toothaches, wrinkles, aches and pains, and yeast infections. The internal cleansing can also assist in faster healing and injury recovery.

Benefits of the Body Balance Footbath Therapy

- Assists in recovery from disease, injury, and surgeries
- Can also assist with headache and pain, joint stiffness, sleep patterns, heavy metals, menstrual and arthritis pain, and the immune system
- May assist with kidney and liver functions
- Energizes red blood cells

Far Infrared Sauna

The far infrared sauna therapy is perhaps the most effective method of removing toxins from the body. Regular whole body detoxification will assist the body's natural elimination, leading to a balanced, healthful life.

Exposure to chemicals and heavy metals often exceeds the body's ability to detoxify. The High Tech Health Thermal Life Far Infrared Sauna removes heavy metal toxins (including mercury), fat-stored (lipophilic) toxins, and metals trapped in connective tissue and the brain. It also increases the detoxifying and cleansing capacity of the skin by stimulating the sweat glands.

When the liver, kidneys, and lungs have been damaged by chronic exposure to environmental toxins, the body's ability to eliminate toxins becomes impaired. The Thermal Life sauna assists the body in

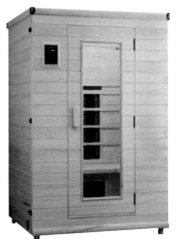

eliminating the toxins and promotes the restoration of those organs so they can properly address future toxins.

Because infrared penetrates safely and comfortably up to three inches inside your body, your deep tissues and organs are stimulated. Hard to reach impurities are eliminated through your skin

Creating Energy for Balanced Living

using lower, comfortable temperatures. As your body increases sweat production to cool itself, your heart works harder, pumping more blood and achieving the conditioning benefits of continuous exercise. The process widens your blood vessels and enriches your blood with oxygen. You feel more energetic and your skin gets a beautiful, youthful glow.

Conditions Relieved by Using Infrared Sauna

Acne/blackheads	Heavy metal toxicity
Arthritis	Hemorrhoids
Asthma	Hepatitis
Backache	Hypertension
Bell's palsy	(high blood pressure)
Benign prostatic hypertrophy	Hypotention (low blood pressure)
Brain damage	Inflammatory conditions
Bronchitis	and infiltrates
Bursitis	Keloids
Cancer	Leg and decubital ulcers
Cancer pain	Low core body temperature
Children's overtired muscles	Lyme borreliosis
Crohn's disease	Nervous tension
Chronic fatigue syndrome	Neurasthenia
Cirrhosis	Neuritis
Colds/flu	Nosebleeds
Cold hands and feet	Obesity
Cholecystitis	Pediatric pneumonia
Cystitis	Pelvic infections
Dandruff	Peripheral occlusive disease
Diabetes	Post-surgical infections
Diarrhea	PMS and menopausal symptoms
Duodenal ulcers	Pneumonia
Ear diseases	Rheumatoid arthritis
Ear infections	Sciatica
Eczema with infection	Short-term memory loss
Edema	Skin tone
Electromagnetic pollution	Sore throats
Exudates	Strained muscles
Fibromyalgia	Stretch marks
Gastritis	Tinea (fungal infection)
Gastroenteric problems	Tinnitus (ringing in the ears)
Gout arthritis	TMJ
Headaches	Varicose veins

Vitamin D Therapy with Collagen & Healthy Tanning

Vitamin D is an essential nutrient that can make a world of difference for your heart health, bones, skin, immunity, and even your mood. Your body produces it naturally when your skin comes in contact with sunlight. In reality, you are your own vitamin-D-producing machine!

But without enough outdoor sun exposure, it is difficult to maintain adequate levels of vitamin D year-round. For lack of an effective, convenient solution, most people take the problem of vitamin D deficiency lightly.

The best way to regulate our vitamin D is not through intake of supplements. Instead, exposure to real ultraviolet A & B rays is the best course. That is why tanning beds can be useful, especially in the winter.

Before you head out to a tanning salon, know these potential problems with commercial tanning beds: some tanning beds use bulbs that emit hazardous x-rays; electromagnetic rays may also cause problems. I was against tanning beds for 20 years until I learned of ESB Tanning Systems. The ESB tanning bed's electronic RT ballast is low in electromagnetic radiation. Their beds are safe and can be a great way to get the light that we need.

Esthetician & Spa Services

The Spa Services are provided by our esthetician, Marion Hoover. As a military spouse, she traveled the world for 20 years while raising three amazing daughters. She received most of her training in Germany. In recent years, she has added new services that include essential oils and tuning forks. Her mission is to provide each client a relaxing and beneficial experience—using her training and intuition for what is most needed each time.

As a fully trained esthetician and massage therapist, she offers a variety of treatments.

- **Facials,** such as acne treatments,
- **European facials,** and
- **The Ultimate Facial**—which includes microdermabrasion and oxygen treatment.

Microdermabrasion removes layers of dead skin cells and leaves the skin feeling smooth and better able to absorb anti-aging skin products.

The oxygen treatment supplies the skin with pure oxygen, enhanced with essential oils, selected for their anti-aging and healing benefits. This treatment is an extremely soothing and relaxing experience you don't want to miss!

All facials include deep pore cleansing and relaxing massage. The products she uses are fully organic and healthy for your skin—no harsh or harmful ingredients.

Further esthetician services include:
- **Waxing** (any body parts)
- **Brow & lash tint**
- **Raindrop therapy**
- **Relaxing full-body massage** (no deep tissue)
- **Full body scrubs** with light massage
- **Hot stone massage**

Furthermore, the beautiful vibrations of Solfeggio and Ohm **tuning forks** have been added to most treatments. The vibrations are deeply relaxing and healing on different levels. She applies them as guided and needed—no two treatments are the same.

Raindrop Massage Therapy

Raindrop Therapy is a light-touch massage technique using Young Living Essential Oils on the spine.

The 7 Powerful Benefits of Raindrop Massage Therapy

- Reduces Pain: Massage is a significant component, with a particular focus on the spinal muscles.

- Reduces Inflammation: Several essential oils are used as powerful anti-inflammatory agents. These include wintergreen, thyme, and peppermint.

- Improves Circulation: Helps to improve overall blood circulation, leading to balancing of the autonomic nervous system and regulation of gastrointestinal functions.

- Asists in the healing of Spinal Misalignment (Scoliosis, Kyphosis, etc.): Influences the body and the spine for healing.

- Relieves Stress: Promotes conscious and subconscious "letting go" so normal body function can be restored.

- Improves Immune Function: Increases dopamin levels and lymphocytes to help reduce bacterial and viral infections.

- Facilitates the Release of Pent-Up Emotions: Helps activate and release subconscious emotional stress. Severe emotional stresses can produce subconscious neuroses, (stored in the subconscious parts of the brain). Inhaling essential oils stimulates the brain. Also helps reduce depression and anger.

During the Raindrop Therapy session, *seven therapeutic-grade essential oils are sprinkled on the spine (hence the name Raindrop) and also worked into the spinal reflexology area of the feet. Raindrop Technique should not be mistaken for conventional body or deep-tissue massage.*

The purpose of Raindrop Therapy is to stimulate every organ, muscle, and bone at a cellular level, support the immune system, release toxins and disease, and bring the body into structural and electrical balance. It works on both physical and emotional levels, and emotional release may be experienced, depending on the client's ability and willingness to let go of stored issues.

The therapist applies seven oils and two blends (Valor, Oregano, Thyme, Cypress, Basil, Wintergreen, Majoram, Peppermint, Aroma Siez). Other oils may be added as needed for specific complaints. The properties of the oils are highly antibacterial, antiviral, anti-inflammatory, and immune-supporting; and some are relaxing, while others are stimulating. The overall working pressure is from feather-light to medium, no deep-tissue work is required.

Raindrop Technique's objective is to stimulate the receiver's internal healing powers, and at the end of the session, to achieve a state of balance and receptivity to healing energies. Illness is usually the result of accumulated toxins over many years and/or physical, mental, or spiritual trauma. Raindrop Therapy can potentially correct something, but to return completely to a state of perfect health may take several sessions and permanent lifestyle changes to eliminate the source of ill conditions.

Benefits of Raindrop Therapy may not be immediately apparent following a session, but the oils continue to work for several days and adjustments can still occur. Sometimes benefits will be felt right away; other times they may be subtle and not be noticed for a while.

Raindrop Massage Therapy can also be customized to address different health issues. Always remember, the client is his or her own best healer; we only support you with insight, love, and compassion.

Properties of the Oils Used in Raindrop Therapy

Basil—relaxes voluntary muscles, antibacterial, antispasmodic, anti-inflammatory. Used for migraine, throat/lung infections, insect bites.

Cypress—good for circulation, strengthens blood capillaries, antispasmodic, discourages fluid retention. Used for diabetes, circulatory disorders, cancer, grounding, stabilizing.

Majoram—relaxes involuntary muscles, relieves body and joint discomfort, helps sooth the digestive tract, antibacterial, antifungal, vasodilator, lowers blood pressure, expectorant, mucolytic. Used for arthritis, nerve and muscle pain, headaches, PMS, fungal infections, ringworm, shingles.

Oregano—anti-aging, antiviral, antifungal, antibacterial, anti-inflammatory, immune stimulant. Used for arthritis, respiratory disease, digestive problems.

Peppermint—anti-inflammatory, antitumoral, antiparasitic, antiviral, antifungal, gallbladder stimulant, pain reliever, curbs appetite. Used for rheumatoid arthritis, respiratory infections, obesity, cold sores, herpes, back problems, nausea.

Thyme—highly antimicrobial, antifungal, antiviral. Used for respiratory problems, digestive complaints, gastritis, bronchitis, pertussis, asthma, tonsilitis.

Wintergreen—anticoagulant, antispasmodic, anti-inflammatory, vasodilator, anesthetic, reduce blood pressure, reduces all pain. Used for rheumatoid arthritis, muscle and nerve pain, hepatitis, fatty liver.

Aroma Siez—energy balancing blend

Valor—chiropractor in a bottle

Other great oils:
Patchouli—nausea, queasy stomach, motion sickness, morning sickness, antimicrobial, prevents wrinkles, relieves itching. Used for hypertension, skin conditions (eczema, acne), fluid retention.

Lavender—antiseptic, analgesic, antitumoral, anti-inflammatory, sedative. Used for burns, dandruff, allergies, herpes, headaches, indigestion, insomnia, menopausal conditions, nausea, tumors, PMS, acne, dermatitis, eczema.

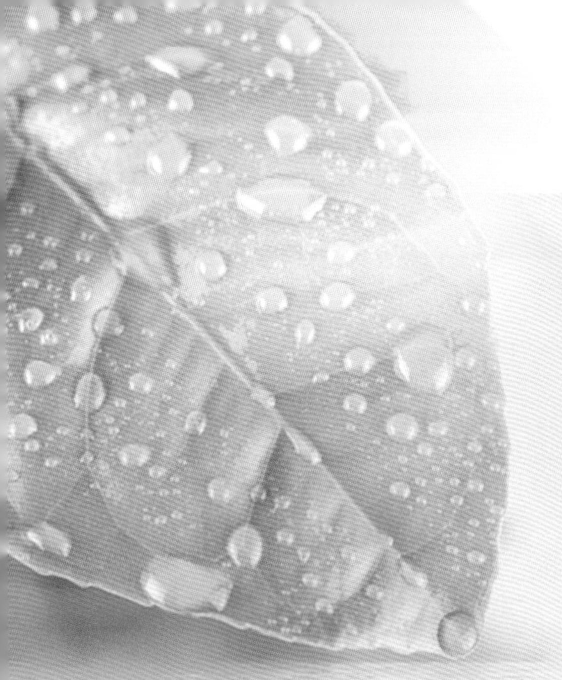

Resources

Books, DVDs & Websites

Testimonies

NUTRITION

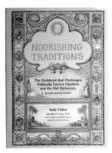

Nourishing Traditions
by Sally Fallon

I am so grateful to the friend that gave me *Nourishing Traditions* as a gift in 2004. Sally has taught me so much about how to prepare food correctly. These lost culinary arts can be learned in your own kitchen. After reading her book, I read Dr. Price's book *Nutrition and Physical Degeneration* which is the foundation of what I teach nutritionally in my practice today. Please purchase your own copy of *Nourishing Traditions*. You will not be disappointed and every recipe is gourmet and amazing!

I prefer using sprouted grains and flours vs. soaking flours and grains as many of Sally's recipes recommend. Both are good methods. Using sprouted flours are easier, some people do both.

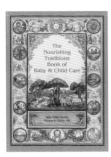

The Nourishing Traditions Book of Baby and Child Care
by Sally Fallon Morell and Thomas S. Cowan, MD

The Nourishing Traditions Book of Baby & Child Care makes the principles of traditional nutrition available to modern parents. The book provides holistic advice for pregnancy and newborn interventions, vaccinations, breastfeeding and child development, as well as a compendium of natural treatments for childhood illnesses, from autism to whooping cough. The work of Rudulf Steiner supports the book's emphasis on the child's spiritual requirement for imaginative play.

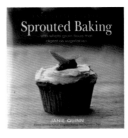

Essential Eating Sprouted Baking
by Janie Quinn

Janie does an amazing job of explaining the benefits of sprouted whole grain flours. Sprouted flour is flour milled from grain that has been sprouted into a plant and therefore digests as a vegetable. You can enjoy sprouted flour in breads and desserts that make for guiltless pleasure. You will soon realize that eating sprouted baked goods is very light and you can actually lose weight.

Every recipe is wonderful! You will be amazed by how easy it is to bake your own delicious healthful desserts and breads. Your family will love them, too.

She uses a lot of maple sugar, which is delicious, but costly. I substituted Rapunzel whole cane sugar for the maple sugar, except for one recipe for sugar cookies. They are amazing with the maple sugar!

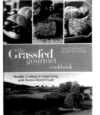

The Grassfed Gourmet Cookbook
by Shannon Hayes

I love this cookbook! This book is well worth buying for all the great information on how to cook pasture-raised foods, as well as the awesome recipes. Some of the recipes call for ingredients that I do not recommend.

Below is a substitute list:

Sugar/brown sugar	Rapunzel whole cane sugar
All purpose flour	Sprouted spelt flour
Shortening	Lard or butter
Breadcrumbs	Homemade Breadcrumbs recipe (p. 158)
Cornstarch	Organic cornstarch
Cheeses	My recommended dairy list

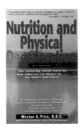

Nutrition and Physical Degeneration
by Dr. Weston A. Price

This book is written based on the research of Weston A. Price. It is a comparison between the traditional, nature-based diet and the more modern diet. It reveals how what we eat affects our health and quality of life.

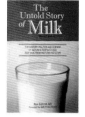

The Untold Story of Milk
by Ron Schmid, ND

The history, politics, and science of nature's perfect food: raw milk from pasture-fed cows. I met Dr. Ron a few years ago at a Weston A. Price conference. He has been a naturopath for 30 years, using nutrient-dense foods in his practice. He is a mentor and a friend. Great book!

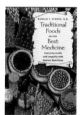

Traditional Foods are Your Best Medicine: *Improving Health and Longevity with Native Nutrition*
by Ron Schmid, ND

Modern medicine now recognizes that the present-day Western diet is responsible for many of today's chronic illnesses. In this book, Ron Schmid explains how a return to a traditional diet can help you reduce your risk of heart attack by 50 percent; fight allergies, chronic fatigue, arthritis, skin problems, and headaches; recover from colds and flu in a day or two; and increase life expectancy.

Healthy 4 Life
by Weston A. Price Foundation

Are you confused about what to eat? Do you have trouble choosing foods to buy for your family—foods that are both healthy and delicious? This book is an alternative to the USDA Food Pyramid Guidelines. *The Healthy 4 Life* dietary guidelines are easy to follow.

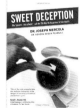

Sweet Deception:
Why Splenda®, NutraSweet® and the FDA May Be Hazardous to Your Health
by Dr. Joseph Mercola

Supported by extensive studies and research, Dr. Joseph Mercola exposes the fact that Splenda® actually contributes to a host of serious diseases. *Sweet Deception* will lay out how the FDA really works for big food companies and should not be trusted when it comes to your health.

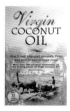

Virgin Coconut Oil: *How it Has Changed People's Lives, and How it Can Change Yours*
by Brian & Marianita Shilhavy

This is the most practical book written on the health benefits of coconut oil. With over 100 personal stories and over 85 recipes, it is a bestseller.

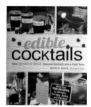

Edible Cocktails by Natalie Bovis

Whether you want to learn how to become a better bartender for your own cocktail parties or you want to experience the journey of creating a cocktail that you plan from planting to pouring, this book teaches you how to put both thought and care into what you drink as well as elevate your cocktails to new earth-friendly, culinary-focused, health-conscious heights. Some of the recipes call for ingredients I do not recommend. Example white sugar—replace with a natural sugar. (pp. 223-234)

Genetic Roulette: *The Documented Risks of Genetically Engineered Foods*
by Jeffrey M. Smith

The biotech industry's claim that genetically modified (GM) foods are safe is shattered in this groundbreaking book. Sixty-five health risks of the foods that Americans eat every day are presented in easy-to-read two-page spreads. The left page is designed for the quick-scanning reader; it includes bullet points, illustrations, and quotes. The right side offers fully referenced text, describing both research studies and theoretical risks. The second half of *Genetic Roulette* shows how safety assessments on GM crops are not competent to identify the health problems presented in the first half. It also exposes how industry research is rigged to avoid finding problems.

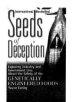

Seeds of Deception: *Exposing Industry and Government Lies About the Safety of the Genetically Modified Foods You're Eating*
by Jeffrey M. Smith

Worldwide industry manipulation and political collusion, rather than sound science, have brought genetically engineered food into our daily diet. *Seeds of Deception* reveals that company research is rigged, alarming evidence of health dangers is covered up, and that political and corporate bullying form the seedy background to the spread of GM crops.

Pasture Perfect: *How You Can Benefit from Choosing Meat, Eggs & Dairy Products from Grass-Fed Animals*

by Jo Robinson.

Jo explores the new grass-fed phenomenon. She explains why tens of thousands of people are saying "no" to factory farming, and buying their meats, eggs, and dairy products from pasture-based ranchers. You'll learn why grass-fed beef, pork, lamb, bison, and dairy products are safer, healthier, and more beneficial for you, the farmers, the animals, and the environment.

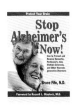

Stop Alzheimer's Now!

by Dr. Bruce Fife

This book outlines a program using ketone therapy and diet that is backed by decades of medical and clinical research and has proven successful in restoring mental function and improving both brain and overall health. You will learn how to prevent and even reverse symptoms associated with Alzheimer's disease, Parkinson's disease, amyotrophic lateral sclerosis (ALS), multiple sclerosis (MS), Huntington's disease, epilepsy, diabetes, stroke, and various forms of dementia.

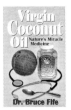

Virgin Coconut Oil:
Nature's Miracle Medicine

by Dr. Bruce Fife

In this book, you will discover how people are successfully using virgin coconut oil to prevent and treat high cholesterol, high blood pressure, arthritis, fibromyalgia, candida, ulcers, herpes, allergies, psoriasis, influenza, diabetes, and much more.

Dr. Bruce Fife is considered an expert on the health benefits of coconut oil and has written many other books on the subject. To see his other books, visit Energetic Wellness or go to www.coconutresearchcenter.org.

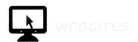

Weston A. Price Foundation

www.westonaprice.org

The Weston A. Price Foundation is a nonprofit, tax-exempt charity founded in 1999 to disseminate the research of nutrition pioneer, Dr. Weston Price, whose studies of isolated non-industrialized peoples established the parameters of human health and determined the optimum characteristics of human diets. Dr. Price's research demonstrated that humans achieve perfect physical form and perfect health generation after generation only when they consume nutrient-dense whole foods and the vital fat-soluble activators found exclusively in animal fats. The Foundation is dedicated to restoring nutrient-dense foods to the human diet through education, research, and activism. To become a member, go to website and click "Join Now."

Price-Pottenger Nutrition Foundation
Your Trusted Guide to Optimal Health

www.ppnf.org

This is one of the most unique health resource organizations in the world. They have been disseminating reliable, unbiased information about nutrition, food preparation, natural healing, and environmental issues for more than half a century.

Real Milk

www.realmilk.com

A Campaign for Real Milk is a project of The Weston A. Price Foundation. Find sources for safe, healthy, real milk in your area. And learn that real milk is from real cows that eat real food.

EatWild

www.eatwild.com

A source for safe, healthy, natural, and nutritious grass-fed beef, lamb, goats, bison, poultry, pork, dairy, and other wild edibles. EatWild provides comprehensive, accurate information about the benefits of raising animals on pasture. A direct link to local farms that sell all-natural, delicious, grass-fed products. Support for farmers who raise their livestock on pasture from birth to market and who actively promote the welfare of their animals and the health of the land.

Tropical Traditions—
America's Source for Coconut Oil

www.tropicaltraditions.com

Brian and Marianita Shilhavy established Tropical Traditions in 1998 in the Philippines. They began making coconut oil using the traditional methods used by Marianita's grandparents. They have a strong commitment to family farming and organic standards and stand firmly against genetically modified foods. Today when you buy Tropical Traditions Gold Label Virgin Coconut Oil, you are buying the highest quality coconut oil they have to offer, and it is still made by hand benefiting families in the rural areas of the Philippines where the coconuts grow.

Farm to Consumer Legal Defense Fund

www.farmtoconsumer.org

Defending the rights and broadening the freedoms of family farms and protecting consumer access to raw milk and nutrient-dense foods.

Vital Choice Seafood

www.vitalchoice.com

Vital Choice is a trusted source for fast home delivery of the world's finest wild seafood and organic fare, harvested from healthy, well-managed wild fisheries and farms.

Jovial Foods – Inherently Good

www.jovialfoods.com

The Jovial Foods mission is to create authentic, unique and satisfying foods you can trust, with a time-honored taste that embraces the heritage of our ancestors. Their crops are lovingly cultivated by small-scale farmers and their products are masterly crafted by Italian artisans, resulting in the finest nutrient-rich, distinctly flavorful foods.

GNOWFGLINS — Enjoying "God's Natural, Organic, Whole Foods, Grown Locally, In Season"

www.gnowfglins.com

One of the best websites that teaches traditional cooking. Great recipes, menu plans, ebooks, etc. Well worth visiting this site.

Salt of the Earth

www.saltoftheearth.com.au

The mission at Salt of the Earth is to supply consumers with the best possible quality hand-harvested sea salt available while educating people on the benefits of natural sea salt and how it can assist in a healthy well-balanced diet essential for well being. This website has some excellent educational information about salt.

Dr. Mercola – Take Control of Your Health

www.mercola.com

Dr. Mercola began this website in 1997 and it is now the world's most visited natural health site. His passion is to transform the traditional medical paradigm in the United States. I have been following Dr. Mercola's website for nearly 15 years. He provides a huge amount of research. Great articles, videos and up-to-the-minute news on natural health.

The Institute for Responsible Technology (IRT)

www.responsibletechnology.org

The Institute for Responsible Technology is a world leader in educating policy makers and the public about genetically modified (GM) foods and crops. Founded in 2003 by international bestselling author and GMO expert, Jeffrey Smith, IRT has worked in more than 30 countries on 6 continents, and is credited with improving government policies and influencing consumer buying habits.

Non-GMO Shopping Guide

www.nongmoshoppingguide.com

You can print off a free shopping guide from this website.

Coconut Oil Research Center

www.coconutresearchcenter.org

The purpose of this website is to dispel the myths surrounding coconut and palm products and to present a more accurate and scientific viewpoint. The health benefits of coconut and palm are so numerous and so remarkable that this information needs to be available to all. For this purpose, the Coconut Research Center was established. It is operated by Bruce Fife, ND, an internationally recognized expert on the health and nutritional aspects of coconut and related products.

Traditional Foods

www.traditional-foods.com

Easy, fuss-free — This is one of my new favorite sites with amazing traditional food recipes.

Slow Food, USA — Supporting Good, Clean & Fair Food

www.slowfoodusa.com

Slow Food is an idea, a way of living and a way of eating. It is part of a global, grassroots movement with thousands of members in over 150 countries, which links the pleasure of food with a commitment to community and the environment. Slow food aims to be everything fast food is not.

We Have the Right to Know

www.justlabelit.org

Most Americans haven't been told about some of the ingredients that are in the food they eat. So it is no wonder that 92% of Americans want the FDA to label genetically engineered foods. If more of us speak out about why we care about the food we put in our own bodies and in our children's bodies, then we can convince the FDA to change its policy.

Heal Your Body and the World…With Food

www.foodrevolution.org

Discover the most cutting-edge information, startling facts, and inspirational wisdom that will heal you and have you celebrating life!

CleanPlates – Enjoy Eating Healthier

www.cleanplates.com

At CleanPlates, their mission is to make it easier and more enjoyable for you to eat healthy, sustainable food without sacrificing an ounce of taste. They have restaurant reviews, news and tips to help boost your health and keep your taste buds happy. *Note: the sole purpose of recommending this site is for restaurant guidance, it does not necessarily mean that I agree with all statements and health recommendations.*

Local Harvest—
Real Food, Real Farmers, Real Community

www.localharvest.org

The best organic food is what's grown closest to you. Use this website to find farmers' markets, family farms, and other sources of sustainably grown food in your area.

Eat Well Guide – Local, Sustainable, Organic

www.eatwellguide.org

This website is a free online directory for anyone in search of fresh, locally grown and sustainably produced food in the United States and Canada.

U.S. Wellness Meats

www.uswellnessmeats.com

This company is a thriving family owned business. Their grass-fed beef is recognized for its exceptional taste, quality and health benefits by chefs, health experts, professional athletes, and many others. In addition, U.S. Wellness has joined with like-minded small family farms across the country to expand its offerings to include grass-fed lamb, bison, and goat, as well as grass-fed butter and cheese, free-range poultry, honey, organic nuts, and other wellness products.

To Your Health Sprouted Flour Company

www.organicsproutedflour.net

To Your Health Sprouted Flour Co. is a family-owned business in rural Alabama. They specialize in sprouted whole grains and whole grain flours to meet all of your cooking and baking needs.

Restoring Ancient Einkorn Farro

www.einkorn.com

Einkorn, recently discovered, is the world's most primitive form of wheat. Purchase the grain directly from them or try the many wonderful recipes provided.

Deland Bakery

www.delandbakery.com

Home of the authentic millet bread. It is kosher & gluten-free certified. Their wonderful bread can be purchased at Energetic Wellness or direct from the website.

The Bulk Herb Store

www.bulkherbstore.com

The Bulk Herb Store provides herbs, homemade herbal concoctions, and articles about the use of herbs from their research and experience.

YouTube Video

Sugar: The Bitter Truth: http://goo.gl/g5Xy2a

Robert H. Lustig, MD, UCSF Professor of Pediatrics in the Division of Endocrinology, explores the damage caused by sugary foods. He argues that fructose (too much) and fiber (not enough) appear to be cornerstones of the obesity epidemic through their effects on insulin.

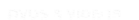

Food, Inc., A Robert Kenner Film

This documentary exposes our nation's food industry and how a handful of corporations put profit ahead of health. It reveals the truth about what we are eating and the horrible treatment of the animals we are consuming.

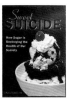

Sweet Suicide, Nancy Appleton, PhD

Nancy Appleton uncovers the health issues caused by sugar consumption. This DVD exposes medical groups that recommend sugar for patients with heart disease, cancer, and diabetes. Also, it reveals the emotional and physical wellbeing created when sugar is eliminated.

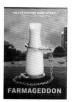

Farmageddon, Kristin Marie Productions, LLC

This DVD shows the violent acts of shutting down family farms by the government. The farms are providing safe, healthy foods but are forced to stop, and this documentary seeks to figure out why.

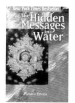

The Hidden Messages in Water
by Dr. Masaru Emoto

This book explores water's susceptibility to human words, emotions and thoughts. It has the potential to profoundly transform your worldview.

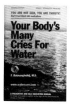

Your Body's Many Cries for Water
by Fereydoon Batmangheidj, MD

A self-help book that reveals the new knowledge of the amazing health values of natural, simple water in maintaining personal health.

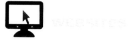

Find A Spring
www.findaspring.com

A community and user-created database of natural springs around the world. Choose your state to find the nearest spring to you.

Water Filters Online
www.waterfiltersonline.com

Water filters online has a large selection of replacement water filters, reverse osmosis membranes, testing kits and water filter system repair parts. Low prices and fast shipping since 1999. 99.5% of all items in stock for same-day shipping.

Pure Water Freedom
www.purewaterfreedom.com

Take control of your water supply today and enjoy the infinite health benefits of pure, clean water with a filter from Pure Water Freedom. This source offers a wide variety of filters from filtered water bottles to whole house filtration systems.

The Water Cure
www.watercure.com

The Water Cure does not sell water or purification systems or any related products. They offer insights and information; both free and in books that give you easy-to-understand scientific explanations on why water is vital to your wellbeing.

APEC
www.freedrinkingwater.com

Ultra fresh drinking water right at home. Shower and bath ball filters, Reverse Osmosis—whole house units and 5-stage filter system under-counter units.

Water Websites and Filtration Systems
www.thankwater.net

A link to other good websites on water and filtration systems.

ECOsmarte
www.ecosmarte.com

Manufacturer of non-salt, non-chemical water technology for whole house, swimming pool, spa, and numerous applications for commercial water. Their natural oxygen and ionic copper systems have root technology from NASA and have been installed in all 50 U.S. States and over 100 Countries since 1994. They offer a non-salt softening and treatment system that gives you premium water that is safe and sustainable for people and the planet. ECOsmarte® is the world's leading rainwater treatment developer.

YouTube Videos

Interview with Dr. Masaru Emoto about the Magic of Water:
http://goo.gl/vZFtlr

Water Consciousness and Intent: Dr. Masaru Emoto:
http://goo.gl/bqkO1d

Dr. Emoto is a Japanese researcher whose astonishing discovery about water, documented photographically, changed most of what we didn't know and led to a new consciousness of Earth's most precious resource.

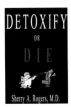

Detoxify or Die by Sherry A. Rogers, MD

Dr. Rogers is a leading environmental medicine authority. She explains why we need to detoxify the body and the best tool to do so is the High Tech Health Infrared Sauna. She has also authored many other books like *The High Blood Pressure Hoax* and *The Cholesterol Hoax*.

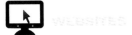

High Tech Health Far Infrared Sauna

www.hightechhealth.com

We live in a very toxic world adding to our toxic exposure daily. Saunas are very effective in helping to detoxify your body. You can purchase a far infrared sauna to be used in the privacy of your own home. Contact High Tech Health and tell them Dr. Menzel sent you.

Body Balance System

www.bodybalancesystemonline.com, 877-296-2228

Provides advanced health & wellness devices, utilizing advanced technology, highest quality, ultimate safety, and maximum value for users and practitioners. You can purchase your own Detox Footbath to be used in the comfort of your own home.

Heal Your Body
by Louise L. Hay

This handy "little blue book" offers positive new thought patterns to replace negative emotions. It includes an alphabetical chart of physical ailments, the probable causes, and healing affirmations to help you eliminate old patterns.

You Can Heal Your Life
by Louise L. Hay

This New York Times Bestseller has sold over 30 million copies worldwide. Louise's key message in this powerful work is: "If we are willing to do the mental work, almost anything can be healed."

Falling Upward: A Spirituality for the Two Halves of Life
by Richard Rohr

In *Falling Upward*, Fr. Richard Rohr seeks to help readers understand the tasks of the two halves of life and to show them that those who have fallen, failed, or "gone down" are the only ones who understand "up." Most of us tend to think of the second half of life as largely about getting old, dealing with health issues, and letting go of life, but the whole thesis of this book is exactly the opposite. This important book explores the counterintuitive message that we grow spiritually much more by doing wrong than by doing right—a fresh way of thinking about spirituality that grows throughout life.

Flower Essence Repertory
by Patricia Kaminski & Richard Katz

A comprehensive guide to North American and English flower essences for emotional and spiritual wellbeing.

Power vs. Force: *The Hidden Determinants of Human Behavior*
by David R. Hawkins, MD, PhD

Dr. Hawkins details how anyone may resolve the most crucial of all human dilemmas: how to instantly determine the truth or falsehood of any statement or supposed fact.

Everyday Miracles by Gods Design: *Manifesting the More Abundant Life*
by Dr. David Jernigan

Dr. Jernigan's work transcends and bridges the gaps between science and faith so that everyone can discover the power of their Maker through a truly miraculous life.

Feelings Buried Alive Never Die
by Karol K. Truman

Karol not only tells you why you feel the way you feel, but how these feelings all started. She then goes on to tell you how *you* can easily transform these undesirable feelings so that they no longer hinder your growth. What a gift!

Defy Gravity
by Caroline Myss

Caroline Myss draws from her years as a medical intuitive to show that healing is not only physical; it is also a phenomenon that transcends reason.

Inspired by ordinary people who overcame a wide array of physical and psychological ailments—from rheumatoid arthritis to cancer—Caroline dived into the works of the great mystics to gain a deeper understanding of healing's spiritual underpinnings. Based on these studies, she demonstrates how conventional and holistic medicine often fall short in times of need. Both systems rely upon a logical approach to curing illness when there is nothing reasonable about the emotional, psychological, or spiritual influences behind any ailment.

German New Medicine®
www.learninggnm.com

German New Medicine® is the research and studies of Dr. Ryke Geerd Hamer. After over 35 years of research, Dr. Hamer's discoveries of the cause of cancer and every condition of the human body is the answer we've been looking for. His 5 Biological Laws explain how the human body was designed. With this knowledge, we can understand our symptoms and why they happen.

GNM is one of the foundations of Dr. Menzel's practice.

Hay House
www.hayhouse.com

Hay House was founded in 1984 by Louise L. Hay as a way to publish her first two books. Today Hay House is committed to publishing products that have a positive self-help slant and are conducive to healing Planet Earth.

Ten Thousand Waves
www.tenthousandwaves.com

Ten Thousand Waves is a unique mountain spa near Santa Fe, New Mexico that feels like a Japanese hot spring resort.

Meditation & Relaxation CDs
Learning Strategies, by Paul Scheele, PhD
www.learningstrategies.com

Release the untapped power of your mind quickly; make changes fast, and benefit immediately. With degrees in biology, psychology, and adult learning, Paul ardently mastered three powerful technologies of human development.

- Neuro-Linguistic Programming (NLP) imparts a unique understanding of how the human brain works.
- Accelerated learning provides keys to learning 5 to 50 times faster than traditional techniques.
- Preconscious Processing gives access to the vast capacity of the mind to accomplish virtually anything.

Neurologists tell us that the human brain is more powerful than the most powerful computer on earth. Paul's expertise makes it possible for you to experience that power and use it to make a difference in your life, whether you want better grades, new skills, wealth, or wellness.

I listen to these CDs almost daily. They have changed my life. Several years ago when sitting before the board for my board certification, I listened to the *Memory Supercharger* CD. It really helped me get through the long tests! I still listen to that one, as I have to recall lots of information all of the time. Most of the time I fall asleep while listening—it doesn't matter, you are still learning.

We plan to start carrying these CDs through our online store, but for now you can go to their website and order. For your convenience, you can download the CD or CDs of your choice immediately to your mobile device.

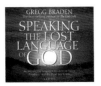

Speaking the Lost Language of God
by Gregg Braden
www.greggbraden.com
This mix of CDs offers a new and deeper understanding of the unseen forces of thought, feeling, and emotion, and how they relate to the web of energy that connects you to the world.

Gregg has also written many wonderful books which can be found on his website. He is probably my new favorite author and lecturer as I have learned a great deal from him. I love that he continues his purpose of bringing science and spirituality together.

The Cause & Natural Healing of Breast Cancer, *Including an introduction to the Five Biological Laws*
Order on EW online store or download from learninggnm.com.

Healing Rejection and Abandonment
Including an introduction to the Five Biological Laws
Order on EW online store or download from learninggnm.com.

Virus Mania: The Truth about Infectious Diseases
Order on EW online store or download from learninggnm.com.

The Living Matrix: Beyond Distribution
www.thelivingmatrixmovie.com
The Living Matrix is a provocative, full-length feature documentary on healing and the nature of human health. The film uncovers innovative breakthroughs and discoveries that will transform your understanding of how we heal. The most significant revelation is how energy and information fields are as influential as genetics in determining human health, physiology, and biochemistry. The film illustrates the undeniable benefits of integrating alternative healing modalities into conventional healthcare and advocates shifting from a disease-centered system to a healing-centered model. A film on the new science of healing.

The Language of the Divine Matrix
by Gregg Braden
www.greggbraden.com
Groundbreaking experiments were done between 1993 and 2000 that revealed evidence of a web of energy that connects everything in our lives and our worlds. This includes healing of our bodies, success, relationships, and peace between nations. This DVD demonstrates that we hold the power to speak directly to the force that links all of creation.

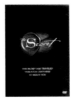

The Secret
The Secret reveals the single most powerful law in the universe. Rhonda Byrne's discovery of *The Secret* began with a glimpse of the truth of life within a 100-year old book. She went back through the centuries, tracing and uncovering *The Secret* that lay at the core of the most powerful philosophies, teachings, and religions in the world. What Rhonda discovered is now captured in *The Secret,* a film that has changed millions of people's lives across the planet. No matter *who* you are, no matter *where* you are, you can change your life.

The Urban Rebounder
www.urbanrebounding.com
JB Berns started this company 15 years ago after a severe knee injury. He needed a workout system of rehabilitation that was gentle yet strengthening. I purchased my first rebounder 10 years ago. About 4 years ago I found Urban Rebounder online and ordered one to experience the quality. The rebounder came with several workout DVDs and I was hooked. This is an amazing workout. Probably the #1 overall best way to heal, restore, and strengthen every organ and tissue in the body. 30 minutes on a rebounder is worth one hour on a treadmill. Love it!

Needak Rebounders

www.needakrebounders.com

Robert Sanders began selling rebounders in late 1985 and soon found that the rebounders available did not meet his standards. Mr. Sanders knew rebounders, or mini-trampolines, were one of the most efficient and pleasurable forms of modern exercise available. He determined he would build the best rebounder in the world.

ReboundAIR

www.reboundair.com

Albert Earl Carter, founder of AIR, Inc., is the pioneer of Rebound Exercise, bestselling author and the lead designer of the "best-built, most innovative rebounders on the planet." As a lecturer and educator, Carter has shared his findings on health and rebound exercise all over the world. In 1983, Carter and a team of Hong Kong engineers developed the first Half-Fold rebounder.

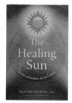

The Healing Sun: Sunlight & Health in the 21st Century

by Richard Hobday, MSe, PhD

Explains how and why we should welcome sunlight into our lives. It shows how sunlight was used to prevent and cure diseases in the past and how it can heal us now and in the future.

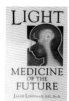

Light, Medicine of the Future: How We Can Use it to Heal Ourselves Now

by Jacob Liberman, OD, PhD

This book challenges the modern myth that the sun is dangerous to our wellbeing and claims that technological advancements, such as most fluorescent lighting, sunglasses, tanning lotions, and our indoor lifestyles, may be more harmful than helpful.

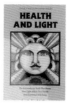

Health and Light: The Extraordinary Study That Shows How Light Affects Your Health and Emotional Well Being

by John N. Ott

The story of John Ott's discovery of the role light plays in sustaining physical health is one of the true scientific breakthroughs of the last half century. *Health and Light* has led many people to a greater understanding of the subtle role light plays in maintaining physical and emotional health.

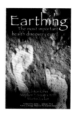

Earthing: The Most Important Health Discovery Ever

by Clinton Ober, Stephen T. Sinatra, MD, Martin Zucker

Beneath your feet is not just a mere patch of grass, dirt, sand, or concrete. It is an omnipresent source of natural healing energy. Simply walking or sitting barefoot on the earth may be the solution for chronic inflammation, which is the leading trigger of chronic pain and most major health disorders. After you read this book, you will never look at the ground the same way.

The Earth Was Flat: Insight into the Ancient Practice of Sungazing

by Mason Howe Dwinell, LAc

For centuries, people and researchers believed that it was impossible for human beings to live their lives without sustenance, and that their vision would be destroyed by looking straight at the sun. Based on science, human eyes are not strong enough to resist the damage of direct sunlight while the human body has a natural cycle of hunger that has to be curbed. But for author Mason Howe Dwinell, people can overcome such obstacles and even achieve the impossible. He elaborates deeply on these in this groundbreaking book.

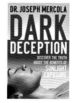

Dark Deception

by Dr. Joseph Mercola

Debunks the widespread myth that sunlight is harmful to your health and demonstrates how sunlight exposure can improve your quality of life.

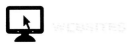

Earthing Institute
www.earthinginstitute.net

The mission of the institute is to disseminate knowledge about the benefits of Earthing, coordinate Earthing research, facilitate the development of effective Earthing products, and to train experts in the practical applications of Earthing for home and workplace use.

Coconut Oil
www.coconutoil.com

Type "skin" in the search bar to find all the benefits of coconut oil for your skin. CoconutOil.com is managed by Brian and Marianita Shilhavy. Marianita grew up on a coconut plantation in the Philippines and in a culture that consumed significant amounts of coconut fat in their diet.

Sungazing
www.sungazing.com

This is a practical, easy-to-follow website about how to sungaze and the benefits of sungazing.

Eat the Sun

Mason is a modern-day sungazer and subject of Peter Sorcher's award-winning and suspenseful documentary film that follows Mason on an unbelievable and often hilarious cross-country tour into the little-known world of sungazing, an ancient practice of looking directly at the sun for a range of physical and spiritual benefits.

Throughout his journey, Mason is riddled with uncertainty. Will he damage his eyes? Is the man who inspires thousands lying? Will Mason succeed in his quest to uncover the truth? This captivating documentary will challenge your deepest-held beliefs.

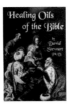

Healing Oils of the Bible
by David Stewart, PhD

Healing by prayer and anointment with oils as practiced by Jesus' disciples and early Christians is made practical for us today in this book. Based on both science and scripture.

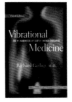

Vibrational Medicine: The #1 Handbook of Subtle-Energy Therapies
by Richard Gerber, MD

Explores the actual science of etheric energies, replacing the Newtonian worldview with a new model based on Einstein's physics of energy.

Young Living Essential Oils
www.youngliving.com

D. Gary Young is the founder of Young Living. His commitment to understanding the remarkable therapeutic power of plants has resulted in the world's largest line of essential oils and blends. Gary has traveled the globe discovering how to best support both physical health and emotional wellness.

To become a distributor: Go to the website and select "Member sign up" at top of page. Follow step-by-step instructions. Sponsor ID & Enroller ID #1047977.

GIA Wellness

www.mygiawellness.com/menzel

GIA carries products designed to neutralize the effects of your exposure to electromagnetic radiation (from cell phones, TVs, computers, etc.) and an i-H2O Activation system that restructures the water molecules making them easily absorbed into your cells.

To become a distributor: Go to the website and select "Join GIA." Follow step-by-step instructions. Sponsoring Consultant ID #48342

Thrive

www.thrivemovement.com

Foster Gamble, the host of the *Thrive* movie, explains his journey of discovery in what it will take to thrive on Earth.

Natural News Network

www.naturalnews.com

The Natural News Network is a nonprofit collection of public education websites covering topics that empower individuals to make positive changes in their health, environmental sensitivity, consumer choices, and informed skepticism. They have no particular religious affiliation and are considered religion-neutral. They also have no particular political affiliation and do not endorse political candidates.

YouTube Videos

Leadership Lessons from the Dancing Guy

http://goo.gl/8YmBts

We're told we all need to be leaders, but that would be really ineffective. The best way to make a movement is to courageously follow and show others how to follow.

What Is HAARP? (full documentary)

http://goo.gl/Q0CgcB

HAARP (High-frequency Active Auroral Research Program) is a major Arctic facility for upper atmospheric and solar-terrestrial research. Principal instruments include a high-power, high-frequency (HF) phased array radio transmitter (known as the Ionospheric Research Instrument, or IRI), used to stimulate small, well-defined volumes of ionosphere, and an ultra-high frequency (UHF) incoherent scatter radar (ISR), used to measure electron densities, electron and ion temperatures, and Doppler velocities in the stimulated region and in the natural ionosphere.

What in the World Are They Spraying (chemtrails, full documentary)

http://goo.gl/Wk8kgl

The Chemtrail/Geo-Engineering Cover-up Revealed, DVD to be released about the same time as this book goes to press.

DVDS & VIDEOS

Thrive: What on Earth Will It Take?

This is an unconventional documentary that lifts the veil on what's really going on in our world by following the money upstream—uncovering the global consolidation of power in nearly every aspect of our lives.

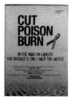

Cut, Poison, Burn

by Nehst Out

This film shows the grueling truth of how the FDA tries to control treatment options and how the government tries to suppress alternative treatments. The documentary is based on a family, the Navarros, who are fighting to keep their son alive. *Cut, Poison, Burn* expresses the hope that we can create a new paradigm of prevention, have a choice in the type of therapy, and medical freedom.

What If?

www.whatifthemovie.tv

This movie is an inspiring documentary created by James A. Sinclair.

Have you ever sensed that who you really are is far greater than what you are currently experiencing? Within you sits the power to move mountains, manifest instantly, live in the Divine Reality of unconditional love, and be, do, and have everything you could ever want. Why? It's already who you are, you've just learned to limit it.

Testimonies

I would like to share my testimony concerning my past experience of *The Transformation*. This will be my third time completing the process. Each time I participated, I felt my health was improving after the 48 days. During this process, I lost weight, and the compliments began to come from family, friends, and acquaintances. Their comments were: "You just look healthy." I began to gain more and more energy. It had been a long time since I felt like doing something other than sitting on the couch. Dr. Menzel has given those participating lots of education on nutrition—most of all, encouragement and inspiration to pursue a healthy lifestyle. I am looking forward to the new changes in *The Transformation*—to further my pursuit of a better quality of life. I know making healthy choices for my body is the key.

For the last several years, I have felt older than my age (or thought I did) and it bothered me deeply. I remember my mother when she was my age—big difference—and my grandmother when she was my age—an even bigger difference. I wondered what to do and where to turn. I knew eating different was the answer but that was too overwhelming. I liked eating my junk food, funny as it seems. The foods I ate were considered *comfort foods*, yet I got very little comfort and a whole lot of misery later. I had talked and talked about doing something. So in April 2010, I did.

My girls and I went to Michele's open house. She had samples of good organic whole foods. I was very surprised how good everything tasted—truly I was shocked at such flavor! After thinking it over, I decided to call and set up an appointment. I have had two appointments, and I am feeling better every day. The bonus is that I have lost 23 pounds so far.

The decision I had to make was this: I needed to make a lifestyle change. I was so tired all the time. Was I willing to change in order to feel better? Yes! Yes! Yes! The neat part of this is that I am not hungry all the time like I used to be. I have been on diets before and was hungry all the time (I was hungry whether dieting or not). I have even been on diets with no sugar and was still hungry. Now I am eating whole, organic foods, lots of water, and no sugar or high-fructose corn syrup. I feel terrific! Michele is the best!

Michele told me that the big difference between me and my mother and grandmother was this: I was the third generation raised on high-fructose corn syrup and pro- cessed foods like white flour and white sugar. My grand- mother lived to be almost 90; all but two years were good and strong. At 74, my mother can hardly get around. She is extremely overweight. I wanted to do something about my health now. I wanted to be strong, healthy, and feel great as I age.

By this time I have lost 54 pounds. I feel so good. Words cannot describe just how terrific I feel! Thank you so much, Michele!

P.S. In one year, I lost a total of 70 pounds!

My husband and I had always considered ourselves healthy eaters. But after meeting Michele about a year ago and attending her health awareness classes, I dis- covered how much I really didn't know! So we have been implementing changes to our shopping and eating habits one at a time—sprouted grains, raw milk, the right meats, and organic produce.

Because of toxic overload due to his job, my husband

had been taking many whole-food supplements (along with sauna therapy). When the last 48 Day group began, I decided to jump on board. Though dreading giving up grains for 30 days, it wasn't nearly as tough as I thought it would be. Such delicious foods to enjoy!

During *The Transformation*, I think the biggest change for me was giving up my Diet Dr. Pepper! I was so addicted, starting at a young age, and couldn't imagine a day without one. Mentally, I told myself to just do it for the 48 days—that was an attainable goal. I did, and then kept going! I've learned to enjoy other delicious drinks instead.

My encouragement to others would be to just start making healthy changes, however small they may seem. And, before you know it, those little 1-degree course corrections will add up. I'm not to 180° yet, but I'm not finished with the journey either.

In October 2011, I decided I was finished with the allopathic medical system. For years they put me on one medication after another and never once suggested I might come off one! I took myself off a proton pump inhibitor which I took for 11 years. After two weeks, I learned I should not have done it cold turkey but I wasn't turning back.

I visited Dr. Menzel in early December because I wanted guidance and someone to hold my hand while I dropped more prescriptions and to tell me I wasn't going to die on the spot if I did so.

She scanned me with the SpectraVision™ and discovered sensitivities to seven different foods/substances and many areas of improper functioning in my body. She taught me how to eat and cook properly (forget the white sugar, white flour, and processed foods) and gave me homeopathic remedies and supplements. I was able to

reintroduce butter and animal fats as well as coconut oil into my diet. Wonders never cease! Not only did I not get fatter, I lost weight! I learned that "fat doesn't make you fat; sugar does."

I went from seven prescriptions down to two since that time and I am working with an osteopathic physician to get off those two. I dropped 18 pounds without even trying and feel healthier than I have in years. I now test sensitive to no foods/substances! My family is astounded, as am I.

I try to attend Dr. Menzel's classes every other week. She teaches us good nutrition, her 7 Laws of Wellness, and shows us how to make healthy food. She keeps a store of products in her office to save us having to hunt them down. I used that often until I felt secure in making my purchases at other places.

At the end of July, I completed *The Transformation*, a process whereby you drop many food categories from two to four weeks at a time, gradually adding them back in to see how they affect your system. I now know that sugar in almost any form, even healthy, is not my friend. You can do a body cleanse with it, which I did, to get your system back on track. *The Transformation* can be done twice a year.

I look forward to the day I am totally free of prescription drugs. Meanwhile, I continue to drop a pound here and there and I have more energy, clarity of thinking, and stamina than I can remember. She encourages me to be patient with myself and says to expect at least one month of healing for every year I lived with a disease.

Thank you, Dr. Menzel!

*See www.energeticwellnessok.com
for more testimonies!*

Source Acknowledgments

This book compiles my personal research and cites the works of many others—I am grateful for their work and assistance. Their books, articles, and websites have been a wealth of information and wisdom for me. I am grateful for their part in educating the world on natural living. Citing these resources does not imply complete agreement with everything written therein.

Books

Combining Old and New: Naturopathy of the 21st Century, Robert J. Thiel, PhD
..... Introduction to the 7 Laws, Nutrition, Exercise

The Chemistry of Man, Bernard Jensen, PhD, ND
.... General Health, Nutrition

Nourishing Traditions, Sally Fallon
General Health, Nutrition, Recipes, Fats & Oils, Dairy, Fermented Foods, Bone Broth, Whole Grains, Salt

Nutrition and Physical Degeneration,
Weston A. Price, DDS......... General Health, Nutrition

The Genie in Your Genes,
Dawson Church, PhD.................... Rest, Faith

You Can Heal Your Life, Louise Hay............. Faith

Detoxify or Die, Sherry Rodgers, MD..... Detoxification

Your Body's Many Cries for Water,
Fereydoon Batmanghelidj, MD.............. Hydration

The Hidden Messages in Water,
Dr. Masaru Emoto........................ Hydration

The Blue Zones, Dan Buettner............. Rest, Dairy

The Untold Story of Milk, Ron Schmid, ND....... Dairy

Pottenger's Cats, A Study in Nutrition,
Francis M. Pottenger, Jr., MD................. Dairy

Sprouted Baking, Janie Quinn.......... Whole Grains

The Mood Cure, Julia Ross, MA............... Sugar

Lick the Sugar Habit, Nancy Appleton, PhD...... Sugar

Heal Your Body, Louise Hay.................. Sugar

Sweet Addiction, Joseph Mercola, DO.......... Sugar

Salt Sugar Fat, Michael Moss.................. Salt

Your Energy Manual, Dori Luneski, ND.... General Health

The Maker's Diet, Jordan Rubin, NMD, PhD
.... General Health, Recipes

Articles

"Seven Strategies to Detoxing Your Body," Jeffrey Rossman, PhD, rodalenews.com, July 2012........ Detoxification

"Lack of Forgiveness Can Affect Our Health," Sheryl Walters, www.naturalnews.com........... Faith

"Menopause Transformation—a Case in History," Laura Coniver, MD, earthinginstitute.net.. Sunshine & Outdoors

"Hippocrates and the Water Cure," "History of the Water Cure," Jethro Kloss, watercure2.org/hippocrates.htm
.... Sunshine & Outdoors

"Negative Ions for the Brain," Pierce J. Howard, PhD negativeionsinformation.org..... Sunshine & Outdoors

"Negative Ions Create Positive Vibes," Pierce J. Howard, PhD, rabbitair.com............. Sunshine & Outdoors

"The Natural Healing Properties of Marine Environments," www.aqua4balance.com........ Sunshine & Outdoors

"The History of Crisco," crisco.com........ Fats & Oils

"Agave Nectar: Worse Than We Thought," Sally Fallon Morell and Rami Nagel, westonaprice.org....... Sugar

"Raw Sugarcane Juice Nature's Perfect Wonder Food" and "The Truth about Evaporated Cane Juice," Dee McCaffrey, CDC, processedfreeamerica.org...... Sugar

Brochures & Booklets

The Weston A. Price Foundation, Principles of Healthy Diets Booklet.......................... Nutrition

The Weston A. Price Foundation, Butter is Better Brochure
.... Fats & Oils

The Weston A. Price Foundation, 2013 Shopping Guide Foods for Life, Healthy Foods, Foods to Avoid for Life

The Weston A. Price Foundation, Cod Liver Oil: Our Number One Superfood............. Wild-Caught Fish

Websites

Take Control of Your Health, mercola.com
. . . General Health, Exercise, Sunshine & Outdoors, Fats & Oils, Dairy, Sugar

The Weston A. Price Foundation for Wise Tradition in Food, Farming and the Healing Arts, westonaprice.org
. . . . General Health, Nutrition, Sugar, Dairy

Real News Powered by the People Naturally, naturalnews.com . . . . . . General health, Hydration, Dairy

Morning Star Minerals, morningstarminerals.com
. . . . .Hydration

Office of Masaru Emoto, masaru-emoto.net/english
. . . . .Hydration

The Water Cure, watercure.com . . . . .Hydration

Fiji Water, fijiwater.com. . . . . .Hydration

Artisan Water from Norway, vosswater.com . . .Hydration

Health & Harmony Products, wellcarehealthproducts.com
. . . . . . .Detoxification, Suggested Supplement Plan

Gregg Braden, greggbraden.com . . . . Rest

Urban Rebounding, urbanrebounding.com . . . . .Exercise

ReboundAir, rebound-air.com . . . . .Exercise

The Mayo Clinic, mayoclinic.com . . . . .Exercise

Aqua for Balance, aqua4balance.com
. . . . Sunshine & Outdoors

Sun Gazing Limitless Potential, sungazing.com
. . . . Sunshine & Outdoors

Earthing Institute, earthinginstitute.net
. . . . Sunshine & Outdoors

Halotherapy Center, salinair.com . . Sunshine & Outdoors

Vitamin D Council, vitamindcouncil.com
. . . . Sunshine & Outdoors

Eat Wild—Getting Wild Nutrition from Modern Food, eatwild.com . . . . .Grass-Fed Beef

A Campaign for Real Milk, realmilk.com . . . . Dairy

Raw Milk Institute, www.realmilkinstitute.net. . . . . . Dairy

Vital Choice Wild Seafood & Organics, vitalchoice.com
. . . . .Wild-Caught Fish

Jovial Inherently Good, jovialfoods.com . . .Whole Grains

iloveindia.com . . . . .Sugar

The Worlds Healthiest Foods, whfoods.com . . . . . .Sugar

Salt of the Earth, saltofthehearth.com.au . . . . Salt

Saltworks, saltworks.us . . . . Salt

Redmond Trading Company—Real Salt, realsalt.com, redmondtrading.com . . . . Salt

WellCare Technology, home of the SpectraVision™, wellcaretechnology.com. . . . . .Therapies

German New Medicine®, learninggnm.com . . . .Therapies

Body Balance System, bodybalancesystemonline.com
. . . . .Therapies

High Tech Health Int'l, hightechhealth.com . . . .Therapies

ESB Tanning Systems, esbtans.com . . . . .Therapies

Young Living Essential Oils, youngliving.com . .Therapies

Written Material

Rachel Lawrence Mor, Third Street Yoga Studio, Edmond, Oklahoma, Yoga . . . . .Exercise

Daren Kosters, CPT, MAT Specialist, Body Rock Fitness, Oklahoma City, Oklahoma . . . . .Exercise

Lee G. Woolley, CBP, BPA, BMD, Founder & Inventor, WellCare Health Services & Technology, Atlanta, Georgia
. . . . Sunshine & Outdoors, Suggested Supplement Plan, Therapies

Photography

Virginia Boyles Photography . . . . . . .Menzel family, yoga

Juli Bowen, Oliphaunt Photography . . . Walnut Creek Farms, Waynoka, OK (grass-fed beef, pastured chickens, pork)

The EW Store

Shop online at energeticwellnessok.com

- Recommended whole-food supplements to assist in *The Transformation*
- Recommended personal care items
- Other misc. items include teas, books, cookbooks

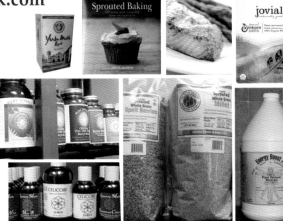

In the Oklahoma City area, our store is open six days a week with additional products available for local pick-up. Please check our website for hours.

- Organic free-range chicken & eggs, grass-fed beef & lamb, wild-caught fish
- Dairy—yogurt, raw cheeses, butter, kefir
- Sprouted whole grains—Einkorn, spelt, rye, oats, rice, bread

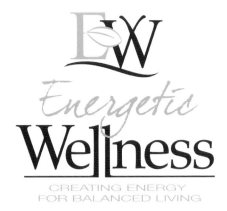

Many patients come from out-of-town for an initial wellness appointment and SpectraVision™ scan. This is such valuable information to target your body's specific needs with the most helpful whole-food supplements and homeopathic remedies!

Services include:

- Wellness Appointments with Michele Menzel, ND, D.PSc
- SpectraVision™ Bionetic Stress Assessments
- IL360 Low-Level Light Therapy
- Flower Essence Therapy
- Emotox (for allergic sensitives)
- Emotional CPR
- German New Medicine® Appointments
- Body Balance Foot Bath / Far Infrared Sauna / Vitamin D Therapy
- Esthetician & Spa Services

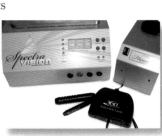

For more information visit energeticwellnessok.com.

Follow us on Facebook, Twitter, and sign up for our eNewsletter.

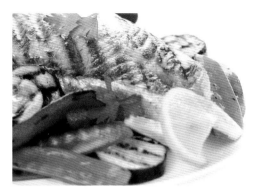

My Transformation
Journal

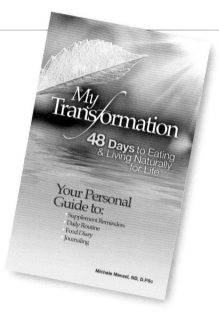

Your Personal Guide to 48 Days of:

- Supplement Reminders—easy daily checklists

- Daily Routine—healthy reminders throughout the day

- Food Diary—record what you eat, new recipe ideas, etc.

- Journaling—thoughts, feelings...your personal journey

Order online at energeticwellnessok.com

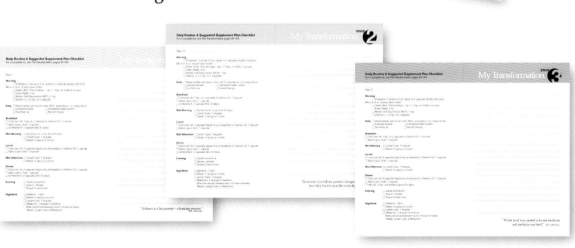

Index

Notes